FORENSICS II

Books by Harry A. Milman, PhD

A Death at Camp David

Soyuz: The Final Flight

Forensics: The Science Behind the Deaths of Famous People

FORENSICS II

The Science Behind the Deaths
of Famous and Infamous People

HARRY A. MILMAN, PHD

To order additional copies of this book, contact:
Xlibris
844-714-8691
www.Xlibris.com
Orders@Xlibris.com
840094

CONTENTS

Introduction ix

Chapter 1   George Washington 1
             President of the United States

Chapter 2   Napoleon Bonaparte 17
             French Military Leader and Politician

Chapter 3   Grigori Rasputin.............................33
             Russian Mystic

Chapter 4   Umberto "Albert" Anastasia 49
             Boss of the Anastasia Crime Family

Chapter 5   Charles Whitman................................59
             The University of Texas Tower Shooter

Chapter 6   Brian Jones 75
             Member of the Rolling Stones

Chapter 7   Sonny Liston..................................87
             *Former Heavyweight Boxing Champion of
             the World*

Chapter 8   Bruce Lee 97
             Actor and Martial Artist

Chapter 9   Jim Jones 111
             Key Figure in the Jonestown Massacre

Chapter 10   David Koresh.................................133
             Key Figure in the Waco Siege

Chapter 11   Vince Foster..................................153
             Deputy White House Counsel

Chapter 12 John Candy 163
            Actor-Comedian

Chapter 13 Kurt Cobain.................................... 171
            Member of Nirvana

Chapter 14 Jerry Garcia 181
            Member of the Grateful Dead

Chapter 15 Mickey Mantle................................193
            Professional Baseball Player

Chapter 16 Marshall Applewhite 203
            Key Figure in the Heaven's Gate Mass Suicide

Chapter 17 Chris Farley 217
            Actor-Comedian

Chapter 18 Eric Harris and Dylan Klebold....................225
            The Columbine High School Massacre Shooters

Chapter 19 Timothy McVeigh............................243
            The Oklahoma City Bomber

Chapter 20 George Harrison...........................257
            Member of the Beatles

Chapter 21 Dee Dee Ramone...........................267
            Member of the Ramones

Chapter 22 Maurice Gibb................................277
            Member of the Bee Gees

Chapter 23 John Ritter 287
            Actor in Three's Company

Chapter 24 Bobby Hatfield 293
            Member of the Righteous Brothers

Chapter 25 Johnny Carson 303
            Host of The Tonight Show

Chapter 26 Ken Lay 313
            Former CEO of Enron

Chapter 27   Alexander Litvinenko..................................325
Former Officer of the Russian Federal
Security Service

Chapter 28   Evel Knievel 345
Stunt Performer

Chapter 29   Dawn Brancheau 357
SeaWorld Trainer

Chapter 30   Andrew Breitbart..........................369
Conservative Journalist

Chapter 31   Tamerlan Tsarnaev 379
One of the Boston Marathon Bombers

Chapter 32   Tom Petty 395
Member of Tom Petty and the Heartbreakers

Chapter 33   Anthony Bourdain.........................403
Celebrity Chef

Chapter 34   Aretha Franklin 413
Singer-Songwriter

Chapter 35   Jeffrey Epstein...............................423
Financier and Convicted Sex Offender

Chapter 36   Naya Rivera...................................435
Actor in Glee

Chapter 37   Conclusions 443

Formulary..455

Glossary 475

Notes 529

Index 739

INTRODUCTION

EDMOND LOCARD'S EXCHANGE principle, proposed in the early nineteenth century, stated, "It is impossible for a criminal to act, considering the intensity of the crime, without leaving a trace."[1] Thus, trace evidence, no matter how infinitesimal, tells a story that could be helpful in a crime investigation.[2]

Forensics is a scientific tool that helps identify and evaluate evidence in support of criminal and civil investigations. Forensic toxicology, a subset of toxicology, a branch of chemistry, includes the detection and quantification of chemicals and drugs in biological fluids and tissues, and an understanding of the mechanism of toxicity—how toxic substances, sometimes referred to as poisons, affect people.

Since poisons must enter the bloodstream before they can exert their toxic effects, forensic toxicologists employ scientific principles dealing with absorption, distribution, metabolism, and elimination to determine the harmful effects caused by drugs and chemical toxicants.[3] The most common analytical techniques to detect poisons in bodily fluids are immunoassays using antibody reactions. These screening methods are fast, but they do not quantify and are subject to false-positive and false-negative results.[4] Any presumptive positive finding in a screening test must be verified by a second confirmatory test that not only identifies and quantifies but also is specific for the presumed substance.[5] Unlike immunoassays, confirmatory tests take longer, are more expensive, and require specialized equipment, such as gas chromatography and mass spectrometry.

Blood is the biological specimen of choice to establish whether a drug has caused impairment or death.[6] Urine is the biological fluid most often examined during random drug testing in the workplace. However, while a positive result in a urine test indicates prior drug use, it does not correlate with impairment at the time of sampling.[7]

In postmortem forensic investigations, blood, urine, and tissue specimens are collected at the autopsy and then analyzed by forensic toxicologists.[8] Results obtained using postmortem blood, however, may be difficult to interpret, as postmortem redistribution, a time during which the concentration of a drug in blood could rise, sometimes by as much as threefold, may have taken place.[9]

After the toxicology tests are completed, forensic toxicologists evaluate their findings and provide a scientific, fact-based explanation of how a chemical, drug, injury, or disease caused death. Manner of death, of which there are five categories—natural, accident, suicide, homicide, and undetermined—is a medicolegal opinion provided by a medical examiner-coroner based on a review of the forensic findings, as well as the circumstances surrounding the death and other relevant information, such as police reports and medical history.

Occasionally the public disagrees with the coroner's conclusions, suggesting, for example, that Marilyn Monroe's death was a homicide and not a suicide. As can be seen in this example, the disagreement is nearly always regarding the manner of death; rarely, if ever, is it about cause of death, which in the Marilyn Monroe example was generalized depression of nerve activity in the brain, a drop in blood pressure (hypotension), depression of heart muscle contractility, and respiratory arrest due to an overdose of chloral hydrate and pentobarbital, two sedative and hypnotic medications.[10] This is because when determining manner of death, different opinions can arise if they are based on incomplete information, intuition, suspicion, or inadequate or incomplete understanding or appreciation of the forensic evidence, unlike cause of death, which is an objective determination based on scientifically proven facts.

As a PhD pharmacologist and toxicologist with substantial experience reviewing medical records, autopsy and toxicology reports, and the scientific literature, I have assisted in more than 350 civil, criminal, and high-profile cases and have provided expert testimony at trials and depositions. In the first book in this series—*Forensics: The Science Behind the Deaths of Famous People*—I researched the deaths of twenty-three famous people in the entertainment industry.[11] In the current sequel, I investigated the deaths of thirty-six famous and infamous people in a variety of occupations. In the course of determining the immediate cause and manner of death, I reviewed the circumstances surrounding the deaths, as well as publically available autopsy findings, toxicology testing results, death certificates, published lay articles, and the scientific literature. To assist the reader, I have included a formulary of medications and a glossary of medical terms mentioned in the book, as well as notes citing appropriate references.

Forensics II: The Science Behind the Deaths of Famous and Infamous People is not a textbook or an exposé of never-before-described salacious revelations about famous and infamous people. It is not even a platform for undermining the conclusions reached by medical examiners-coroners. On the contrary, the book reads like a mystery novel, presenting biographical and scientific information that helps readers understand how medical examiners-coroners utilized forensic analysis to determine the causes and manners of death of thirty-six famous and infamous people.

CHAPTER 1

George Washington

Died December 14, 1799
President of the United States

WITH THE TEMPERATURE hovering close to thirty degrees Fahrenheit, Mount Vernon in Fairfax County, Virginia, was cold and blustery on Thursday morning, December 12, 1799, with light snow, hail, frigid rain, and sleet.[1] Nonetheless, as was his usual practice at about ten o'clock every morning, George Washington, the now retired first president of the United States, went riding for several hours on his plantation, supervising activities on his vast estate.[2]

Washington's two terms as president had ended thirty months earlier, and he was happy to be riding his horse—most likely Nelson, since his other favorite horse, Blueskin, a half Arabian with great endurance, had been given to Colonel Benjamin Tasker Dulany after he married Elizabeth French, Washington's ward.[3] Priding himself on being punctual, Washington returned home at 3:00 p.m., sitting down for dinner without changing out of his wet clothes.[4]

By the next morning, Washington had developed a painful sore throat, a cough, a runny nose, and mild hoarseness.[5] A heavy snow prevented him from riding out in the morning, but in the afternoon, after the weather had cleared, he went out again to mark some trees that needed to be cut down.[6] That evening, after drinking a hot cup of tea, Washington spent time in his library, writing until eleven o'clock or midnight, after which he went to bed, the pain in his throat having not improved.[7] His chief aid, Colonel Tobias Lear, suggested that Washington take something for his cold, but Washington refused.[8] "No, you know I never take anything for a cold. Let it go as it came," he protested.[9]

Around 2:00 a.m. on the morning of December 14, Washington awoke with a terribly painful throat, suffering shortness of breath and clutching his throat.[10] Seeing her husband in great distress and unable to speak or swallow, Washington's wife, Martha, asked Lear to summon Dr. James Craik, Washington's sixty-nine-year-old personal physician, as well as George Rawlins, the estate's overseer, who was well versed in the art of bloodletting, a common practice in the eighteenth century believed to rid the body of disease-causing pathogens by draining it of "bad blood."[11]

By 6:00 a.m., Washington had a high fever and a raw throat, and his breathing was much more labored.[12] Lear gave him a tonic of molasses with butter and vinegar, which Washington found difficult to swallow, almost choking because of his inflamed throat.[13] An hour and a half later, Rawlins began to remove twelve to fourteen ounces of blood from Washington.[14] Washington's wife begged Rawlins not to bleed her husband too much, but Washington, a strong believer in bloodletting, encouraged Rawlins not to stop, exclaiming, "More, more."[15]

Craik arrived at the Mount Vernon mansion at 9:00 a.m.[16] Born in Scotland, he received his medical training at the prestigious University of Edinburgh, at the time the acknowledged international center of medicine.[17] Craik had joined the Virginia Provincial Regiment in 1754, where he met Washington, the regiment commander.[18] Twenty years later, he worked closely with Washington as assistant director of the Middle Department in the Continental Army.[19] When the American War of Independence ended, Craik opened a medical practice in Alexandria, Virginia, and became Washington's personal physician.[20]

After taking Washington's medical history, Craik applied an agonizingly painful "blisters of cantharides" to Washington's throat.[21] Consisting of broken dried remains of the emerald-green Spanish fly beetle, the blistering agent was believed to draw out inflammation and was a popular but painful remedy in the eighteenth century.[22] A half hour later,

Rawlins removed an additional eighteen ounces of blood from Washington, repeating the procedure at 11:00 a.m.[23]

At noon, Washington was administered an enema.[24] When he attempted to gargle with sage tea and vinegar, he almost suffocated.[25] Although able to walk around the room and sit up in an easy chair for two hours, Washington found it difficult to breathe when he lay down on his back.[26]

Dr. Elisha Cullen Dick, a thirty-seven-year-old physician, arrived at Mount Vernon at 3:00 p.m.[27] Dick objected to further bloodletting, claiming, "He needs all his strength—bleeding will diminish it."[28] Despite Dick's objections, Craik overruled the younger doctor and ordered another bleeding, this time of thirty-two ounces; the blood was viscous and flowed slowly owing to Washington's significant dehydration.[29] At 4:00 p.m., Dr. Gustave Richard Brown, a fifty-two-year-old physician who, like Craik, had also been trained at the University of Edinburgh, arrived at Washington's bedside.[30] Brown ordered that Washington receive a dose of calomel (mercurous chloride) for constipation and tartar emetic (antimony potassium tartrate) to induce violent vomiting, but neither treatment improved Washington's symptoms.[31]

Washington's swallowing seemed to improve by five o'clock in the evening, but not long thereafter, he began to struggle to breathe, and his condition deteriorated further.[32] "Doctor, I die hard, but I am not afraid to go," Washington told Craik.[33] "I believed from my first attack that I should not survive it. My breath cannot last long."[34] Three hours later, blisters of cantharides were again applied, this time to Washington's feet, arms, and legs, as well as "wheat-bran poultices," a moist concoction similar to plaster, to his throat, but neither preparation was successful in improving Washington's ailment.[35]

At 10:20 p.m., Washington calmly took his pulse, and then, dropping his fingers from his wrist, he took his final breath and died.[36] He was sixty-seven years old.[37] When Washington's wife was informed that her husband had died, she said, "'Tis well. All is now over. I shall soon follow him. I have no more trials to pass through."[38]

Later that night, Dr. William Thornton arrived.[39] Thornton had planned to recommend performing a tracheotomy, a procedure Dick had proposed after his suggestion to stop further bloodletting was overruled by Craik and Brown.[40] "I proposed to perforate the trachea as a means of prolonging life and of affording time for the removal of the obstruction to respiration in the larynx [voice box], which manifestly threatened speedy resolution," Thornton later explained.[41] Rarely done as elective surgery in the eighteenth century, let alone on an emergency basis, this new, revolutionary, and risky method to circumvent the obstruction in Washington's larynx potentially could have prolonged his life.[42]

Sometime after Washington died, Lear described his final moments. "With perfect resignation and in full possession of his reason, he closed his well-spent life."[43]

The Autopsy

No autopsy or toxicology testing was done after Washington died.[44]

Cause and Manner of Death

There has been much debate over the years about the exact cause of Washington's death, including the possibility his death was due to therapeutic complications from bloodletting.[45] "Old people cannot bear bleeding as well as the young," wrote Dr. James Brickell six weeks after Washington died, adding, "very few of the most robust young men in the world could survive such a loss of blood."[46] Paul Leicester Ford, a lay critic, wrote, "There can be scarcely a doubt that the treatment of his last illness by the doctors was little short of murder."[47]

By all accounts, Washington was physically fit, weighing approximately 230 pounds and measuring six feet three inches tall.[48] Based on his height and weight, I estimated his total blood volume to have been six and a half liters. Removing eighty to eighty-two ounces (two and a half liters) of blood in less than eight hours was equivalent to reducing Washington's total blood volume by 38.5 percent.[49]

Generally, if a person loses too much blood, he will experience a rapid heart rate and a drop in blood pressure (hypotension), and his breathing will become rapid as the body tries to compensate for the loss of blood and ensure the brain receives enough oxygen to maintain life.[50] Most adults can lose up to 14 percent of their total blood volume without experiencing any side effects, while mild side effects, such as nausea, can occur at a blood loss of 15 to 30 percent.[51] As blood loss increases to 30 to 40 percent of total blood volume, signs of confusion and disorientation can develop, and breathing often becomes more rapid and shallow.[52] At a blood loss greater than 40 percent, the body may not be able to maintain adequate circulation; death often occurs at a blood loss of 50 percent of total blood volume.[53] Considering Washington's height, weight, and physical health, as well as that he died almost eight hours after his last bloodletting, I concluded it is unlikely his death was due to the loss of nearly 40 percent of his total blood volume.[54]

Treating Washington with an enema and emetics that cause severe vomiting further depleted Washington's body of fluids, leading to dehydration and electrolyte imbalance.[55] Along with his significant loss of blood, these treatments only further aggravated Washington's ability to fight his underlying disease. In addition, application of blisters of cantharides and the feeling of suffocation due to his infection ensured that Washington's dying hours were agonizingly painful.[56]

Craik insisted Washington died from "quinsy," a painful, pus-filled inflammation of the tonsils and surrounding tissues, the most common deep infection of the head and neck whose symptoms usually include fever, sore throat, dysphagia (difficulty swallowing), trismus ("lockjaw,") and a muffled voice.[57] However, quinsy is almost exclusively seen only in children or young adults, and it causes unilateral neck swelling, which was not present in Washington.[58] In addition, at sixty-seven years old, Washington was at an age considered extremely old in the late eighteenth century, when the average life expectancy for a man was thirty-eight years.[59] After reviewing the available medical evidence, Dr. White McKenzie Wallenborn of the University of Virginia concluded that Washington's symptoms were not consistent with quinsy.[60]

Dick suggested three alternative diagnoses: "stridular suffocates," a blockage of the larynx or throat; "laryngeal diphtheria," an inflammation and suppuration (the process of pus formation) of the larynx; and "cynanche trachealis," an inflammation and swelling of the larynx, the upper trachea, and the glottis—the part of the larynx consisting of the vocal cords and the opening between them—that can block airflow into the lungs, a diagnosis the three doctors eventually embraced.[61]

In 1778, William Cullen, professor of medicine at the University of Edinburgh, wrote that cynanche trachealis "frequently produces such an obstruction of a passage of air as suffocates, and thereby proves suddenly fatal. Bleeding … has often given almost immediate relief, and by bleeding repeatedly has entirely cured the disease. Blistering … has been found useful … Vomiting … sometimes removes the disease … the frequent use of laxatives [is necessary]."[62] It is no wonder that Craik and Brown, both of whom were graduates of the University of Edinburgh, followed Cullen's treatment advice.[63]

Dr. James Jackson offered a different opinion in 1860. According to Jackson, Washington had suffered from "acute laryngitis" in which the inflammation extended beyond the mucous membrane of the larynx into the surrounding tissues.[64] In 1927, Dr. Walter A. Wells diagnosed Washington with streptococcal laryngitis, a diagnosis with which Drs. Fielding O. Lewis and Creighton Barker both concurred in 1932 and 1936, respectively.[65] However, Drs. F. A. Willius and T. E. Keys both argued in 1942 that "laryngitis is not fatal … the course of the illness was too short for quinsy … and the possibility of [laryngeal] diphtheria was untenable because of probable immunity by previous infection and … diphtheria seldom is found in a person of sixty-seven."[66] They concluded, "The modern American physician in all probability would sign the death certificate in the following manner—'septic sore throat, probably of streptococcus origin, associated with acute edema of the larynx.'"[67]

In 1997, Wallenborn reported, and Dr. David M. Morens of the University of Hawaii and Dr. Howard Markel of the University of Michigan both agreed, that all of Washington's symptoms were a "classic textbook" case of acute epiglottitis, a severe and rapidly progressing infection causing sudden airway obstruction leading to a very painful and frightening death.[68] It is this diagnosis, which I support, that has held strong through the test of time as more and more physicians have accepted the diagnosis.

After I reviewed the circumstances surrounding Washington's death, as well as relevant information obtained from published articles and the scientific literature, I concluded that the immediate cause of death more likely than not was epiglottitis, an infection of the airways causing blockage and suffocation. The manner of death was natural.

Life and Career

Washington was born in 1732 to a middle-class family on a plantation at Pope's Creek in Westmoreland County, Virginia.[69] His father, Augustine, was a justice of the county court.[70] In 1735, Washington's family moved to Little Hunting Creek Plantation, later renamed Mount Vernon.[71] Three years later, they again moved, this time to Ferry Farm, a plantation on the Rappahannock River near Fredericksburg, Virginia, where Washington spent his early years.[72]

Between the ages of seven and fifteen, Washington was homeschooled, studying with the local church sexton and then learning math, geography, Latin, and English with a schoolmaster.[73] When he was eleven years old, Washington's father died, leaving most of the family's property to Washington's adult half-brothers.[74]

By his early teens, Washington learned how to survey land, grow tobacco, and raise livestock.[75] His surveying skills were put to good use in 1748 when he began plotting land in Virginia's western territory.[76] The following year, Washington was appointed the official surveyor of Culpeper County, Virginia.[77]

In 1752, Washington's half-brother, Lawrence, died from tuberculosis, thereby making twenty-year-old Washington the apparent heir to the family's fortune, including the vast estate at Mount Vernon.[78] Shortly thereafter, Washington was appointed major in the Virginia militia by Virginia's lieutenant governor.[79]

On October 31, 1753, Washington was sent to Fort LeBoeuf to warn the French military to vacate land previously claimed by Britain.[80] When the French refused to leave, Washington and 150 of his troops attacked the French post of Fort Duquesne, killing the commander and nine others and taking the remaining French troops as prisoners.[81] The French retaliated by regaining the fort and taking Washington prisoner, but he was soon released and later promoted to colonel.[82] Two years later, Washington became a volunteer aide to Edward Braddock, a general in the British army stationed in Virginia.[83] Unfortunately, Braddock was killed when British soldiers attacked the French forces at Fort Duquesne, Fort Niagara, and Crown Point.[84] Although Washington fought with utmost bravery, he could do little except return the defeated army to safety.[85] Nevertheless, in August of the same year, at the young age of twenty-three, Washington was given command of Virginia's entire military force, patrolling nearly four hundred miles of border with a few hundred lackluster troops.[86]

Sometime in late 1755, Washington returned to his home in Mount Vernon suffering from dysentery, but three years later, he and his men recaptured Fort Duquesne and full control of the Ohio Valley.[87] After resigning his commission in late 1758, Washington was elected to Virginia's House of Burgesses.[88]

A month after leaving the military, Washington married twenty-seven-year-old Martha Dandridge Curtis, whose dowry included an eighteen-thousand-acre estate.[89] Within two years of his marriage, Washington not only received land in appreciation of his military service but also inherited his family estate when his half-brother's widowed wife died, thereby making Washington one of the wealthiest landowners in Virginia.[90]

At the start of the American Revolution in 1775, Washington was appointed major general and commander-in-chief of the colonial forces.[91] Two years later, the French aligned themselves with the Americans in their fight for independence against the British.[92] The battle at Valley Forge followed in the winter of 1777 with its thousands of deaths, mostly from disease, but by December 23, 1783, the Americans finally won their independence from the British.[93]

The Constitutional Convention, held in Philadelphia, Pennsylvania, began on May 14, 1787, with Washington as its president.[94] By September 17, the Constitution of the United States had been adopted and distributed to the states for ratification.[95] In late 1789, Washington took his oath of office as the first president of the United States.[96]

In March 1797, after eight years as president, Washington turned over the powers of the government to John Adams.[97] "It shall be my part to hope for the best," Washington said, "to see this country happy whilst I am gliding down the stream of life in tranquil retirement."[98] Determined to live his remaining years as a gentleman farmer on his Mount Vernon estate, Washington enjoyed his retirement for thirty months until, on one cold and snowy December day in 1799, he spent too much time outside and caught a "cold."[99]

Conclusions

Washington was not only the first president of the United States but was also a very wealthy landowner who could afford the best medical care that money could buy.[100] Craik and Brown were both well qualified to treat Washington, having been trained at Edinburgh University.[101] As for Dick, he received his medical training at the University of Pennsylvania, an excellent reputable school in nearby Philadelphia.[102]

It would not be appropriate to criticize the treatment provided to Washington by his three physicians based on current standards of medical practice.[103] "The truth of the matter is that they did the best they could against a pathologically implacable foe, using now antiquated and discredited theories of medical practice," Markel of the University of Michigan proclaimed.[104] "Nearly all men die of their remedies and not of their illnesses," Moliére wrote one hundred years prior to Washington's death.[105] That sentiment was still applicable in the eighteenth century.

Bloodletting, a common practice in Washington's time, was discredited as a treatment for most infections only in the late nineteenth century.[106] At that time, the more serious the illness, the more blood was withdrawn.[107] Doctors in the 1700s knew very little about blood volume and blood replacement, thinking the process of blood replenishment took only a few hours.[108] In fact, while the body can replace plasma, the liquid portion of blood, within forty-eight hours, it takes four to eight weeks to completely replace the blood's oxygen-carrying red blood cells.[109] As for Washington's treatment with laxatives and emetics, these medicines did more harm than good, dehydrating and weakening Washington so he could not muster enough energy to fight off his infection.[110] Also, the blistering agents undoubtedly caused Washington severe chemical burns, inflicting excruciating pain and suffering and providing little, if any, measureable relief.[111]

It has been suggested that had Craik performed a tracheotomy, as was recommended by the younger physician, Dick, Washington would have survived his infection; however there is no evidence to support that notion.[112] At most, a tracheotomy might have temporarily prolonged Washington's life, but not saved it.[113] "[Washington's] physicians were totally fixated on repeating futile treatments and could not comprehend the need for a radical alternative, like tracheotomy," Dr. Ahmad K Abou-Foul of the Imperial College Healthcare NHS Trust in London, UK proclaimed in one of his publications.[114] Morens of the University of Hawaii agreed, noting, "Undoubtedly, the specter of failure with a grisly, painful, and untried surgical experiment on the former president weighed heavily in Craik's decision to veto this radical suggestion."[115]

As is sometimes the case, the leadership model under which Washington was being treated was based on a hierarchy rather than a competency scale.[116] Thus, the two elder physicians, Craik and Brown, were reluctant to accept advice from the junior doctor, Dick, to perform a tracheotomy.[117] Instead they continued to perform bloodletting and to apply blisters of cantharides, causing Washington agonizing pain and allowing suffocation from his infection to progress until death finally relieved him of the suffering he had endured throughout his treatment.[118]

The science of bacteriology was not known in the eighteenth century, and the pathways of disease transmission were beyond imagination.[119] Except for quinine, against malaria, and mercury, for syphilis-related sores, there were no specific treatments against most infections.[120] In the absence of modern-day antibiotics, the only line of defense Washington had was his immune system, which had been significantly compromised by the bloodletting. "Delayed presentation, prolonged Class IV hemorrhagic shock, acute respiratory failure, and probable septic shock even today has a high mortality rate … and [it] would have been irreversible in 1799," Dr. Michael L. Cheatham of Orlando, Florida proclaimed.[121]

Had Washington lived past the second half of the nineteenth century, when the modern pharmaceutical industry came into existence, his physicians not only would have performed a tracheotomy but also would have prescribed aspirin for his pain and the antibiotic penicillin, discovered in 1928 by Sir

Alexander Fleming, a Scottish physician and microbiologist, to combat the bacteria causing his infection.[122] Doomed to die from his disease in the eighteenth century, Washington would have been well on the road to recovery had he been infected fifty years later.[123]

Nowadays, treatment of epiglottitis, the infection with which Washington is believed to have been afflicted, involves ensuring the patient receives enough oxygen as well as intravenous treatment with a broad-spectrum antibiotic, possibly followed by a more targeted antibiotic regimen.[124] This treatment regimen is readily available at all major hospitals in the United States.

Within fifteen years of Washington's death, Craik and Brown both died and Dick was elected mayor of Alexandria, Virginia.[125] As for Thornton, he became an architect, designing the Capitol of the United States and developing the city of Washington.[126]

CHAPTER 2

Napoleon Bonaparte

Died May 8, 1821
French Military Leader and Politician

WHEN NAPOLEON BONAPARTE, a former emperor of France who some consider to be one of the greatest military generals in history, was defeated at the Battle of Waterloo in 1815, he was sent into exile to St. Helena, a small, isolated island in the South Atlantic Ocean, once described as "further away from anywhere else in the world."[1] As his ship approached the rising black rocks, Bonaparte saw the jagged cliffs and the desolation of St. Helena and remarked, "I should have stayed in Egypt."[2] Although his boat arrived at the island on October 15, Bonaparte was unable to disembark until the night of October 17.[3]

Two months after his arrival at St. Helena, Bonaparte and his entourage of about thirty people moved from a small, temporary cottage into a large, dilapidated house on a fifteen-hundred-acre estate called Longwood, which stood at eighteen hundred feet above sea level.[4] Hot and dry for part of the year, Longwood was cold and damp for the remainder.[5] Bored on the lonely island and stripped of his political and military powers, Bonaparte filled his days with gardening, reading, and writing his memoirs.[6] "To die is nothing, but to live defeated and without glory is to die every day," he lamented.[7]

Soon after settling in at Longwood, Bonaparte began to complain of assorted aches and pains, insomnia, diarrhea, and occasional constipation.[8] His headaches became more frequent and severe, and a rash appeared on his legs and feet, which were swollen and painful.[9] In June 1816, he developed an inflammation with pustules on his lips and mouth that was diagnosed as scurvy.[10]

Throughout 1816, Bonaparte experienced insatiable thirst, difficulty hearing, and nausea.[11] By December of that year, he became jaundiced and had three severe attacks of "involuntary spastic movements" and transient loss of consciousness.[12] Nevertheless, by early 1817, Bonaparte's health seemed to improve.[13]

On September 25, 1817, Dr. Barry O'Meara, a thirty-year-old British naval surgeon and Bonaparte's private physician, diagnosed Bonaparte with severe pain in the right abdomen; a swollen, palpable, tender liver; poor appetite; occasional vomiting; fever; and profuse night sweats.[14] O'Meara labeled the ailment "chronic hepatitis," an affliction that at the time was believed to be caused by a poor climate.[15] But in July 1818, the British government, mindful that O'Meara's diagnosis could lead the French to accuse them of mistreating Bonaparte by confining him to a desolate island, ordered O'Meara to leave Longwood, eventually discharging him from military service.[16]

After O'Meara left, Bonaparte seemed to recover his health, but in late December 1818, he again became seriously ill with the same abdominal symptoms he had previously experienced.[17] When he lost consciousness on the night of January 16, 1819, the British sent Dr. John Stokoe, another naval physician, who spent nearly a week examining and treating Bonaparte.[18] Unfortunately for Stokoe, he, too, diagnosed Bonaparte with chronic hepatitis, so like O'Meara before him, Stokoe was court-martialed on trivial charges and discharged from the navy.[19] Not wanting the British to send another naval doctor, Bonaparte's mother and his uncle, Cardinal Fesch, quickly selected Dr. Francesco Antommarchi, a thirty-year-old Corsican anatomist and pathologist with little clinical experience, to become Bonaparte's new personal physician.[20]

By mid-1819, Bonaparte became cheerful and pleasant, waking up at 4:00 a.m. and supervising a landscaping project until 10:00 a.m.[21] But in September 1820, his health again deteriorated, and he suffered persistent and recurring violent upper abdominal pain and loss of appetite.[22] Although he occasionally underwent periods of remission, the pain and vomiting substantially increased, and he lost weight.[23] "Why did the cannon-balls spare me, only to die in this deplorable manner?" he bemoaned to Antommarchi.[24]

On March 22, 1821, Antommarchi gave Bonaparte a dose of emetic tartar, which promptly caused violent vomiting.[25] The following day, Bonaparte received a second dose of the emetic, causing him to writhe on the floor in agony and convulsions and to refuse to take any more of the doctor's medications.[26] To assist Antommarchi, the British sent Dr. Archibald Arnott, an army physician.[27] Determined to avoid a fate similar to O'Meara's and Stoke's, Arnott diagnosed Bonaparte with stomach ulcers.[28]

For weeks Bonaparte teetered between life and death, calling Antommarchi "a blockhead, an ignoramus, a fop, a sneak."[29] One of Bonaparte's most loyal companions, Louis-Étienne Saint-Denis, said, "We expected to see him pass away every moment. One or another of us was continually going to his bed to make sure he was still breathing."[30]

With the end near, Bonaparte began to write his will, in which he requested to be buried in France, "on the banks of the Seine, among the French people I have loved so much."[31] As if by a premonition, he added, "I die before my time, murdered by the English oligarchy and its assassin."[32] He signed the last of the many codicils on April 24, 1821.[33]

On May 1, an extremely weak Bonaparte was deaf, bothered with labored breathing, and persistently hiccupping and vomiting.[34] Two days later, having had no bowel movements for three days, he was administered a large dose of calomel, after which he passed several large black, tarry stools.[35]

Bonaparte's illness entered its final stage by daybreak on May 5.[36] General Henri Bertrand recalled, "From three o'clock until half-past four there were hiccups and stifled groans. He appeared to be in great pain" and was speaking incoherently.[37]

Bonaparte died in the early evening of May 5, 1821.[38] He was fifty-one years old.

The Autopsy

Bonaparte's body was shaved and washed at midnight on the same day he died, using a dilute cologne solution.[39] At 2:00 p.m. the following day, Antommarchi conducted the autopsy at Longwood, assisted by five to seven British doctors, including Arnott.[40] Nine other witnesses were also present— six Frenchmen from Bonaparte's entourage and three British officers.[41]

Across Bonaparte's abdomen was an inch and a half layer of fat.[42] Later, an examination of twelve pairs of Bonaparte's pants obtained from various European museums determined that Bonaparte's waist size had shrunk in the last six months of his life from forty-three inches down to thirty-eight inches.[43] This is equivalent to Bonaparte having lost twenty to thirty pounds and suggests that he had probably been suffering from a chronic debilitating disease, such as cancer.[44]

The autopsy of the cardiovascular system revealed a "heart in good condition enveloped in its pericardium and covered with a small amount of fat."[45] After removing the heart, Antommarchi examined the stomach and then placed both organs in separate silver vessels filled with wine.[46] A British plumber hermetically sealed and soldered shut both vessels, which were entrusted to Arnott for safekeeping.[47] They were later placed inside Bonaparte's coffin for burial.

The spleen was enlarged, as was the liver, which was hardened and congested and affected by chronic hepatitis, the left lobe adhering to the diaphragm and the stomach.[48] Since Antommarchi's liver diagnosis of chronic hepatitis was not acceptable to the British government, the British doctors prepared their own separate autopsy report, noting the liver had "no unhealthy appearance."[49] As for the respiratory system, there were pleural adhesions (fibrotic bands) over the left lung, a few ounces of citrine-colored fluid in each pleural cavity, and some pitted scars in the upper lobe of the left lung.[50] These findings could have been an indication of a previous bout of tuberculosis or possibly of "pseudotubercles," nodules histologically similar to a tuberculous granuloma due to schistosomiasis, a disease caused by parasitic worms.[51] The British doctors, however, wrote in their report, "The lungs [are] quite sound."[52]

Of special significance to the identification of cause of death was the appearance of the stomach. It was perforated throughout the center and contained a considerable amount of dark material resembling coffee sediment, "which exhaled an infectious odor."[53] Antommarchi reported, "Having removed the said liquid, I observed a very extensive cancerous ulcer occupying the stomach and extending from the cardiac orifice [the area where the contents of the esophagus empties into the stomach] to about an inch from the pylorus [the lower section of the stomach that empties the stomach contents into the duodenum]."[54] Surprisingly, the British physicians agreed, writing in their report, "The internal surface of the stomach to nearly its whole extent was a mass of cancerous tissue or hardened portions advancing to cancer; this was particularly noticed in the pylorus."[55]

Two ulcerated lesions complicated with bleeding were identified in the stomach—a large ulcerated lesion in the stomach and a smaller one that had pierced through the stomach wall and had reached the liver.[56] "It was a huge mass from the entrance of his stomach to the exit," Dr. Robert Genta of the University of Texas Southwestern Medical Center in Dallas, Texas said in 2007 after he reviewed the autopsy results.[57] "It was at least ten centimeters long. Size alone suggests the lesion was cancer."[58] Genta labeled Bonaparte's tumor as "stage IIIA gastric cancer" based on the presence of several enlarged and hardened regional lymph nodes and the absence of distant metastasis.[59]

Louis-Joseph Marchand, Bonaparte's valet and one of the witnesses at the autopsy, described the end of the autopsy in his diary as follows: "The inside of the body was wiped and washed with an aromatic fluid. As Sir Hudson Lowe had declared his government opposed to any kind of embalming, needle stitching by Dr. Antommarchi restored everything to its original state."[60]

Cause and Manner of Death

Bonaparte's symptoms and the autopsy findings strongly suggested he had been suffering with stomach cancer: abdominal pain, nausea and vomiting, night sweats, progressive weakening, rapid weight loss, and a stomach with a four-inch tumor that was filled with a grainy substance, suggesting gastrointestinal bleeding.[61] Without the benefit of a microscopic examination, Antommarchi and the British doctors concluded the cause of Bonaparte's death was advanced gastric cancer.[62] However, the examining physicians could not agree on the diagnoses related to the lungs and liver.[63] When his conclusions of chronic hepatitis and lung abnormalities were stricken from the autopsy report, Antommarchi refused to sign the final report.[64] Nevertheless, he signed the death certificate declaring that Bonaparte died from stomach cancer.[65]

After I reviewed the circumstances surrounding Bonaparte's death, the death certificate, the autopsy findings, published lay articles, and the scientific literature, I concluded that the immediate cause of death was advanced gastric cancer associated with upper gastrointestinal bleeding.[66] The manner of death was natural.

Life and Career

Bonaparte, the son of a lawyer, was born on August 15, 1769, on the French island of Corsica.[67] His parents were not wealthy, although they were members of the minor Corsican nobility.[68]

When he was nine years old, Bonaparte attended College d'Autun, a religious school in mainland France.[69] In May 1779, he transferred to a military academy at Brienne-le-Château.[70] Upon completing his studies in 1784, Bonaparte was admitted to the École Militaire in Paris.[71] After graduating in one year, he was commissioned a second lieutenant in an army artillery regiment.[72]

Four years after the French Revolution broke out in 1789, Bonaparte gained military success at the Siege of Toulon.[73] Promoted to brigadier general, he secured a political victory when he stopped an uprising against the republic.[74] For his successes, Bonaparte was promoted to major general and "Commander of the Army of the Interior."[75]

Between 1796 and 1799, Bonaparte was engaged in a series of military conflicts against Australia, Egypt, and the Ottoman Empire.[76] He is reported to have said, "Never interrupt your enemy when he is making a mistake."[77]

In November 1799, Bonaparte took part in a successful overthrow of the French Directory and became the first consul and a leading political figure in the three-member Consulate.[78] While in office, he instituted the "Napoleonic Code," forbidding privileges based on birth, allowing freedom of religion, and providing government jobs based on merit.[79] "The only way to lead people," Bonaparte said, "is to show them a future; a leader is a dealer in hope."[80] His reforms proved so popular that in 1804, Bonaparte crowned himself emperor of France.[81]

One of Bonaparte's greatest military victories occurred in 1805 when he defeated the Austrian and Russian armies at the Battle of Austerlitz.[82] His luck ran out in 1812, however, when he invaded Russia, losing approximately a half a million men and having to retreat.[83]

In 1813, Bonaparte was defeated at the Battle of Leipzig. A year later, he was forced to abdicate his throne and was exiled to Elba, an island in the Mediterranean. But the following year, Bonaparte escaped, sailing to mainland France with hundreds of his supporters.[84] Upon his return to France, he began his "Hundred Days" campaign, raising a new army and invading Belgium, where British and Prussian troops were stationed.[85]

Bonaparte defeated the Prussians at the Battle of Ligny on June 16, 1815, but within two days, the end of his reign began when he was defeated at the Battle of Waterloo.[86]

Conclusions

The cause of Bonaparte's death from stomach cancer came into question in 1961 when Dr. Sten Forshufvud, a Swedish dentist, noticed that Bonaparte's symptoms were similar to those caused by the toxic, noncancer effects of arsenic poisoning.[87] While the exact biochemical mechanism by which arsenic causes noncancer toxicity is not known, the chemical can cause cell injury and death by interfering with cellular respiration.[88] At a biochemical level, arsenic can replace phosphate, and it can react with critical sulfur-containing molecules in proteins to inhibit many critical reactions in the body.[89]

Using neutron activation methodology, Forshufvud was able to detect more than ten parts per million of arsenic, about ten times more than normal, in samples of Bonaparte's hair.[90] The distribution of arsenic along the hair strand suggested that the highest levels formed between September 1820 and January 1821, the years Bonaparte had been exiled at St. Helena.[91] Other investigators soon found arsenic levels in Bonaparte's hair as high as forty times more than normal.[92] With such elevated arsenic concentrations, three questions immediately came to my mind: Was Bonaparte's exposure to arsenic incidental, or was it a deliberate act of poisoning? Was Bonaparte's death caused by arsenic poisoning? And, lastly, did arsenic cause or contribute to Bonaparte's stomach cancer?

In the nineteenth century, arsenic was commonly present in medicine, various food products, weed killers, rat poisons, and hair tonic.[93] It was also popular as a brilliant green pigment in paints, fabrics, and wallpaper, including in the wallpaper at Longwood, a sample of which was tested in the 1990s and found to contain arsenic.[94] Some have implied that Bonaparte's incidental exposure to any of these products while exiled at St. Helena most likely was responsible for the elevated arsenic levels in his hair but in my opinion, that is unlikely. Six years of incidental low exposure to one or more of these arsenic-containing products while contributory, would not have been sufficient to achieve the high arsenic levels detected in Bonaparte's hair.

Others have suggested Bonaparte was deliberately poisoned with arsenic, with Charles Tristan, the Count of Montholon, Bonaparte's trusted companion, being the most likely suspect.[95] Tristan had access, opportunity, and motive— he was a beneficiary of two million francs in Bonaparte's will, and his wife was Bonaparte's mistress.[96] While this theory is intriguing, it has been disproven by historians.[97] "There is no proof, only presumptions," Jean-Claude Damamme, a French historian, said.[98] Moreover, for Bonaparte to have died from arsenic poisoning, he would have to have been given a single massive dose of arsenic. Small doses over many years would not have killed him, although they could have caused abdominal discomfort and possibly his gastric cancer.

A 2008 study conducted at the Italian Institute of Nuclear Physics conclusively disproved the "arsenic poisoning at St. Helena as a cause of death" hypothesis. The Italian scientists discovered that although hair samples taken at four different periods of Bonaparte's life—as a young boy in Corsica, while in exile in Elba, and on the day of and the day after Bonaparte's death—showed arsenic levels approximately one hundred times higher than those in hair specimens from people living in 2008, the year the Italian study was conducted, the amount measured in Bonaparte's hair after he died was similar to levels found in his hair at other periods of his life as well as in the hair of Bonaparte's son and his first wife.[99] The results "undoubtedly reveal a chronic exposure that we believe can be simply attributed to environmental factors, unfortunately no longer easily identifiable, or habits involving food and therapeutics," the Italian scientists concluded.[100] Moreover, if such arsenic levels could cause death by poisoning, then Bonaparte should have died long before he was exiled to St. Helena.

A report from the Mayo Clinic casts additional doubt that the levels of arsenic detected in Bonaparte's hair the day he died were substantial enough to have caused his death. According to the Mayo Clinic, the highest concentration of arsenic ever detected in their laboratory in hair of someone who had died from chronic exposure to arsenic was 210 parts per million; this is more than twice the amount detected by the Italian scientists in Bonaparte's hair.[101]

Unlike other organs, hair is a metabolic end product believed to incorporate trace elements, such as arsenic, during its growing phase.[102] However, for hair analysis to become more than a screening tool, difficulties inherent in determining exogenous versus endogenous deposition of arsenic must first be resolved.[103] Also, sample collection and precleaning methodologies to remove external contamination must be standardized.[104] Without suitable reference ranges for arsenic in hair, interpreting the meaning of any observed finding is almost impossible.[105]

In 2004, Dr. Francesco Mari and his coworkers at the University of Florence, Italy proposed that the immediate cause of Bonaparte's death was torsades de pointes, a form of ventricular tachycardia, a fast pumping of the heart ventricle chambers associated with a prolonged QT interval, an electrical abnormality that is seen on an electrocardiogram.[106] Mari claimed it was caused by a combination of calomel and tartar emetic administered to Bonaparte in the final days of his life, combined with his incidental exposure to arsenic.[107] Mari concluded, "Had Napoleon not been given calomel and tartar emetic, arsenical effects on cardiac conduction would have remained balanced [and] he would then have lived to die a natural death, probably from gastric carcinoma."[108] He classified Bonaparte's manner of death as "medical misadventure."[109] Mari's theory, however, has little support in the scientific community.

While Bonaparte's death may not have been caused by the toxic effects of arsenic poisoning, the question still remained whether arsenic caused or contributed to his gastric cancer. Gastric or stomach cancer is one of the most common cancers in the world. Some risk factors for developing gastric cancer include a family history of stomach cancer (genetics), smoking, obesity, a diet high in salt or low in fruits and vegetables, an infection with *Helicobacter pylori* bacteria, as well as ingestion of alcohol and exposure to certain chemicals.[110] However, while risk factors indicate an increased likelihood of developing cancer, they are not causes of cancer.

There is little doubt Bonaparte had a genetic predisposition for gastric cancer. A 1938 study concluded that Bonaparte's father died of stomach cancer.[111] In addition, Bonaparte's diet was rich in salt-preserved foods and was sparse in fruits and vegetables.[112] In 2007, Genta, of the University of Texas Southwestern Medical Center, reaffirmed that Bonaparte died from stomach cancer after he cross-referenced the description of the stomach lesions, as presented in Bonaparte's autopsy report, with photographs of fifty benign and fifty cancerous stomach lesions.[113] Bonaparte's stomach lesions did not resemble any of the benign lesions; they only resembled the cancerous ones.[114] "He would have been unlikely to be saved, even if he had been seen at Sloan-Kettering today," Genta declared.[115] The most likely cause of Bonaparte's gastric cancer, Genta concluded, was a chronic infection with *Helicobacter pylori* bacteria.[116] However, while the US National Toxicology Program (NTP) has categorized a chronic *Helicobacter pylori* infection as "a known human carcinogen," the bacteria have never been detected in Bonaparte's system, and he has never been diagnosed with an infection caused by this microorganism.[117]

In my opinion, there is no mystery to what caused Bonaparte's death. He died from gastric cancer, the cause of which was his long-term exposure to arsenic, possibly contributed to by a chronic *Helicobacter pylori* infection. According to the NTP and the International Agency for Research on Cancer (IARC) of the World Health Organization (WHO), arsenic is a known human carcinogen that causes digestive tract cancer, including stomach cancer.[118] This is supported by oral studies in a second species, rats, where arsenic exposure caused stomach cancer in these laboratory rodents.[119] Equally important, studies of Bonaparte's hair confirmed he was exposed to high levels of arsenic for over forty years, a more than adequate latency period for the development of gastric cancer.[120] Undoubtedly, Bonaparte's demise began long before he arrived at St. Helena. The manner of his death was natural. This, however, does not preclude the possibility that at some point while at St. Helena, Bonaparte may also have been intentionally poisoned with low, non-fatal doses of arsenic.

CHAPTER 3

Grigori Rasputin

Died December 30, 1916

Russian Mystic

THE YEAR WAS 1916, right in the middle of World War I. The Allied Powers of Great Britain, France, Russia, Italy, Romania, and Japan were fighting the Central Powers of Germany, Austria-Hungary, Bulgaria, and the Ottoman Empire in what became known as the "Great War."[1] At first the United States remained neutral, but in April 1917, after German U-boats sunk several commercial and passenger vessels, including both American ships and the *Lusitania*, a British ocean liner, America finally declared war and joined the Allied Powers.[2] By the time World War I ended, more than sixteen million people had perished.[3]

When Tsar Nicholas II assumed command of the Russian Army on the Eastern Front, his German-born wife, the tsarina Alexandra, took over responsibilities for domestic policy, with Grigori Rasputin as her advisor.[4] A self-proclaimed monk who Alexandra was convinced had special healing powers, Rasputin became a powerful member of her entourage after he helped her son, Alexei, recover from internal bleeding caused by hemophilia.[5] Alexander Kerensky, a Russian lawyer and a key political figure, lamented, "The Tsarina's blind faith in Rasputin led her to seek his counsel not only in personal matters, but also on questions of state policy."[6] Michael Rodzianko, president of the Duma, the Russian assembly, was also concerned. "No one opens your eyes to the true role which this man [Rasputin] is playing," Rodzianko wrote Nicholas II.[7] "His presence in Your Majesty's court undermines confidence in the Supreme Power and may have an evil effect on the fate of the dynasty and turn the hearts of the people from their Emperor."[8]

Rasputin made many political enemies when he opposed the tsar's decision to have Russia join the war against the Central Powers of Germany and its allies.[9] "God willing there won't be a war, and I'll get busy on that score," he told an Italian journalist in early 1914, just before World War I began.[10]

With Russian defeats on the battlefield and domestic food shortages at home, there was growing discontent and outright hostility among the Russian citizenry toward the imperial regime of Tsar Nicholas II, Tsarina Alexandra, and Rasputin's meddling in governmental affairs and his dismissal of ministers of whom he was not fond.[11] "The aristocrats can't get used to the idea that a humble peasant should be welcome at the Imperial Palace," Rasputin told Prince Felix Yussupov, the richest man in Russia, "but I'm not afraid of them."[12] Little did Rasputin know that at that very moment, a sinister plot was being hatched against him in which Yussupov was an ardent and willing participant.

Rasputin was not new to assassination attempts. In 1914, a thirty-three year old peasant woman named Chionya Guseva stabbed him in the stomach outside his home in Pokrovskoye.[13] Despite losing a lot of blood, Rasputin survived.[14] A year later, another plot to kill him was thwarted just before it could be carried out.[15]

Rumors began to circulate that Alexandra and Rasputin were seeking a separate peace with Germany.[16] Some were convinced that the only way of restoring Nicholas's dependence on his extended family, the nobility, and the Duma was to eliminate Rasputin's influence on Alexandra.[17] "I'm terribly busy working on a plan to eliminate Rasputin," Vladimir Purishkevich, deputy of the Duma and leader of the monarchists in the Russian assembly, wrote Yussupov.[18] "[Grand Duke] Dmitri Pavlovich Romanov knows all about it and is helping. You, too, must take part in it."[19]

By December 29, 2016, five coconspirators had joined the plot to murder Rasputin, their method of choice being poisoning with potassium cyanide.[20] Yussupov, the leader of the conspirators, thought killing Rasputin would help restore the legitimacy of the monarchy.[21] Purishkevich, a right-wing politician, agreed, believing Rasputin's influence over the tsarina was threatening the empire.[22] Other participants included Pavlovich, first cousin of Tsar Nicholas II, Lieutenant Sergei Mikhailovich Sukhotin, an officer in the Preobrazhensky Regiment, and Stanislaus de Lazovert, a doctor whose responsibility it was to provide the poison and to dispose of Rasputin's body once the deed was done.[23]

To reduce the likelihood Rasputin would become suspicious of their plan to "kill the scoundrel," as Rodzianko declared upon hearing of the assassination plot, Yussupov pretended to befriend Rasputin.[24] On the pretense that his attractive wife and the tsar's only niece, Princess Irina, expressly wanted to meet him, Yussupov invited Rasputin to spend the evening of December 29 at his Moika Palace in Saint Petersburg.[25] "He had long wished to meet my wife," Yussupov wrote in his memoir, so "believing her to be in St. Petersburg … he accepted my invitation."[26] In fact, Irina was in Crimea, and her name was mentioned only to encourage Rasputin to accept Yussupov's invitation, which he promptly did.[27]

Shortly after midnight on December 30, Yussupov and Lazovert, wearing a chauffeur's uniform, arrived at Rasputin's apartment.[28] After climbing up the back stairs to avoid being seen by police monitoring the front rooms, Yussupov and Lazovert picked up Rasputin, and the three drove to the Moika Palace.[29] "I looked behind us to see whether the police were following, but there was no one, the streets were deserted," Yussupov later recalled.[30]

Upon reaching the palace, Yussupov, Lazovert, and Rasputin went down to the basement apartment, which Yussupov had hurriedly furnished, while upstairs the other conspirators played "Yankee Doodle Went to Town" on the gramophone.[31] When Rasputin asked whether someone was having a party, Yussupov lied, "[It's] just my wife entertaining a few friends; they'll be going soon."[32]

Over the next two hours, Yussupov offered Rasputin Maderia wine, his favorite, that had been laced with potassium cyanide, as well as chocolate cream cakes and other "dainties" that had been sprinkled with the poison.[33] "I stood watching him drink, expecting any moment to see him collapse," Yussupov wrote in his memoir.[34] Instead, the cyanide had no effect and Rasputin's only complaints were a "heavy head," a burning sensation in his stomach, and occasional belching.[35] "There was something appalling and monstrous in his diabolical refusal to die," Yussupov bemoaned in his memoir.[36]

"It's impossible!" Pavlovich cried out when Yussupov went upstairs and informed the other conspirators that despite ingesting the poison, Rasputin had not died.[37] "He drank two glasses filled with poison, ate several pink cakes and as you can see, nothing has happened," Yussupov exclaimed.[38] Taking Pavlovich's Browning revolver, Yussupov went back down to the apartment and, finding Rasputin struggling to breathe, aimed the gun at his heart and pulled the trigger.[39]

Leting out a piercing, wild scream, Rasputin fell to the floor, a bloodstain beginning to form on his silk shirt.[40]

Hearing the gunshot, the other conspirators rushed downstairs. Seeing Rasputin on the floor, Lazovert declared him dead. Surprisingly, Rasputin soon opened his eyes, leapt to his feet and, foaming at the mouth, ran up the stairs and then to the courtyard, where Purishkevich shot at him twice, missing him both times.[41] Purishkevich shot at Rasputin two more times, hitting him in the back and in the forehead, after which Rasputin collapsed in the snow, showing no sign of life.[42] It was then that in a fit of anger, Yussupov and his coconspirators savagely beat Rasputin's dying body with a club.[43]

"I heard revolver shots," a passing policeman told Yussupov. "What has happened?"[44]

"Nothing of any consequence," Yussupov replied with an offhand lie. "I gave a small party this evening and one of my friends who had drunk a little too much amused himself by firing his revolver at a dog."[45]

Having disposed of the policeman around 3:00 a.m., Pavlovich, Sukhotin, and Lazovert tied up Rasputin's body, wrapped it in a sheet, shoved it into the car, and drove off to Petrovski Island, where they hurled it off Petrovski Bridge and through an ice hole, directly into the Malaya Nevka River.[46] Meanwhile, back at Moika Palace, Yussupov washed away all traces of blood, ensuring that no evidence was left to implicate him or his coconspirators in what had transpired that night.[47]

On the afternoon of December 30, blood was found on the railings of Petrovski Bridge, and a brown boot was retrieved from the frozen river.[48] A couple of days later, a policeman noticed a fur coat trapped beneath the ice.[49] Soon Rasputin's body was discovered approximately two hundred meters away from the bridge.[50] He was forty-seven years old.

The Autopsy

At 10:00 p.m. on January 2, Professor Dmitrii Kosorotov, the city's senior autopsy surgeon, conducted the autopsy at the mortuary room of Chesmenskii Hospice.[51] "The body is that of a man about fifty years old, of medium size, dressed in a blue embroidered hospital robe, which covers a white shirt," Kosorotov wrote in the autopsy report.[52] "His legs, in tall animal skin boots, are tied with a rope, and the same rope ties his wrists."[53]

Rasputin's hair was light brown and disheveled, as were his long moustache and beard, both of which were soaked with blood, as was his face below the forehead.[54] There was a strong smell of alcohol emanating from the head.[55] "At the moment of death, the deceased was in a state of drunkenness," Kosorotov concluded.[56] "Rasputin was already dead when he was thrown into the water," he emphatically declared upon seeing no evidence of drowning, such as water in the lungs.[57]

The stomach contained about "twenty soup spoons" (ten ounces) of liquid smelling of alcohol, which was consistent with Rasputin having spent his final hours drinking wine.[58] "The examination reveals no trace of poison," Kosorotov said, which is different from Yussupov's account of the events the night Rasputin was murdered during which he was served cakes laced with potassium cyanide along with poisoned wine.[59]

Three bullet wounds were identified on the body, two of which were inflicted when Rasputin was standing, and a third, to the forehead, when he was already on the ground.[60] The first bullet penetrated the left side of the chest, traveling through the stomach and the liver.[61] The second entered the right side of the back and went through the right kidney.[62] And the third bullet wound to the forehead occurred at close range, presumably because gunpowder residue was found around the entrance wound, penetrating the brain.[63] "The mortal blow had been shot from a distance of twenty centimeters," Kosorotov explained.[64] Kosorotov concluded that the three bullet wounds came from different revolvers of different calibers.[65]

What is especially interesting about Rasputin's bullet wounds is that his liver and kidney wounds were caused either by a Browning handgun, which was in Yussupov's possession on the night of the assassination, or by a Sauvage gun, owned by Purishkevich.[66] However, according to Kosorotov and several ballistic experts, the fatal gunshot wound to the head could only have come from a British-made .455 Webley revolver, a favorite gun of Oswald Rayner, a close friend of Yussupov who was a British agent working for MI6, the British Secret Intelligence Service.[67] A proposed theory, based in part on Russia's importance to Britain and

40

the Allies in the war against Germany, was that Rayner shot Rasputin in the head; however, this theory has not received much support among historians.[68] Keith Jeffrey, an MI6 historian, said he found no evidence MI6 was involved in Rasputin's assassination.[69] This does not mean there wasn't any evidence, but only that he could not find it.

Besides the bullet wounds, there was ample evidence Rasputin had been brutally attacked. A slicing type of wound was on the left side of his body, as if from a sword or a knife. The right eye, whose membrane was torn, was out of its socket and hanging down on his face. The right ear was torn and hanging down. The face and torso showed signs of blows by a supple but hard object. The neck had a wound seemingly caused by a rope. And the genitals were crushed.[70]

Cause and Manner of Death

A toxicology report was not available for review. However, in his memoir, Yussupov wrote, "I took from the ebony cabinet a box containing the poison and laid it on the table. Dr. Lazovert put on rubber gloves and ground the cyanide of potassium crystals to powder."[71] The potassium cyanide was dissolved in wine, so after it was ingested, it undoubtedly was rapidly absorbed.[72]

Ten ounces of alcohol were found in Rasputin's stomach, confirming that Rasputin drank several glasses of wine in the early morning hours of December 30. However, no mention was made in the autopsy report of finding fragments of partially eaten cakes.[73] In her book, Rasputin's daughter,

Maria, wrote that her father did not like sweets and would never have eaten a platter of cakes.[74] Historian Douglas Smith agreed, saying, "He did not eat too much or rich, heavy foods. He kept a simple table."[75] The absence of undigested food in Rasputin's stomach is consistent with claims made by Maria and Smith, but it does not confirm them.

Yussupov noted that "lifting the top of each cake, he [Lazovert] sprinkled the inside with a dose of poison which, according to him, was sufficient to kill several men instantly."[76] If true, then Rasputin should have died from potassium cyanide poisoning within ten to twenty minutes, assuming he had ingested a lethal dose of the poison (one hundred to two hundred milligrams). However, two hours after he consumed at least three cakes laced with potassium cyanide and drank several glasses of poisoned wine, he was still alive.[77] With the possible exception of a burning sensation in his stomach, which may have been caused by gastritis, a stomach inflammation often present in people who overindulge in alcohol, something Rasputin was known to do, Rasputin did not exhibit any of the classic symptoms of cyanide poisoning, such as an odor of almonds, dizziness, red-colored skin, or convulsions. This appears to lend some support to the possibility that Rasputin did not ingest the poisoned cakes at all.[78]

It is possible that the potassium cyanide Rasputin ingested had lost its potency. With improper storage, the poison could have reacted with carbon dioxide, forming the nontoxic chemical cyanocarbonate.[79] Another possibility is that Yussupov substituted an inert, harmless substance for potassium cyanide or purposely embellished the story surrounding the assassination to make Rasputin seem like a menacing, "demonic, and superhuman figure whose malign hold over the Tsarina was proving disastrous for Russia."[80]

Some have suggested Rasputin died by drowning, but that is unlikely. His lungs were free of fluid, a recognized sign of drowning that is present in at least 50 percent of drowning victims. What is also abundantly clear is that Rasputin did not die from potassium cyanide poisoning. Instead his death was caused by a gunshot wound to the forehead that penetrated his brain. Although Rasputin was severely bludgeoned, it is impossible to say whether the violent beating occurred before or after he died. Nonetheless, the beating did not cause or contribute to his death. Also, while Rasputin had two other gunshot wounds—one to the liver and stomach and the other to the right kidney, both of which could have caused him to bleed to death within approximately twenty minutes—it was the third bullet to the head that was the fatal shot.[81]

After I reviewed the circumstances surrounding Rasputin's death, the autopsy findings and results of toxicology testing, published lay articles, and the scientific literature, I concluded that the immediate cause of death was a gunshot wound to the head. The manner of death was homicide.

Life and Career

Rasputin was born in 1869 in Pokrovskoye, a small peasant village along the Tura River in Siberia.[82] With no formal education, he remained illiterate until early adulthood.[83] In 1886, Rasputin entered the Verkhoture Monastery in the middle of the Ural Mountains with hopes of becoming a monk, but his dreams were dashed when he met a peasant girl named Praskovya.[84] "She was plump with dark eyes, small features and thick blonde hair," Rasputin later recalled.[85] "Though short, she was strong, an important asset in a wife expected to bear children while tackling the harvest."[86]

Three weeks after his eighteenth birthday, Rasputin left the monastery and married Praskovya. In time, they had many children, but only three survived to adulthood.[87]

Rasputin developed a strong interest in religious mysticism and soon began to visit holy sites, making short pilgrimages to the Holy Znamensky Monastery in the village of Abalak and to Tobolsk's cathedral.[88] Living on charity, he traveled to Greece and Jerusalem, sometimes leaving his family for months at a time.

Rasputin had a magnetic personality, an oval face, a long nose, a heavy black beard, thick eyebrows, and small gray eyes.[89] Never ordained and always dressed in dirty monks' clothing, he slowly built a reputation as a holy mystical man with unusual powers of healing.[90] By the early 1900s, he had acquired a small following.[91]

In 1903, after years of wandering and religious teaching, Rasputin arrived in Saint Petersburg, the seat of power, where he met Hermogenes, the bishop of Saratov, probably the most widely respected figure in the Russian Orthodox Church.[92] Two years later, impressed with Rasputin's healing powers,

Hermogenes introduced Rasputin to the tsar and tsarina, whose only son and heir to the throne, Alexei, had been suffering from hemophilia.[93]

When Alexei became very ill in 1908 and his physicians could not stop his bleeding, Tsarina Alexandra sent Rasputin a telegram asking for his help.[94] "God has seen your tears and heard your prayers," Rasputin cabled back.[95] "Do not grieve. The little one will not die. Do not allow the doctors to bother him too much."[96] Alexandra followed Rasputin's advice, and within two days, Alexei improved and his bleeding stopped.[97] Confident in Rasputin's healing powers, the tsar and tsarina made Rasputin an integral part of their royal entourage and Alexandra's closest confidante.[98] However, when Rasputin's influence in domestic affairs became too much to endure and he began to dismiss important ministers, a group of men led by Yussupov decided he had to be killed.[99]

Conclusions

In 1782, Swedish chemist and pharmacist Carl Wilhelm Scheele discovered hydrogen cyanide.[100] Cyanide had "a taste which almost borders slightly on sweet and is somewhat heating in the mouth" and "a peculiar, not unpleasant smell," Scheele reported at the time.[101] When it was discovered the chemical was readily available and could kill within minutes, it became an ideal poison for suicide and murder.[102]

Cyanide has a bitter, burning taste, and its odor of bitter almonds can be detected by only about 50 percent of the population.[103] Once absorbed, the poison inhibits the enzyme cytochrome c oxidase, thereby preventing the production of adenosine triphosphate (ATP), a compound in the body that provides energy and drives many biochemical processes in cells, leading to hypoxia (a low oxygen level) and metabolic acidosis, an increase in the acidity of blood due to increased anaerobic respiration (respiration in the absence of oxygen).[104]

Side effects of cyanide poisoning, which are directly related to dose and route of exposure, include headache, anxiety, agitation, confusion, low blood pressure, convulsions, coma, and death.[105] A telltale sign of cyanide exposure is a red color of the skin and mucous membranes, a skin color that has not been reported in Rasputin.[106]

Today murder by cyanide poisoning is rare, mainly because the chemical is heavily regulated and difficult to obtain.[107] However, the poison has had a long history of use, including in Russian KGB assassinations, suicides by Nazi leaders, the mass suicide in Jonestown, Guyana, and the 1982 unsolved murders of seven people who ingested cyanide-laced acetaminophen (Tylenol).[108]

According to Yussupov, Rasputin was unaffected by potassium cyanide despite having ingested so much of the poison it was "sufficient to kill several men instantly."[109] It is understandable, therefore, why some people may be skeptical whether Rasputin had ingested the poison at all. Frederick Dillon concluded, "There seems to be no doubt that he swallowed some substance assumed to be potassium cyanide but by far the most likely solution of the mystery is that the powder, whatever its nature, was not what it purported to be."[110] G. A. Wilkes agreed.[111] "Before we assume that the debauched and unsavory body of Rasputin was protected against large quantities of potassium cyanide by natural immunity, alcoholic gastritis, or supernatural agency, we must be sure that he consumed and retained the poison. Of this there is no certain evidence," Wilkes said.[112]

Professor R. J. Brocklehurst pointed to several of Rasputin's symptoms as possible indications he had, in fact, ingested potassium cyanide—a bitter taste, an obstruction in Rasputin's throat when he swallowed, drowsiness, headache, extreme thirst, a burning sensation in the stomach, and a "dull appearance of the eyes."[113] Brocklehurst failed to mention that with the exception of a burning sensation in the stomach, all of the other symptoms are fairly common and not specific to cyanide poisoning. As for the burning sensation, it could have been caused by preexisting gastritis.[114]

If Rasputin did consume potassium cyanide, then the poison must have lost some of its potency. Brocklehurst described a study in which 75 percent of the cyanide had "disappeared" after three hours from wine containing 2 percent potassium cyanide and 8.5 percent sugar, a substance that can bind to cyanide, rendering it inactive.[115] However, while Rasputin ingested copious amounts of sweetened wine the night he died, the alcoholic beverage was not spiked with potassium cyanide until shortly before Rasputin arrived at Moika Palace, which may not have been sufficient time for the sugar in the wine to inactivate the poison. As for the sweetened cakes, no evidence of digested cake was found in

Rasputin's stomach, so it is impossible to verify whether he ate the poisoned cakes or not.

Whether Rasputin ingested potassium cyanide the night he died remains a mystery. However, of one thing there is no doubt—his death was caused by a bullet wound to the head and not by cyanide poisoning.

CHAPTER 4

Umberto "Albert" Anastasia

Died October 25, 1957

Boss of the Anastasia Crime Family

"I WAS SITTING at my table, facing the door," said Jean Wineberger, a manicurist at the Park Sheraton Hotel on Seventh Avenue and Fifty-Fifth Street in Manhattan, "[when] I saw [Albert] Anastasia, at about ten a.m., leaning on the counter of the ticket booth."[1]

Wineberger was being interviewed by two detectives about what she saw on Friday, October 25, 1957, the day Anastasia was murdered at the barbershop of the hotel. "Anastasia came in and took chair number four," she said, "and this short man came in with him and took chair number five."[2] The short, thin man was later identified as Vincent Squillante,

Anastasia's protégé.[3] Squillante had a dark complexion, dark brown wavy hair, and thick eyebrows, and he appeared to be Italian.[4]

Anastasia was a burly, balding, fifty-five-year-old boss of the Anastasia crime family, although his business card said "Sales Representative for the Convertible Mattress Corporation."[5] Formerly known as Umberto Anastasio, police claimed Anastasia always ranked high in the criminal hierarchy, but had never been the top man.[6]

Anastasia, who never patronized the same shop twice in a row, on this particular day decided to get a haircut and a shave at his favorite barbershop, owned by Arthur Grasso, at the Park Sheraton Hotel.[7]

Anastasia's veteran chauffer and bodyguard, Anthony Coppola, dropped Anastasia off at the hotel's lobby level and then went to park the car in an underground garage.[8] Instead of meeting his boss in the barbershop, however, Coppola took a walk outside, leaving Anastasia completely unprotected.[9]

At about 10:20 a.m., Anastasia entered the barbershop and hung up his blue topcoat, gray hat, and the jacket of his brown suit and sat down in a barber's chair, facing the window so he could look out onto the corner of Fifty-Fifth Street and Seventh Avenue.[10] As he leaned back in his chair, absorbed in conversation with Grasso, Joseph Bocchino, the other barber, placed a hot towel on Anastasia's face before giving him a shave.[11] Unexpectedly, two gunmen wearing fedoras entered the barbershop from the hotel lobby, their faces obscured by scarves and aviator sunglasses with dark green lenses.[12] Walking around a partition, they approached chair number four and, pushing Bocchino and Grasso aside, began to shoot.[13]

Two bullets ripped through Anastasia's left hand as he tried to shield himself.[14] A third bullet tore into his left hip.[15] As Anastasia stumbled onto chair number three, a fourth bullet entered the back of his head.[16] The final bullet was aimed at Anastasia's back as he fell, dead, between chairs numbered two and three.[17]

"It seemed to be three flurries of shots," said Constantine Alexis, manager of the hotel's flower shop.[18] "It sounded like one shot, then a pause, then two or three shots, another pause, and then two or three more shots."[19]

Police arrived on the scene within minutes, but the killers were long gone, having escaped through the hotel's lobby door.[20] They have never been apprehended.[21] In Anastasia's pockets, police found over nineteen hundred dollars.[22] In the corridor outside of the barbershop, they recovered a .38 caliber Colt handgun.[23] Later, a .32 caliber Smith & Wesson revolver was discovered at the bottom of a baling machine used to gather refuse deposited in litter baskets at a nearby metro stop.[24]

"There was one grand guy," Coppola said of Anastasia when he heard his boss had been murdered.[25] "Lots of people will cry, now that he is dead."[26] That remained to be seen.

The Autopsy

The autopsy was conducted the following day at Bellevue Hospital by Dr. Milton Helpern, the chief medical examiner-coroner of New York City.[27]

Of special significance for the identification of cause of death were the several bullet wounds—a .38 caliber gunshot wound at the back of the head that lodged in the left side of the brain, two .38 caliber gunshot wounds on the left hand, and a .32 caliber wound through the right hip.[28] On the back of the neck was a "slap wound" caused by a ricocheted bullet.[29] In addition, a .38 caliber wound was found on the upper left side of the back, near the midline; the bullet took a downward course and lodged in the left flank after penetrating the kidney, lung, and spleen.[30]

The only powder marks were those on the barber's apron; the apron was found in the barbershop, near Anastasia's left hand.[31]

Three bullets were recovered at the scene.[32] One bullet was in Anastasia's underwear, a second was in his brain, and a third bullet was located in his left flank.[33]

No other autopsy findings were available for review; nor was there a publically available toxicology report.

Cause and Manner of Death

Since the complete autopsy report was not available, the path of the projectile through the head or the internal organs could not be evaluated. In addition, it was not possible to determine whether Anastasia had been suffering from any ailment, such as cirrhosis of the liver, atherosclerosis due to an accumulation of plaque in his coronary arteries, or heart disease.

Helpern, the chief medical examiner-coroner, concluded, "Death resulted either from the bullet in the back or the bullet in the head."[34] According to the American Association of Neurological Surgeons, gunshot wounds to the head are fatal in about 90 percent of the time.[35] A bullet wound to the head causes destruction of important centers in the brain, such as the respiratory center responsible for breathing, with death occurring almost immediately.

As far as whether Anastasia died as a result of a bullet to his back is difficult to say. However, if so, death would have been due to penetration and destruction of major organs, such as the heart and lungs.

After I reviewed the circumstances surrounding Anastasia's death, the autopsy findings, and published lay articles, I concluded that the immediate cause of death was gunshot wounds to the head and back. The manner of death was homicide.

Life and Career

Anastasia was born on September 26, 1902 in Tropea, a small town on the east coast of Calabria, in Southern Italy, a region known for its prized onions, clifftop historic center, and pristine beaches.[36] The son of a railroad worker and one of twelve siblings, Anastasia illegally immigrated to the United States in 1919 and settled in Brooklyn, working as a longshoreman.[37] His life of crime began as soon as he arrived in New York.

In March 1921, Anastasia was arrested for killing an Italian longshoreman in a brawl.[38] He was convicted of murder in July of that year and sentenced to die in the electric chair, but his attorneys appealed the verdict.[39] By the time a retrial was granted on technical grounds, key state witnesses disappeared or changed their stories. Anastasia was released for lack of evidence.[40]

Anastasia was again arrested for homicide in August 1922. Eight months later, he was arrested for felonious assault.[41] In both cases, the charges were dropped for lack of evidence or because the state's witnesses changed their stories.[42] However, in June 1923, Anastasia was convicted for illegal possession of a firearm, for which he spent two years at New York's Blackwell's Island Penitentiary, now known as Roosevelt Island.[43]

By the late 1920s, Anastasia's criminal activities were centered on the waterfront, having gained control of local unions of the International Longshoremen's Association.[44] By some accounts, Anastasia was one of the gunmen ordered by Charles "Lucky" Luciano in April 1931 to kill Joe "the Boss" Masseria, the self-styled "Boss of Bosses," at a seafood restaurant called Nuova Villa Tammaro on Coney Island.[45]

Upon Masseria's death, Salvatore Maranzano immediately declared himself "Boss of Bosses," but the other Mafia bosses were not impressed.[46] Maranzano was killed in his Park Avenue office in September 1931.[47]

After Maranzano's death, a "National Crime Syndicate," known as "The Commission," of top Mafia bosses from across the country and of the five New York crime families was formed to resolve future interfamily disputes.[48] It was then that Anastasia became an underboss of the Vincent Mangano crime family and an intermediary between the Commission and Murder Inc., a Brooklyn-based enforcement group of veteran assassins.[49]

In 1936, Anastasia married Elsa Bargneti, an Italian Canadian woman twelve years his junior.[50] A year later, she gave birth to a baby boy.[51] In time, Elsa would bear Anastasia two sons and two daughters.[52] In the mid-1940s, the Anastasia family relocated to Fort Lee, New Jersey, eventually settling into a sixty-five-hundred-square-foot mansion with twenty-five rooms, including seven bedrooms and seven and a half bathrooms, that overlooked rolling hills and the Hudson River.[53]

Three years later, Brooklyn District Attorney William O'Dwyer was ready to convict Anastasia for ordering the murder of Peter Panto, a crusader against racketeering in organized labor.[54] O'Dwyer's star witness was Abe Reles, a Murder Inc. hired killer.[55] Reles had committed the crime but agreed to turn state's evidence in exchange for immunity.[56] While waiting to testify, Reles was held under guard by six armed police detectives at the Half Moon Hotel in Coney Island.[57] However, just before he was to appear in court, Reles was found dead below his fifth floor hotel room window.[58]

After his death, he became known as "The canary who sang, but couldn't fly."[59]

Following the unwelcome publicity of the O'Dwyer case, the Commission disbanded Murder Inc.[60] Looking to escape further scrutiny by O'Dwyer, Anastasia enlisted in the US Army.[61] Luckily for him, Congress enacted a special act granting a speedy naturalization to aliens who served in the US armed forces, so on June 29, 1943, Anastasia became a US citizen.[62]

In 1951, Philip Mangano of the Mangano Crime Family was found dead in a swamp with three bullets in the back of his head and two in each cheek.[63] At the same time, his brother, Vincent, disappeared; to this day, he has never been found.[64] Seizing the moment, Anastasia took control of the Mangano Crime Family and renamed it after himself.[65]

In a surprise move, Anastasia took a plea deal in 1955 in which he agreed to plead guilty to tax evasion related to the purchase of his New Jersey home.[66] In exchange, he was fined twenty-five thousand dollars and sentenced to one year in jail, which he served in a federal prison in Milan, Michigan.[67] He was released from prison in 1956.

When Frank Costello, boss of the Luciano Crime Family, retired in 1957, Vito Genovese became head of the Luciano Crime Family.[68] Anastasia was a close friend of Costello, and he opposed Genovese sitting on the Commission.[69] Seeing an opportunity to get rid of the irksome, greedy, and ambitious Anastasia, crime bosses Joe Bonanno and Joe Profaci aligned themselves with Genovese, as well as with the "Mob

Accountant" Meyer Lansky, and Carlo Gambino, Anastasia's underboss who later became the most powerful Mafia boss in US history.[70] Their expectations were realized in late October when Anastasia went for a haircut and a shave at Grasso's barbershop in the Park Sheraton Hotel.

Conclusions

It is ironic that while Anastasia escaped the electric chair in 1921, his life ended in a barber's chair approximately thirty-five years later.[71] Although the thugs who carried out his execution were never apprehended, several theories have been proposed as to who ordered the assassination and why.[72] But the simple fact is that Anastasia had gotten too big for his britches.

After Anastasia's death, Lansky, Luciano, Costello, and Gambino conspired against Genovese by bribing a drug dealer to testify he had worked for Genovese.[73] As a result, Genovese was convicted in 1959 on a narcotics charge and sentenced to fifteen years in prison.[74] In 1969, while still in prison, Genovese suffered a heart attack and died at the United States Medical Center for Federal Prisoners in Springfield, Missouri.[75]

In February 1957, Anastasia's wife returned to Canada.[76] Later that year, comedian Buddy Hackett purchased Anastasia's Fort Lee, New Jersey, home at auction for $64,000.[77] The mansion changed hands a couple of times and in 2017, it sold for $6.9 million.[78]

After Anastasia's murder, the management of the Park Sheraton Hotel broke Grasso's lease and ordered him to vacate the premises.[79] He refused and took the hotel to court, where Municipal Court Justice Pelham St. George Bissel III ruled in Grasso's favor and allowed him to reopen the barbershop.[80] As for the barber's chair on which Anastasia sat for his final haircut and shave, it eventually was placed on display in the Mob Museum in Las Vegas.[81]

With time, the Park Sheraton Hotel was renamed the Park Central Hotel. Grasso's barbershop was converted into a Starbucks.

CHAPTER 5

Charles Whitman

Died August 1, 1966

The University of Texas Tower Shooter

FOR AMERICA'S AIR transportation system, Sunday July 31, 1966, was expected to be a very important day. Twenty-three days earlier, thirty-five thousand members of the International Association of Machinists had gone out on strike against five airlines, grounding 60 percent of commercial air traffic and causing massive confusion.[1] However, after President Lyndon Baines Johnson intervened, an end to the strike seemed imminent, the ratification of which was all but assured.[2]

Much to everyone's surprise, after all the votes were counted, union members overwhelmingly rejected the resolution.[3] It would take another twenty days before union rank and file would agree to the settlement package.[4] Nevertheless, as difficult as the disruption in air travel was, it paled in comparison to the shock and sorrow generated by events that unfolded in Austin, Texas, on that last day in July.

It all began on a beautiful sunny morning. It was then that Charles Whitman, a handsome, blond twenty-four-year-old architectural engineering student at the University of Texas in Austin went shopping, first at a 7-Eleven convenience store, where he purchased Spam, and then at Davis Hardware, where he bought a hunting knife and a pair of binoculars.[5] After picking up his wife, Kathy, from her summer job as a telephone operator, Whitman met his mother for lunch at the Wyatt Cafeteria.[6] Their lunch date ended at 4:00 p.m., which left plenty of time for Whitman and his wife to visit with their close friends, John and Fran Morgan, before Kathy's six o'clock shift at the telephone company.[7]

At 6:45 p.m., Whitman returned to the small duplex apartment in south Austin he shared with his wife and started to type a letter. "I don't quite understand what it is that compels me to type this letter," he began. "Perhaps it is to leave some vague reason for the actions I have recently performed."[8] Whitman was interrupted when two of his friends unexpectedly dropped by for a visit.[9]

Shortly after midnight, after his friends had finally left, Whitman drove to his mother's fifth-floor luxury apartment near downtown Austin. When he arrived, he shot his mother in the back of the head and bludgeoned her to death.[10] Before leaving the apartment, Whitman placed a handwritten letter next to his mother's body in which he admitted killing her and claiming to have "relieved her of her suffering here on earth."[11]

As brutal as the death of his mother was, Whitman's murderous rampage wasn't over. About three hours after leaving his mother's apartment, he returned home and stabbed his twenty-three-year-old wife several times in the chest while she slept.[12] He then calmly sat down and finished the letter he had started the previous evening, only this time, he finished it in longhand.[13] In the letter, Whitman noted, "The prominent reason [for killing my wife] in my mind is that I truly do not consider this world worth living in, and am prepared to die, and I do not want to leave her to suffer alone in it."[14] Besides the half-typed, half-handwritten letter, he also wrote short notes to each of his brothers.[15]

Just before seven o'clock on Monday morning, August 1, Whitman contacted his wife's supervisor at Bell System to say she was ill and wouldn't be coming to work that day.[16] At about eleven, he made a similar phone call to his mother's workplace, after which he went to three separate stores and purchased canned food, water, a portable radio, a Universal M1 carbine rifle, and a 12-gauge semiautomatic shotgun.[17] Wearing overalls to look like a maintenance man, Whitman placed the items in a footlocker, along with other supplies, guns, and equipment, and headed to the university's main building, known as "the tower," a Texas landmark and Austin's tallest building, located in the center of the University of Texas campus.[18]

Having arrived at the tower at 11:35 a.m., Whitman flashed his old career identification card and told the security guard he was a research assistant delivering equipment.[19] Wheeling the footlocker behind him, Whitman took the elevator up to the twenty-seventh floor and then hauled his arsenal up an additional flight of stairs to the reception area on the twenty-eighth floor.[20] There he knocked out the receptionist with the butt of his rifle. Tragically, she later died of her injuries.[21] When a family of tourists was about to enter the reception area from the staircase, Whitman fired his shotgun, killing two of the family members and severely wounding two others.[22] The two remaining members escaped unharmed.[23]

By 11:48 a.m., Whitman had barricaded himself on the observation deck, nearly 230 feet above ground, and began to randomly shoot passersby.[24] Over the next hour and a half, he fired approximately 150 rounds with his high-powered rifles, killing thirteen people and wounding thirty-one, including an eighteen-year-old female student who was eight months pregnant.[25]

It was only after police shot Whitman dead on the northwest corner of the observation deck that the bloody carnage finally stopped.[26]

The Autopsy

Since Whitman had written, "After my death I wish that an autopsy would be performed on me to see if there is any visible physical disorder," his father gave permission for an autopsy to be conducted.[27] It was performed at the Cook Funeral Home in Austin at 8:55 a.m. on August second, by Dr. Coleman de Chenar, a neuropathologist.[28]

de Chenar had been the resident pathologist at Austin State Hospital, a mental institution, since the 1950s.[29] By the time he died in 1985, he had amassed approximately two hundred brain specimens of mental patients, including Whitman's.[30] According to Linda Campbell, the director of Clinical Support Services at Austin State Hospital, the specimens were a valuable research tool that offered a glimpse into how diseases attack the brain.[31] In 1987, the samples were bequeathed to the University of Texas; by 2014, half of the brain samples, including Whitman's, were missing and presumed lost.[32]

Whitman's body was well nourished and proportionally developed, but his left arm was shortened and deformed, the cause of which was not explained in the autopsy report.[33] More than ten ammunition entry holes were identified between the eyes, in the left temporal region of the skull, an area on the left side of the head, as well as on both sides of the neck, the heart, and in the area called the left axillary region, where the left arm connects to the shoulder.[34]

The internal examination, which began with the cardiovascular system, revealed a collapsed heart due to a penetrating gunshot wound to the right ventricle, the heart chamber that pumps oxygen-depleted blood to the lungs.[35]

The heart valves were smooth, and the coronary arteries and aorta, the main artery that carries oxygenated blood away from the heart to the rest of the body, were normal.[36] The internal cavity, however, was filled with blood, undoubtedly from the gunshot wound to the heart.[37]

While the lungs contained a small amount of blood, the tracheobronchial tree, a system of airways that allows passage of air into the lungs, was filled with frothy, bloody fluid.[38] And although the left chest cavity contained less than two ounces of blood, it had a considerable amount of air due to the penetration of the lungs by the projectiles.[39]

The stomach, small and large intestines, spleen, liver, pancreas, urinary bladder, and gall bladder were all within normal limits and without any pathological changes.[40] Both kidneys, while appearing normal, were relatively large.[41]

Since Whitman had reported having "many unusual and irrational thoughts" and "overwhelming violent impulses," I was especially interested to review the autopsy findings related to the head and brain.[42] The skull was "unusually thin" with numerous fracture lines.[43] As for the brain, while it was symmetrically developed and without anomalies, it was damaged by penetrating fragments of bone created by the gunshot wounds.[44] Nevertheless, despite the limitations caused by the bone fragments, the brain showed evidence of a fairly well outlined pecan-size glioma-type cancerous tumor, the most common brain tumor in humans, which de Chenar labeled "astrocytoma."[45] When tumor tissue was examined under a microscope, it was found to be "just on the borderline to malignant formations."[46] Unlike Robin Williams's brain, whose abnormalities led to a diagnosis of Lewy body dementia, a progressive form of dementia that frequently presents with Parkinson's-like motor symptoms, depression, and hallucinations, de Chenar concluded Whitman's astrocytoma had "no correlation to psychosis or permanent pains," after he reviewed its anatomical location and microscopic properties.[47]

Having reviewed the autopsy findings, I was left with one question: if Whitman's brain tumor did not contribute to his bizarre behavior on August 1, was it possible his conduct was influenced by drugs? The answer would have to reveal itself in the toxicology report, which I was anxious to examine.

Cause and Manner of Death

Toxicology testing was severely limited, since Whitman's body was embalmed, which completely depleted the body of blood and replaced it with formaldehyde.[48] In addition, the urinary bladder was empty, so urine couldn't be tested for the presence of drugs either.[49] Nevertheless, despite these limitations, no drugs were detected in the kidneys, stomach, brain, or liver.[50]

A group of psychiatrists reviewed the toxicology report and concluded that while Whitman had taken central nervous system stimulant medications in the past, including amphetamines, there was no evidence of acute or chronic toxicity from these drugs on August 1, 1966.[51]

John Connolly, the governor of Texas, requested that the University of Texas conduct its own independent review of the Whitman case.[52] Toward that goal, the university assembled a task force of thirty-two scientists and other experts who, after analyzing the facts in the case, issued their final report on September 8, 1966.[53]

Seven pathologists examined the autopsy findings, brain specimens, and histological slides. They determined that while de Chenar was correct in his assessment that Whitman's brain tumor was an astrocytoma, the tumor's characteristics were consistent with "glioblastoma multiforme," the most aggressive grade of astrocytoma, whose median survival rate does not exceed twelve to twenty-four months.[54] People with this type of tumor often exhibit persistent headache, personality changes, difficulties in thinking and learning, nausea and vomiting, blurred vision, and seizures.[55] The pathologists further concluded the autopsy did not provide any evidence of a clinical neurological abnormality or that the tumor interrupted nerve pathways, leading to detectable neurological signs.[56] They conceded, however, that while "abnormal aggressive behavior may be a manifestation of organic brain disease … the application of existing knowledge of organic brain function does not enable us to explain the actions of Whitman on August first."[57]

Next, a team of six psychiatrists was assembled to determine Whitman's state of mind on that fateful day in August.[58] While Whitman's tumor undoubtedly exerted pressure on his brain and very likely accounted for his severe headaches, Dr. Stuart L. Brown, a member of the task force, noted, "The highly malignant brain tumor conceivably could have contributed to his inability to control his emotions and actions."[59] Dr. Michael Koenigs of the University of Wisconsin qualified Brown's remarks, saying, "It is unlikely that a tumor initiated some type of psychotic rage, but it could have tweaked his personality to be a bit more aggressive or a bit less empathetic."[60]

Dr. N. Bradley Keele of Baylor University College of Medicine took a different point of view.[61] He felt that while the tumor was pressing against the amygdala, an area of the brain involved in regulating emotion and aggression, it "could have impacted his bizarre and violent behavior," but it's unlikely to have been the only reason for Whitman's actions or even an important contributing factor in his behavior.[62]

Without a recent psychiatric evaluation of Whitman, the psychiatric team could not make a proper psychiatric diagnosis. However, the team noted that Whitman was under increasing stress and personal dissatisfactions, and that he at times was prone to impulsive actions and loss of control.[63] They were aware Whitman had been deeply concerned about the recent separation of his parents as well as his own marital problems, despite having strong and loving ties to his wife. They were also mindful that four months prior to the shooting, Whitman had consulted a psychiatrist complaining of severe headaches and violent impulses.[64] And yet, despite this revealing information, the team of psychiatrists concluded, "The relationship between the brain tumor and Charles

J. Whitman's actions on the last day of his life cannot be established with clarity. However, the highly malignant brain tumor conceivably could have contributed to his inability to control his emotions and actions."[65]

While people with brain tumors may sometimes present with psychiatric symptoms, the biochemical mechanisms by which the tumors can produce such symptoms are not well understood.[66] In his review article for the *World Journal of Psychiatry*, Subramoniam Madhusoodanan observed that there are no large, double-blind controlled prospective studies examining the relationship between brain tumors and the onset of psychiatric symptoms, something that is needed before conclusions can be drawn about the effects of brain tumors on behavior.[67] Madhusoodanan stated, "Although there may be an association between some tumor locations and psychiatric symptoms, it is difficult to predict the symptoms based on the location or vice versa."[68]

After I reviewed the circumstances surrounding Whitman's death, the autopsy findings and results of toxicology testing, published lay articles, and the scientific literature, I concluded that the immediate cause of death was multiple gunshot wounds and the resulting fatal injuries to the head and heart. There was insufficient information available to determine whether Whitman's brain tumor contributed to his violent behavior. The manner of death was justifiable homicide.

Life and Career

Whitman was born in 1941 to a devout Roman Catholic mother and an abusive perfectionist father who ran a plumbing contracting business.[69] By the time Whitman was six years old, his family had moved eight times.[70]

When he was seven, Whitman began taking piano lessons; at eleven, he joined the Boy Scouts.[71] His father kept pushing Whitman to excel, so by the time he was twelve years old, Whitman had attained the rank of Eagle Scout, the youngest ever do so.[72]

A gun enthusiast, Whitman's father taught his son how to handle firearms from an early age.[73] "Charlie could plug the eye out of a squirrel by the time he was sixteen," Whitman's father declared.[74] Later, when he was in the Marine Corps, Whitman earned a Sharpshooter Badge because of his excellent marksmanship.[75]

With an IQ of 139, Whitman was ranked in the top 10 percent of his high school graduating class.[76] Although he was accepted at the Georgia Institute of Technology, he decided to enlist in the Marine Corps instead.[77]

When he was twenty years old, Whitman was awarded a scholarship to attend The University of Texas in Austin. His scholarship was withdrawn after seventeen months because of his poor academic performance.[78] Nevertheless, while attending the university, Whitman met Kathy, and they married on August 17, 1962.[79]

In February 1963, Whitman returned to active duty in the Marine Corps; in July, he advanced to the rank of lance corporal.[80] But in February 1964, Whitman was court-martialed for gambling and usury, and was demoted back to private.[81]

After his discharge from military service in November 1964, Whitman returned to the University of Texas, where he enrolled in an architectural engineering program.[82] In March 1966, his parents were about to divorce, so Whitman went to Florida to help his mother move to an apartment in Austin.[83]

In 1965, Whitman saw several doctors for his headaches; by the following year, his headaches had become much more severe.[84] Very concerned about his overwhelming violent impulses, he sought psychiatric help on March 29, 1966, at the University of Texas Student Health Center, where he was referred to Dr. Maurice Dean Heatly, the staff psychiatrist.[85] After meeting with Whitman for an hour, Heatly summarized the session as follows: "This massive, muscular youth seemed to be oozing with hostility as he initiated the hour with the statement that something was happening to him and he didn't seem to be himself. Repeated inquiries attempting to analyze his exact experiences were not too successful, with the exception of his vivid reference to 'thinking about going up on the tower with a deer rifle and start shooting people.'"[86]

Whitman was asked to make an appointment with Heatly for the following week, but he failed to do so.[87] Instead, four months later, he went to the observation deck on the twenty-eighth floor of the tower with several guns and numerous rounds of ammunition and began to shoot.

Conclusions

In 1843, the British House of Lords declared that a defendant could be found not guilty because of a "diseased mind" if he didn't know right from wrong at the time he committed the crime.[88] The so-called "insanity defense" is based on the theory that an insane person lacks the intent necessary to commit the crime.[89] It is one of the most controversial, least used, and least successful criminal defense strategies.[90] Two of the most publicized and successful recent cases in which an insanity defense was used include the 1984 acquittal of John W. Hinckley Jr. for his attempted assassination of President Ronald Reagan and the 1994 acquittal of Lorena Bobbitt for hacking off her husband's penis.[91]

Unlike the insanity defense, which is dependent on a psychiatric evaluation, use of neuroscience as a defense strategy is a relatively new concept that is dependent on providing evidence of a linkage between criminal behavior and physical brain damage.[92] Recently, more and more criminal defense lawyers have presented brain scans and other neurological evidence to defend their clients.[93] Three examples of such legal proceedings include a 1991 case of a sixty-eight-year-old man with a large cyst on his brain who strangled his wife and threw her out of their twelfth-floor apartment in Manhattan. Another is a 2002 case of a forty-year-old teacher with a cancerous brain tumor who had secretly started visiting child pornography websites and soliciting prostitutes, activities he had never engaged in before. When his tumor was removed, his sexual obsessions disappeared. And a third example is of a 2018 case of an eighty-year-old man with a benign but inoperable brain tumor who brutally murdered his seventy-one-year-old wife.[94] None of these cases was successfully litigated by defense attorneys, although in other cases, use of neurological evidence has led to plea deals.

According to Stephen Morse of the University of Pennsylvania, "You can't say, 'he has a hole in his head that made him do it.' You have to translate that hole in his head into an excusable condition."[95] Nita A. Farahany of Duke University agreed.[96] "The biggest way in which neuroscience is being used" in the courtroom "is to mitigate punishment in one way or another."[97]

In his article in *Scientific American*, Micah Johnson wrote, "The lesson is that human behavior is complex and a brain lesion is neither necessary nor sufficient for criminal behavior."[98] Johnson added, "Violence can be a symptom of brain disease … and free will can be injured just like other human abilities."[99]

Whitman being the exception, most people with brain tumors do not go out and shoot people. "There are nearly seven hundred thousand people living with brain tumors in the United States, but the known legal cases leading to criminal behavior numbers in the dozens," Johnson noted.[100]

To this day, it is not known what made Whitman go on a violent, bloody rampage on August 1, 1966. Some people think it was due to a chemical imbalance caused by his long-term use of amphetamine.[101] Others suggest it was due to the child abuse he experienced from his dad, the domestic violence he witnessed for many years against his mother, or the training he received as a soldier in the Marine Corps.[102] Still others speculate that his brain tumor was responsible for his aggressive behavior.[103] None of these theories fully explains the underlying cause of Whitman's inexplicable actions on that first day in August.

In my view, the best way to think about the potential contribution of Whitman's glioma to his behavior on August 1, 1966, is to ask whether he would have committed the horrific crimes had he not had a cancerous brain tumor. I believe the answer is decidedly "I don't know." This clearly shows there is still much more to be learned about the possible effect of brain tumors on behavior and reasoning.

The question remains, then, Could the University of Texas massacre have been prevented? In the days, weeks, and even months leading up to August 1, 1966, Whitman showed signs of mental incapacity. He complained of severe headaches and of unusual and irrational thoughts, so much so that he sought professional psychiatric help.[104] "[I'm] thinking about going up on the tower with a deer rifle and start shooting people," Whitman told his psychiatrist at their first and only meeting four months prior to the day he randomly started shooting people from the top of the tower.[105] Shouldn't that have been a red flag to be followed up with the proper authorities? Apparently it wasn't enough, and as a result, numerous people died and many more were severely injured.

CHAPTER 6

Brian Jones

Died July 2, 1969
Member of the Rolling Stones

BRIAN JONES, A founding member of the popular British band the Rolling Stones, had been modernizing Crotchford Farm, the former home of A. A. Milne, author of *Winnie the Pooh*, ever since he bought the eleven-acre estate near Hartfield, in East Sussex, United Kingdom.[1] On July 2, 1969, Jones invited Frank Thorogood, the builder who had been renovating the home, and a twenty-two-year-old nurse, Janet Lawson, to join him and his Swedish girlfriend, Anna Wohlin, for a drink.[2]

Thorogood and Lawson arrived at the farmhouse at about 10:30 p.m.[3] "He had been drinking and he was a bit unsteady on his feet," Lawson later recalled, speaking of Jones.[4] "I attempted a conversation, but it was a little garbled. Jones said it was because he had taken his sleepers [a reference to sleeping pills]."[5]

Sometime before midnight, Jones decided to go for a swim in his heated swimming pool.[6] Lawson warned Jones and Thorogood, both of whom had been drinking, that they were not fit to go swimming, but they disregarded her warning.[7] "Despite his condition, he was able to swim, however he was rather sluggish," Lawson said of Jones.[8]

Wohlin joined Jones and Thorogood in the pool, but when she received a phone call, she left and went inside the house.[9] Later, Thorogood, looking for a towel, also came into the house, leaving Jones alone in the pool.[10]

At about 11:30 p.m., Mary Haddock, Jones's housekeeper, alerted the others that Jones was lying motionless at the bottom of the pool.[11] Thorogood and the two women companions got Jones out of the pool and laid him on his back on the patio deck.[12] Lawson began giving Jones heart massage, and Wohlin, who was a nurse, performed artificial respiration.[13]

An ambulance was summoned, but by the time the doctors arrived, Jones was already dead.[14] He was twenty-seven years old.[15]

The Autopsy

The autopsy was conducted at the Mortuary of Queen Victoria Hospital on July 3, 1969, by Dr. Albert Sachs, a medical pathologist.[16] "[The] deceased apparently went for a swim in a pool at his home with friends. Friends left the pool and the deceased decided to stay in the water. Last seen alive 11:30 p.m., the second of July, 1969. Found dead shortly afterwards," Sachs wrote in the autopsy report.[17]

Jones's body was sixty-nine inches long, "powerfully built, with a tendency to obesity."[18] A little bloodstained fluid was found in the mouth, which, according to Sachs, could have been due to attempts at artificial respiration.[19] Frothy fluid around the nostrils was a sign consistent with drowning.[20]

Compared to an average heart weight of 331 grams, Jones's heart was approximately 25 percent larger, weighing 411 grams, a risk factor for sudden death from an arrhythmia, an electrical abnormality in the heart that causes ventricular fibrillation, an erratic, disorganized firing of impulses from the ventricle chambers of the heart.[21] The myocardium, the muscular tissue of the heart, was fatty and "flabby," but it showed no evidence of vascular (coronary vessels) or valvular (heart valves) disease.[22] The aorta, the large artery through which oxygenated blood is pumped from the heart to the rest of the body was narrowed due to an accumulation of plaque.[23]

The brain was congested, edematous (fluid-containing), and with "punctate hemorrhages" (microscopic hemorrhaging) in the white matter, the cause of which is unknown.[24]

The respiratory tract was congested with a few "flakes" of "glairy mucus," a thick nasal secretion, in the bronchi, but not the viscid, adherent mucus that is normally associated with death due to an asthmatic attack.[25] Frothy bloodstained fluid exuded from both lungs, consistent with drowning, with each lung significantly heavier at 632 grams (left lung) and 643 grams (right lung), respectively, as compared to an average weight of 395 grams (left lung) and 445 grams (right lung).[26]

The spleen, kidneys, and liver were all congested, with the liver significantly enlarged, about twice the weight of a normal liver.[27] Microscopic examination of liver tissue identified architectural loss, extensive fatty degeneration, and liver dysfunction undoubtedly due to chronic abuse of alcohol and illicit drugs.[28] The stomach contained about one ounce of undigested food.[29] Very little urine was present in the urinary bladder.[30]

It is apparent that the autopsy findings were consistent with drowning, with the lungs significantly heavier than normal and frothy fluid exuding from the lungs and nasal passages. In addition, the autopsy indicated that Jones did not suffer an asthmatic attack prior to his death. And while the liver was significantly enlarged and dysfunctional, there was also some narrowing of the aorta, and the heart was fatty, flabby, and enlarged, which put Jones at an increased risk of an arrhythmia. I was anxious to review the toxicology report, hoping it would shed additional light on how Jones died.

Cause and Manner of Death

Alcohol was detected in the blood at a concentration of 140 milligrams per 100 milliliters, equivalent to a blood alcohol concentration (BAC) of 0.140, a level that is 75 percent above the legal limit for driving an automobile in the United

Kingdom and in the United States.[31] That amount of alcohol, however, was not sufficient to cause death.

An unidentified "amphetamine-like" substance was detected in the urine at a concentration of 1.72 milligrams per 100 milliliters indicating Jones consumed the drug sometime prior to his death.[32] Amphetamine has been documented to predispose the heart to electrical instability and a wide range of arrhythmias. However, the drug was not reported as being present in the blood, although it may have been, especially since Jones's death certificate clearly notes that alcohol and drugs contributed to his death.

After I reviewed the circumstances surrounding Jones's death, the autopsy findings and results of toxicology testing, the death certificate, published lay articles, and the scientific literature, I concluded that the immediate cause of death was drowning, possibly in combination with an arrhythmia or some other heart-related event, such as a heart attack. Contributing factors in the death included severe liver dysfunction due to fatty degeneration, as well as ingestion of alcohol and amphetamine.[33] The manner of death, which the coroner of East Sussex, Dr. Angus Sommerville, labeled "death by misadventure," was accidental.[34]

Life and Career

Jones was born in 1942 in the Park Nursing Home in Cheltenham, ninety-eight miles west of London.[35] When he was four years old, an attack of croup left him with lifelong asthma.[36]   Jones's parents were both interested in music.[37] His mother was a piano teacher, and his father was an aeronautical engineer who played the piano and organ and led the choir at the local church.[38]

Jones was sent "to the finest schools," including the Dean Close School and Cheltenham Grammar School for Boys, from which he was suspended twice.[39] Dick Hartrell, a childhood friend, recalled, "He was a rebel without a cause, but when examinations came he was brilliant."[40]

Jones's interest in jazz was inspired in 1957 after he heard the music of Cannonball Adderley.[41] Jones taught himself to play the guitar and harmonica, and in later years, he learned to play the clarinet, eventually mastering the recorder, soprano sax, keyboard, and several string instruments, including the harp.[42]

In the late summer of 1959, Jones's seventeen-year-old girlfriend, Valerie Corbett, became pregnant.[43] Jones encouraged her to have an abortion, but she refused, carrying the child to term and giving it up for adoption.[44] In November of the same year, Jones had a one-night stand with a married woman who also became pregnant. Unlike Corbett, the woman and her husband decided to keep the baby.[45] By 1965, Jones had impregnated four additional women and had fathered a total of seven children.[46]

When Jones discovered rhythm and blues music, his parents bought him his first acoustic guitar as a present for his seventeenth birthday.[47] After traveling for a summer in Scandinavia, Jones returned to England, where he held odd jobs and performed at local blues and jazz clubs.[48]

In 1962, Jones went to London, where he met Mick Jagger and Keith Richards at the Bricklayers Arms, a popular London pub.[49] Together the three formed a band they named the Rolling Stones, with Jones playing rhythm guitar.[50] Eventually they recruited Charlie Watts to join the band on drums, and Bill Wyman, on bass guitar.[51]

Shocked by the appearance, long hair, and rebelliousness of the band members, the press initially was unkind to the Rolling Stones.[52] "These ruddy reporters don't seem to want to take us seriously," Jones said at the time.[53] "Well, that's okay. We'll make them eat their lousy words one day."[54]

Nonetheless, while the popularity of the Rolling Stones increased, hostility between Jones and his bandmates also grew, and Jones's attitude began to change for the worse.[55] He developed a serious drug problem that was in part due to his inability to cope with the rising fame of the Rolling Stones.[56] "There were at least two sides to Brian's personality," Wyman observed.[57] "One Brian was introverted, shy, sensitive, deep-thinking. The other was a preening peacock, gregarious, artistic, desperately needing assurance from his peers. He pushed every friendship to the limit and way beyond."[58]

In May 1967, Jones was charged with marijuana possession.[59] He was given a sentence of nine months in jail that was later suspended and reduced to a year's probation.[60] The following year, Jones was again arrested for possession of marijuana.[61] When Jones was found guilty, the judge fined him and told him, "For goodness sake, don't get into trouble again or it really will be serious."[62]

By 1969, Jones's substance abuse and mood swings had become intolerable. He was "literally incapable of making music; when he tried to play harmonica, his mouth started bleeding," Gary Herman, the author, said.[63] In March of the same year, a company car Jones had been driving was towed by the police when it was parked illegally.[64] In May, Jones crashed his motorcycle into a shop window.[65] And in November, just as the Rolling Stones were getting ready to tour North America, Jones was unable to obtain a work permit because of his drug convictions.[66]

On June 8, 1969, Mick Jagger, Keith Richards, and Charlie Watts fired Jones from the Rolling Stones.[67] According to Wyman, Jones "formed the band. He chose the members. He named the band. He chose the music we played. He got us gigs ... he was very influential, very important, and then slowly lost it — highly intelligent — and just kind of wasted it and blew it all away."[68]

After leaving the Rolling Stones, Jones had aspirations of forming a new band. On July 2, 1969, less than a month after he was fired by Jagger, Richards, and Watts, Jones invited a few friends to his country home in East Essex, where he drank alcohol, ingested pills, and swam in his swimming pool. It was the last time he would do so.

Conclusions

Almost as soon as Jones died, conspiracy theories began to emerge. It was suggested Jones's drowning was due to his asthma. However, no evidence was found at the autopsy to indicate Jones had suffered a recent asthmatic attack. Another proposed theory was that Jones died after having taken a combination of alcohol, sleeping pills, and amphetamines. Based on information presented in the autopsy report, no barbiturates were detected in Jones's blood.[69]

According to some reports, Thorogood, who had been swimming with Jones the day he died, made a deathbed confession in 1993, claiming he had killed Jones, but this was never confirmed.[70]

In August 2009, after receiving new information from Scott Jones, an investigative journalist unrelated to Brian Jones, the Sussex Police Department reexamined the Jones file.[71] When the department completed its review, it decided not to reopen the case, claiming, "There is no new evidence to suggest that the coroner's original verdict of 'death by misadventure' was incorrect."[72]

The author, Paul Trynka, who wrote a biography of Brian Jones, declared in 2014, "I've come to share [the official coroner's] belief that Brian's death was most likely a tragic accident" and that "many of the existing theories that his death was, in fact, murder rely on unreliable witnesses."[73]

In 2019, the Sussex Police Department reaffirmed its position, stating, "The [Jones] case has not been reopened and there are no plans for that to happen."[74]

That Jones died as a result of drowning is clear. His lungs were heavy and filled with fluid, and there was foam around his nostrils—a clear sign of drowning. And while his blood alcohol concentration of 0.140 indicated he drank at least six or seven glasses of alcohol the night he died, which would have made him drowsy, that amount of alcohol was insufficient to cause death.

Of special importance is that Jones was known to be a chronic, heavy user of drugs of abuse.[75] The effect of chronic use of illicit drugs was readily apparent in his autopsy, with significant changes noticeable in the heart and liver. Most illicit drugs have adverse cardiovascular effects and alter heart function.[76] Even "recreational" cocaine abusers often have higher blood pressure, a 30 to 35 percent increase in stiffening of the aorta, and an 18 percent greater thickening of the heart's left ventricle wall.[77]

Interestingly, Jones's death is similar to how the singer and actress Whitney Houston died.[78] Both Jones and Houston died by drowning, Jones in a swimming pool and Houston in a hotel bathtub.[79] However, the most significant finding in the two autopsies is that sometime before they died, Jones had ingested amphetamine and Houston had taken cocaine.[80] The two drugs are central nervous system stimulants that increase heart rate and elevate blood pressure, two risk factors for an arrhythmia, an electrical abnormality in the heart, as well as a heart attack due to blockage of coronary arteries. Since Jones had an enlarged heart with some narrowing of the aorta and Houston had 60 percent narrowing of her right coronary artery, they were both at a significant risk for a heart-related event.[81] By consuming amphetamine or cocaine sometime prior to their deaths, Jones and Houston may have suffered an arrhythmia or a heart attack just before they drowned.

At his death, Jones was only twenty-seven years old, and in his death, he became the first member of the Twenty-Seven Club—a group of musicians who died at the age of twenty-seven.[82] In time, Jones was joined by Jimi Hendrix, Janis Joplin, Jim Morrison, Amy Winehouse, and Kurt Cobain, among others.[83]

CHAPTER 7

Sonny Liston

Died December 30, 1970

Former Heavyweight Boxing Champion of the World

IN 1970, SONNY Liston, the former heavyweight boxing champion of the world, and his wife, Geraldine, were living in a large, split-level home in Paradise Palms, an affluent neighborhood in Las Vegas, Nevada.[1] Sometime in late December, Liston's wife went to St. Louis, Missouri, to visit her mother for the Christmas holiday, leaving Liston home alone.[2] After she was unable to reach Liston for two weeks, Liston's wife became concerned and flew back to Las Vegas on January 5.[3] When she arrived at their residence, she was surprised to find the front door unlocked and a foul odor permeating the air.[4] "I thought he must have cooked and left something on the stove," she later said.[5] Walking up the stairs, the offensive smell became more pronounced.[6]

As she entered the master bedroom, Liston's wife saw her husband's bloated body clad in a T-shirt and boxer shorts, lying at the foot of the bed with blood congealed under his nose.[7] Immediately she called Liston's attorney, and about two to three hours later, she notified the police.[8]

Based on the number of milk cartons and the dates printed on newspapers piled at the front door, police determined that Liston had been dead for about six days.[9] In the kitchen, investigators found a quarter ounce of heroin in a balloon; a half-ounce of marijuana was in a pants pocket, and a glass of vodka was on a nightstand.[10]

"It was common knowledge that Sonny was a heroin addict," Sergeant Dennis Caputo, the first police officer on the scene, said.[11] No syringes or other drug paraphernalia were found at the Liston home. "It wasn't uncommon for family members in these cases to go through and tidy up," former Las Vegas police Sergeant Gary Beckwith explained.[12]

Liston was pronounced dead at the scene.[13] Without an official record of his birth, it was estimated Liston was approximately forty years old when he died.

The Autopsy

An autopsy and toxicology reports were not available for review. However, based on published lay articles, Liston had been suffering from "hardening of the heart muscle" and emphysema, a disease involving the destruction of alveoli, tiny air sacs in the lungs that allow for the exchange of oxygen and exhaled carbon dioxide in blood during the process of respiration.[14] In addition, he had been hospitalized with chest pain (angina) two to three weeks before he died.[15]

Scar tissue, possibly from past needle marks, was identified at the autopsy in the bend of Liston's left elbow, suggestive of past intravenous drug use.[16] Information regarding Liston's medical condition prior to his death indicated he had at least two major risk factors that could have caused his death: emphysema and heart disease. I was anxious to review any available toxicology testing results that might further clarify the cause of Liston's death.

Cause and Manner of Death

Police found no evidence of foul play, signs of a struggle, or forced entry, suggesting that Liston's death was not a homicide.[17]

Clark County coroner Mark Herman reported finding some traces of morphine and codeine, metabolic byproducts of heroin, in the kidneys, but the levels were not sufficiently elevated to be considered an overdose.[18] Since no morphine was identified in the blood, it was unlikely Liston died from respiratory depression, a condition in which there is reduced breathing due to inhibition of the respiratory centers in the brain by the opioid.

After I reviewed the circumstances surrounding Liston's death, as well as published lay articles and the scientific literature, I agreed with the coroner's conclusion that more likely than not, the immediate cause of death was heart failure; lung congestion was a contributing factor.[19] The manner of death was natural.[20]

Life and Career

Liston was born in St. Francis County, Arkansas, the ninth of ten children of Helen Baskin and Tobe Liston, an abusive, alcoholic tenant farmer.[21] "The only thing my old man ever gave me was a beating," Liston once said.[22]

When he was eight years old, Liston began to work in the cotton fields of the Morledge Plantation near Johnson Township.[23] "We hardly had enough food to keep from starving, no shoes, only a few clothes, and nobody to help us escape from the horrible life we lived," Liston later recalled.[24] At thirteen, Liston ran away from home after picking pecans from his brother-in-law's tree and selling them for bus money to go to St. Louis, Missouri.[25]

Unable to read or write, and bullied in school, Liston left school when he was sixteen years old and instead turned to crime, including muggings and armed robberies; he was arrested more than twenty times.[26] In 1950, Liston was convicted of two counts of larceny and two counts of first-degree armed robbery of a gas station, for which he spent more than two years in the Missouri State Penitentiary.[27]

While incarcerated, Liston was introduced to boxing by the prison athletic director, Father Alois Stevens.[28] "He was the most perfect specimen of manhood I had ever seen," Stevens told *Sports Illustrated.*[29] With his powerful arms, big shoulders, large hands, and an iron chin, Liston knocked out all of his opponents.[30]

After he was paroled in 1952, Liston won the Chicago Golden Gloves Tournament of Champions, the Intercity Golden Gloves Championship, and the International Golden Gloves.[31] A year later, he made his professional debut, knocking out Don Smith in thirty-three seconds of the first round.[32] After winning nine straight boxing matches, Liston lost an eight-round split decision to Marty Marshall.[33] However, in a subsequent rematch, he defeated Marshall with a sixth-round knockout.[34]

In 1957, Liston spent six months in prison for assaulting a police officer. The following year, he returned to the ring, winning his next eight bouts.[35] By 1960, having won twenty-six consecutive fights, Liston became the top contender for the heavyweight world championship.[36]

Liston got his shot at a title bout against Floyd Patterson, the heavyweight champion, on September 25, 1962.[37] With his powerful physique and a twenty-five-pound weight advantage over Patterson, Liston had one of the most powerful jabs in boxing history, fifteen-inch fists that were the largest of any heavyweight champion, and an extraordinarily long reach of eighty-four inches.[38] Nevertheless, *Sports Illustrated* predicted Patterson to win, claiming, "Sonny has neither Floyd's speed nor the versatility of his attack."[39]

For the first time in history, the reigning heavyweight champion was knocked out with a powerful left hook to the jaw within the first two minutes of the title fight.[40] Gilbert

Rogin of *Sports Illustrated* wrote, "That final left hook crashed into Patterson's cheek like a diesel rig going downhill, no brakes."[41] In a subsequent match on July 22, 1963, Liston again beat Patterson, knocking him down three times within the first two minutes of the first round.[42]

After he defeated Patterson twice, many presumed that Liston was destined to retain the heavyweight championship for a long time. His quick jabs and brute force made him seem invincible.[43] When he was challenged for the crown by Cassius Clay, a brash, poetry-loving twenty-two-year-old underdog, forty-six sportswriters chose Liston to win by a knockout.[44] Cocky as always, Clay even composed a poem to mark the occasion, reciting it on a CBS television show.[45]

The heavyweight title fight was held on February 25, 1964, with Liston and Clay boxing each other in Miami Beach, Florida.[46] The first round lasted an extra twenty seconds, as neither of the boxers nor the referee heard the closing bell of the round.[47] In the third round, Clay hit Liston with such force that eight stitches were later required to close a cut under Liston's left eye.[48] At the end of the fourth round, Clay complained that a substance used by the "cutman" in Liston's corner had "blinded" him.[49] Enraged, he delivered Liston a combination of devastating punches in the sixth round, after which Liston failed to get up from his stool for the seventh round.[50] The reign of "the ugly bear," as Clay called Liston, had lasted only seventeen months.[51]

In their next bout, on May 25, 1965, in Lewiston, Maine, Muhammad Ali, formerly known as Cassius Clay, knocked out Liston in the first 104 seconds of the first round with a short, chopping right "phantom punch" to the head.[52] "You're supposed to be so bad! Nobody will believe this!" Ali yelled at the twice defeated ex-champion as he lay flat on his back, unable to rise from the canvas.[53] It took several slow-motion replays over the next several days to dispel the notion that the fight was fixed, although many people remained skeptical.[54] The photo of Ali standing over Liston imploring him to "Get up and fight, sucker!" became one of the most iconic pictures in boxing history.[55]

After losing the championship, Liston boxed in Sweden, where he won four consecutive matches, and then in the United States, winning fourteen fights, thirteen by knockouts, including one against fifth-ranked Henry Clark.[56] However, in December 1969, Liston was knocked out in the ninth round by third-ranked Leotis Martin, his former sparring partner. At that moment, all hope for another shot at the title completely vanished.[57] Nevertheless, Liston continued to box, winning his final fight against Chuck Wepner just six months before he died.[58]

Conclusions

Heart failure, also known as congestive heart failure, is a chronic, progressive condition in which the heart muscle is unable to pump enough blood to meet the body's needs for oxygen and nutrients.[59] When left untreated, it can be life-threatening.[60] To compensate for heart failure, the heart may become enlarged, develop more muscle mass, or pump faster.[61]

When the compensatory mechanisms no longer work, fluid can build up in the lungs, causing shortness of breath, fatigue, and swelling in the legs, ankles or feet.[62] Some risk factors for heart failure include coronary artery disease, high blood pressure, diabetes, and obesity.[63] Loss of weight, exercise, and reduced sodium intake can improve the quality of life for those suffering from heart failure.[64] Liston's diagnosis of hardening of the heart muscle and his hospitalization for chest pain two to three weeks prior to his death are consistent with the coroner's conclusion that Liston died from heart failure.

Many people have speculated that Liston's death was the result of a mob hit, although there is no evidence for that.[65] "My inclination is that he was bumped off because he was of no use to the mob anymore," wrote Rob Steen in his biography of Liston.[66] Others have suggested, despite clear evidence to the contrary, that Liston died from a heroin overdose that was not self-administered, claiming Liston was terrified of needles and would never have injected himself with the drug.[67] The fact is that the amount of morphine, the major metabolite of heroin, in Liston's system was low, so the coroner correctly excluded a heroin overdose in his diagnosis.[68] Also, no fresh needle marks on Liston's arms were identified at the autopsy.

In his boxing career, Liston won fifty of his fifty-four fights, thirty-nine of those by knockout. In 1991, he was inducted into the International Boxing Hall of Fame.[69] And yet, because of his race and his ties to organized crime, the press portrayed Liston as "arrogant, surly, mean, rude and altogether frightening … the last man anyone would want to meet in a dark alley," even labeling him with terms such as "gorilla" and "bear."[70] Ali, who defeated Liston twice, admitted, "Of all the men I fought in boxing, Sonny Liston was the scariest."[71]

When he was ready to challenge Patterson for the boxing heavyweight title, President John F. Kennedy urged Patterson to find another opponent—one with "better character."[72] Even the NAACP and civil rights leaders shunned Liston, thinking he was not a good role model for African American youth.[73] In his biography of Liston, Rob Steen wrote, "Liston was about the last person the movement wanted to signify black achievement. He was illiterate, he'd been in prison, and he'd supposedly beaten up striking workers for the mob. He'd sold his soul to the mob in order to get proper fights."[74]

Liston anticipated a warm reception in his adopted hometown of Philadelphia after he won the heavyweight title against Patterson, but he was snubbed instead.[75] Larry Merchant, sports editor of the *Philadelphia Daily News*, wrote, "Emily Post would probably recommend a ticker-tape parade. For confetti, we can use shredded warrants of arrest."[76]

When Liston lost the second heavyweight title fight to Ali, he also lost his remaining fans, the media, and many in the general public who believed he threw the fight.[77] In his final year, Liston's "routine largely involved drinking and … dealing some cocaine out of a casino and also getting involved in heroin," according to Shaun Assael.[78] Michael Green, a professor of history who has studied the mob in Nevada and was a board member at the Las Vegas Mob Museum, agreed. "He appears to have had involvement with drugs and if you're involved with drugs, then you're dealing possibly with the mob," Green said.[79]

It's unfortunate that despite his boxing accomplishments, Liston failed to receive the respect he deserved from the public, the press, and his peers.[80] To many, numerous unanswered questions were left behind by Liston's death.

CHAPTER 8

Bruce Lee

Died July 20, 1973
Actor and Martial Artist

ON MAY 10, 1973, Bruce Lee, the actor and martial artist, was assisting with the dubbing for his latest film, *Enter the Dragon*, at Golden Harvest, a film production, distribution, and exhibition company based in Hong Kong.[1] To cut down on ambient noise, the air-conditioning in the studio had been turned off.[2] Feeling overheated, Lee went to the restroom to put water on his face.[3] Twenty minutes later, he was discovered unresponsive.[4] After being rushed to Hong Kong Baptist Hospital, Lee was found to have a fever of 105 degrees.[5]

Dr. Don Langford, Lee's family physician and a Tulane University-educated American surgeon, diagnosed Lee with cerebral edema, a buildup of fluid on the brain.[6] Dr. Peter Wu, a neurologist, was also consulted, since Lee had experienced seizures while at the hospital.[7]

Lee was treated with mannitol, a diuretic, to reduce the swelling and the pressure on his brain.[8] Aware Lee had consumed hashish (cannabis), made from resin, a secreted gum of the cannabis plant, shortly before his medical emergency, "We gave Bruce a long talk before he was discharged from the hospital, asking him not to eat hashish again," Wu said.[9] "Since he'd already had a very bad time with the drug, we told him that the effects were likely to be worse next time," Wu added.[10]

After Lee recovered, he flew to Los Angeles, where he was given a battery of tests at the Ronald Reagan University of California Los Angeles Medical Center.[11] Declared fit and discharged with a prescription for phenytoin (Dilantin), a drug that prevents seizures, Lee returned to Hong Kong to complete work on his film.[12]

On July 20, 1973, about two months after the cerebral edema episode, Lee was again at Golden Harvest, discussing Australian actor George Lazenby's role in his next film, *Game of Death*, at which time Lee ate a small amount of hashish.[13] After the meeting, he drove to the apartment of Betty Ting-Pei, a Taiwanese actress slated to play Lazenby's love interest in *Game of Death*.[14] Later, Ting-Pei explained why Lee was at her apartment. "I was his girlfriend," she said.[15] At about six o'clock, Raymond Chow, owner of Golden Harvest, also arrived at Ting-Pei's apartment.[16]

Lee performed several scenes from the film in front of Ting-Pei and Chow. But at about 7:30 p.m., after Chow left, Lee began to complain of dizziness and a severe headache, so Ting-Pei gave him a tablet of Equagesic, a prescription pain reliever containing aspirin and meprobamate, a tranquilizer.[17] "Bruce had taken them before," Ting-Pei later declared.[18]

Lee ingested the Equagesic and went to sleep, but at about half past nine, Ting-Pei couldn't wake him for their dinner date with Chow.[19] Ting-Pei called Chow, who rushed over and found Lee unresponsive. Dr. Eugene Chu Poh-hwye, Ting-Pei's personal physician, was summoned, and he immediately rushed Lee to Queen Elizabeth Hospital, arriving at about 10:30 p.m.[20] But despite heroic attempts at resuscitation, Lee was pronounced dead at eleven thirty.[21] He was thirty-two years old.[22]

The Autopsy

Lee's body was identified by his older brother, Peter.[23] Dr. R. R. Lycette, a medical pathologist from New Zealand, conducted the autopsy.[24]

"The body is that of a well-built Chinese male of about thirty years of age and is one hundred and seventy-two centimeters in length," Lycette wrote in the autopsy report.[25] It weighed 128 pounds.[26] There was no evidence of external injuries or foul play.[27]

The scalp was free of bruising, and the skull showed no evidence of fracture or injury.[28] Also, there were no needle marks on the arms or anywhere else on the body.[29]

While the intestines and kidneys were congested, remnants of the Equagesic pill and small traces of cannabis were identified in the stomach.[30]

With respect to the cardiovascular system, the heart and blood vessels were all normal.[31] As for the respiratory system, there was some congestion in the lungs.[32]

What was especially significant for the identification of cause of death was the swelling in the brain.[33] "The brain is very tense beneath the covering dura," Lycette wrote in the autopsy report.[34] At 1,575 grams, it was approximately 13 percent heavier than an average brain as a result of the accumulated fluid.[35]

Cerebral edema is the abnormal accumulation of fluid in the brain.[36] It is a life-threatening medical emergency often caused by traumatic brain injury, the most common of which result from falls, automobile accidents, and assaults, as well as stroke due to blood clots in the brain, certain viral and bacterial infections, brain tumors, high altitudes, and, in rare cases, some pharmaceuticals.[37] Normally, the blood-brain barrier helps maintain the intracranial pressure, allowing entry of certain substances from the blood into the brain.[38] However, when the brain is injured, there is an increase in water movement into the brain, causing swelling and disruption of normal cellular function.[39] This results in higher pressure inside the skull, preventing oxygenated blood to flow into and fluid to leave from the brain, causing symptoms that could include headache, dizziness, vision changes, memory loss, seizures, and loss of consciousness.[40]

In reviewing the autopsy results, it was apparent that the only significant anatomical anomaly detected that could have led to Lee's death was his brain swelling. Whether cannabis or Equagesic caused or contributed to Lee's death remained to be investigated.

Cause and Manner of Death

Police searched Ting-Pei's apartment but found no sign of a struggle or foul play.[41]

Lee's system was tested for the presence of poisons and other toxic chemicals by Dr. Lam King Leung, a government chemist. The tests detected a trace amount of cannabis and Equagesic in Lee's stomach, not enough to be considered an overdose.[42]

Based on the autopsy findings and toxicology results, Lycette concluded, "Congestion and edema of the brain, often referred to as 'cerebral edema,' were the immediate cause of death. The congestion of the lungs and other organs is strongly suggestive of the brain edema first stopping respiratory function, while the heart continued to pump blood into the body's arteries, which were dilating because of lack of oxygen. The edema finally caused failure of cardiac centers in the brain and stopped the heart."[43]

As for the specific cause of the acute cerebral edema, "The findings provide no definitive evidence as to the cause of the cerebral edema," Lycette declared.[44] "It is possible that the edema is the result of some drug intoxication."[45]

On September 3, 1973, a coroner's inquest was held during which none of the experts could agree what caused Lee's cerebral edema.[46] Both physicians—Langford, who had treated Lee's first episode of cerebral edema, and Wu, who had examined Lee in Ting-Pei's apartment after the second episode—were convinced cannabis was responsible.[47] Lycette, who had conducted Lee's autopsy, shared their opinion, writing, "I believe the most likely cause of death is cannabis intoxication, either due to drug idiosyncrasy or massive overdose."[48] However, professor Donald Teare, a highly respected forensic pathologist who had conducted the autopsy on Jimi Hendrix three years earlier and who had been specifically brought in from London by the judge, disagreed.[49] Langford remembered Teare telling the two physicians and the medical examiner, "If one was going to decide that the chemicals in marijuana were dangerous and could be lethal, then that conclusion shouldn't be decided in some little bitty, insignificant backwater like Hong Kong."[50]

When it came time to testify, Langford conceded that the cause of cerebral edema "may or may not have been drug intoxication," while Wu testified, "I am not in the position as an expert to talk about cannabis."[51] Lycette, having learned there were no reliable cases of deaths from cannabis, changed his mind and said the most likely substance to have caused the cerebral edema was one of the ingredients in Equagesic.[52]

Teare testified that, in his opinion, Lee had suffered a severe though "very rare, indeed" allergic reaction to aspirin, meprobamate, or both—two drugs present in Equagesic.[53]

"As far as acute cerebral edema is concerned," Teare said, "taking cannabis or taking a cup of tea or coffee would be identical."[54] Dr. Ira Frank, a physician at UCLA Medical Center, and Dr. David Reisbord, a US neurologist who had examined Lee after his first bout with cerebral edema, both concurred, providing sworn affidavits stating they were not aware of any cases in which marijuana caused a fatality.[55]

It took the three-person lay jury only five minutes to declare that the manner of death was "death by misadventure," similar to "accident" in the United States, with Equagesic, not cannabis, as the likely cause of the cerebral edema and Lee's death.[56]

After I reviewed the circumstances surrounding Lee's death, the autopsy findings and results of toxicology testing, published lay articles, and the scientific literature, I agreed that the immediate cause of death was cerebral edema. However, while cerebral edema is a rare adverse effect of Equagesic, I found it difficult to comprehend how aspirin or meprobamate, the two active ingredients in Equagesic, could have caused Lee's brain swelling.[57]

According to Ting-Pei, Lee had ingested Equagesic in the past without any problem. Also, on July 20, the day Lee suffered his second bout of cerebral edema, he ingested the medication only after he complained of a headache, a symptom associated with cerebral edema, suggesting that Lee's brain swelling had already begun before he consumed the medication. Furthermore, Lee was found unresponsive, and probably dead, only two hours after he ingested

Equagesic, which is inconsistent with published reports that it takes twenty-four to forty-eight hours from the initial brain injury, and in some cases as long as days, to develop clinically significant brain swelling.[58] In addition, at his autopsy, remnants of the Equagesic pill were found in Lee's stomach, which meant that less than a therapeutic dose of the drug was absorbed into Lee's system. Lastly, Lee had suffered a similar bout of cerebral edema only two months prior to his death, at a time when he had not ingested Equagesic.

Chow testified at the inquest that Lee often suffered terrible blows to the head during filming because he wanted to perform all the stunts himself. On the day he died, Lee had been dizzy, a possible sign of cerebral edema, even before he ingested Equagesic.[59] I thought a more likely explanation for the cause of Lee's cerebral edema was that it may have been due to a recent head injury.

In 2006, James Filkins, a Cook County Deputy Medical Examiner in Chicago, suggested Lee died from "sudden unexplained death in epilepsy (SUDEP)," a term coined more than twenty years after Lee died.[60] According to the United States Centers for Disease Control and Prevention (CDC), "SUDP refers to deaths in people with epilepsy that are not caused by injury, drowning, or other known causes."[61] However, since Lee had never been diagnosed with epilepsy, it seems unlikely he died from SUDP.

In his 2008 book, *Bruce Lee: A Life*, Matthew Polly proposed another explanation for Lee's death.[62] Apparently, several months before he died, Lee had an operation to remove the sweat glands from his armpits so he would appear less sweaty on film.[63] Sweating is a way for the body to cool itself down. People suffering from anhidrosis, a severe inability to sweat, could be in serious danger of heat exhaustion, heatstroke, coma, and death if they attempt strenuous activity at high temperatures.[64] Polly points out that Lee's first bout with cerebral edema on May 10, 1973, occurred on a day he had been working in a room with no air-conditioning, and his body temperature had risen to 105 degrees, an obvious sign of heatstroke.[65] And on July 20, the hottest day of the month that year, Lee felt dizzy and had a headache after he exerted himself reenacting several scenes from his upcoming film at Ting-Pei's apartment, two additional signs of heatstroke.[66] According to Polly, since Lee exhibited a sign of heatstroke on May 10 and two signs of heatstroke on July 20, with cerebral edema developing on both occasions, it supports his conclusion that Lee's death from cerebral edema was caused by heatstroke.[67]

Polly's hypothesis may have some merit. Certainly with Lee's body temperature at a reported 105 degrees, the cause of his first bout of cerebral edema is consistent with heatstroke.[68] However, without additional information, including Lee's body temperature the day he died, it is impossible for me to determine whether Lee's second bout of cerebral edema was due to heatstroke.

According to Lisa Leon, an expert in hyperthermia at the United States Army Research Institute of Environmental Medicine, "A person who has suffered one heatstroke is at increased risk for another."[69] This suggests that the cause of Lee's episode of cerebral edema on July 20, the one that claimed his life, may have been related more to his first bout of cerebral edema than to anything else.

In my view, it is clear that Lee died from cerebral edema. He had suffered from brain swelling on a previous occasion, and there was evidence of cerebral edema, a known cause of death, at his autopsy. What is not certain, however, is what caused the cerebral edema. While searching for the answer may be a worthwhile academic exercise, it bears no relevance to the cause of Lee's death, but only to the manner of death, which, depending on the findings, would be natural or accidental.

In the absence of a review of Lee's medical records and additional information about his activities in the days and weeks prior to his death, I concluded that the cause of Lee's death was cerebral edema. As to what caused the cerebral edema, that remains a mystery. I therefore labeled the manner of death undetermined.

Life and Career

Lee was born in 1940, "the Year of the Dragon," at the Jackson Street Hospital in San Francisco's Chinatown.[70] His mother, who came from a wealthy family, was half German and half Chinese; his father was an actor with Hong Kong's Cantonese Opera.[71] In 1941, Lee's family returned to Hong Kong, settling into a second-story apartment in the Kowloon City District.[72]

When Lee was three months old, he made his acting debut in the film *Golden Gate Girl*.[73] At six years of age, he appeared in *The Birth of Mankind* and then in *My Son, Ah Cheun*.[74] All told, Lee appeared as a child actor in approximately twenty Chinese films.[75]

When he was twelve, Lee entered La Salle College, a Christian secondary school where his street fights and his involvement as leader of a gang called "The Tigers of Junction Street," as well as his poor behavior in school, kept landing him in trouble, both with the school and the police.[76] Although very bright, Lee's poor grades and constant fighting led him to transfer to Saint Francis Xavier College, a Catholic secondary school for boys.[77]

A year later, Lee was introduced to Yip Man, a Chinese grand master of the martial art Wing Chun.[78] Focusing all his attention on kung fu and dancing, Lee won the Crown Colony Cha-Cha Championship in 1958.[79] That same year, he entered a boxing championship where he earned a third-round knockout against the reigning title holder.[80]

In April 1959, Lee returned to the United States, living with the Chow family, friends of Lee's parents, in Seattle, Washington.[81] While attending Edison Technical School, later renamed Seattle Central Community College, Lee worked nights as a waiter in Chow's Chinese restaurant, eventually earning his high school diploma. In 1961, he enrolled at the University of Washington, majoring in drama.[82]

Lee opened his first martial arts school in Seattle in 1963. The following year, he dropped out of the university and opened a second martial arts school in Oakland, California.[83] While in Oakland, Lee gave a martial arts demonstration at the Long Beach International Karate Tournament, where Jay Sebring, owner of a Beverly Hills hair salon, was so impressed that he provided a demo tape of the demonstration to television producer William Dozier.[84] Dozier, who was working on a Charlie Chan series titled *Number-One Son*, gave Lee a screen test in February 1965 for the role of Charlie Chan's son.[85] While the project was eventually scrapped, Dozier later cast Lee as Kato in the television series *The Green Hornet*.[86] The show was cancelled after one season, but Lee's fighting scenes became a viewer favorite.[87]

Lee next appeared in small roles in the television shows *Ironside, Longstreet, Here Comes the Bride*, and *Blondie*.[88] To supplement his income, he opened a third martial arts school in Los Angeles and gave private lessons to celebrities, including Steve McQueen, James Coburn, James Garner, and Kareem Abdul Jabbar.[89]

In 1971, Lee returned to Hong Kong, where, much to his surprise, he discovered that *The Green Hornet* was immensely popular and he was a superstar.[90] Not pleased to be dubbed a superstar, Lee said, "The word 'superstar' really turns me off. You would be very pleased if somebody said 'man, you are a super actor!' It is much better than, you know, superstar."[91]

While in Hong Kong, Lee met Chow, a former executive of Shaw Brothers Studio and the owner of Golden Harvest, who immediately signed him to a two-picture deal.[92] After completing filming *The Big Boss* and *Fists of Fury*, Lee and

Chow formed Concord Productions. In May 1972, Chow and Lee began to shoot *The Way of the Dragon*, which marked Lee's directorial debut.[93] The movie was a huge success, so in early 1973, Lee began filming *Enter the Dragon*.[94]

Conclusions

As with other cult figures, such as James Dean, when Lee died at such a young age, many of his fans refused to accept the official explanation of his death. "He was known as the fittest man alive," said Brian Harrison, head of the Bruce Lee Fan Club in the UK.[95] Several theories began to emerge, one of which was that Lee was killed by a "death touch," a fatal martial arts blow, as punishment for teaching Eastern martial arts secrets to Westerners.[96] Another was that he was killed by Hong Kong Triads or Japanese ninjas for refusing to go along with certain financial schemes.[97] Not surprisingly, none of these theories had any evidentiary support or validity.

Lee is listed among *Time* magazine's 100 Most Influential People of the Twentieth Century and is ranked second among the 100 Most Inspiring Asian Americans of All Time by *Goldsea Asian American Daily*.[98] Credited with developing Jeet Kune Do, a system of martial arts that relies on practicality, flexibility, speed, and efficiency, Lee was a master of the "One-Inch Punch," delivering a devastating blow to his opponent with his fist traveling only one inch.[99] "There's no challenge in breaking a board," Lee explained. "Boards don't hit back."[100] Because of his lightning-fast moves and reflexes, the filming of Lee's fight scenes had to be slowed down for fear they would look like they were sped up.[101]

Lee raised the consciousness of people all over the world to martial arts. Although he died at a young age, his contribution to society and the arts will long be remembered. "The key to immortality," Lee once said, "is first living a life worth remembering."[102]

CHAPTER 9

Jim Jones

Died November 18, 1978

Key Figure in the Jonestown Massacre

JIM JONES WAS an immensely charismatic and handsome man who always wore dark aviator sunglasses. "He had that coal-black hair and piercing eyes that would look right through you," recalled Phyllis Wilmore, who had dated Jones in high school.[1] But that was not all. Jones was also a paranoid schizophrenic and a megalomaniac.

A spellbinding reverend of the Peoples Temple, a church Jones founded with nearly one thousand members, Jones had a message that blended evangelical Christianity, New Age spirituality, and radical socialist social justice, attracting a racially diverse, predominantly African American following of all ages.[2]

"[Many] were decent, hardworking, socially conscious people, some highly educated," said Tim Reiterman, a journalist. "[They] wanted to help their fellow man and serve God, not embrace a self-proclaimed deity on earth."[3] Laura Johnston Kohl, a former Peoples Temple member, echoed Reiterman's sentiments entirely. "We all felt that we were a family rather than a church."[4]

Between 1974 and 1976, Jones and his Peoples Temple followers left California and relocated to Guyana, where, despite the oppressive heat, they developed a commune on more than thirty-eight hundred acres of rented densely foliaged jungle east of Venezuela. Known as Jonestown, it was a working agricultural settlement dedicated to building a utopian society free from meddling by the US government and from media scrutiny.[5]

It wasn't long after Jones arrived in Jonestown that his paranoia was on full display. [6] He limited information flow to and from the outside world, encouraged family members to inform on one another, confiscated all medicines, and instituted public punishments and humiliations.[7] In addition, Jones introduced loyalty tests, known as "White Nights," in which he urged his followers to commit mass suicide by drinking from a vat containing what he said was a poisoned fruit drink called Flavor Aid, but which he later claimed wasn't really poisoned.[8] Peoples Temple members were required to spend six days a week in long hours of hard physical labor.

Seniors had to turn over their social security checks, and attendance was mandatory at all night sessions in the main pavilion, where Jones railed against the US government, the media, relatives who wanted to destroy their community, and the inevitability of nuclear war.[9]

"I never thought it would come to this," Philip Blakely, one of the early Jonestown settlers wrote to his ex-wife.[10] "It wasn't until Jones got there that things got bad. If he really wanted to do something for socialism, he couldn't have done anything worse."[11] The writer, Shiva Naipaul, agreed. "[It] was neither racial justice nor socialism, but a messianic parody of both."[12] Leslie Wilson, a former Peoples Temple member, described it best: "It was a slave camp run by a madman."[13]

US Congressman Leo Ryan of San Mateo, California, had heard that followers of the Peoples Temple were being mistreated in Jonestown and were being held there against their will.[14] He decided to fly to Guyana, along with several government officials, nine journalists, and four relatives of Peoples Temple members, to investigate the allegations for himself.[15] At first Jones was reluctant to give Ryan permission to visit the commune, but when Ryan threatened to come anyway, he relented.

Ryan and his congressional entourage arrived in Jonestown on November 17, 2018. Soon thereafter, he was approached by several of Jones's followers who wanted to leave the commune and return to the United States.[16] Much to everyone's surprise, a day after his arrival, Ryan was attacked by a knife-wielding Peoples Temple member. Although he wasn't hurt, Ryan decided to leave Jonestown that afternoon.

While the congressional delegation, along with more than a dozen Peoples Temple members, waited for planes to arrive at the nearby Port Katuma airstrip, gunmen from the commune drove up in a tractor trailer and opened fire, killing the congressman, two photographers, and two journalists, and injuring several others.[17]

Back at the compound, Jones gathered his followers at the main pavilion and told them that Ryan had been murdered and that the Guyanese military would soon come to investigate his death.[18] Jones ordered everyone to drink the fruit punch from the large vat and to commit what he called "revolutionary suicide" as a way of protesting the conditions of an inhumane world.[19]

Unlike in the loyalty tests, this time the punch was spiked with potassium cyanide, a poison that disrupts the body's ability to use oxygen, causing unconsciousness and death by suffocation. Apparently Jones had been planning for this eventuality for a long time, since, having a jeweler's license, he had been stockpiling potassium cyanide for years on the pretext that it was needed to clean gold.[20] "I'd like to choose my own kind of death, for a change," Jones is known to have said.[21] "I'm tired of being tormented to Hell."

Several central-nervous-system-depressant drugs were also added to the poisoned drink, including diphenhydramine and promethazine, two antihistamine medications with sedative properties, as well as chloral hydrate, a tranquilizer, and diazepam, another sedative.[22] To ensure that no one escaped alive, guards carrying guns and crossbows monitored the perimeter of the compound and shot anyone who refused to drink the adulterated brew.[23]

Tim Carter, one of Jones's aides who survived the mass suicide–murder, saw his wife and one-year-old son die a horrible death.[24] "Jones was going to kill everybody, no matter what," Carter later said.[25] "Even those who were making a principled stand of revolutionary suicide probably were influenced a lot by the lies that he was telling them."[26]

The next morning, troops of the Guyanese Army Rescue Forces reached Jonestown and discovered the grounds littered with 909 bodies of members of the Peoples Temple, about a third of whom were children.[27] Near the bodies were plastic cups, packets of Flavor Aid, and syringes.

I distinctly remember the haunting televised images of hundreds of clothed bodies, many lying face down in the grass, scattered throughout the Jonestown grounds, the morning after the massacre. "Smaller bodies under larger bodies and children under those," one reporter said, describing the disturbing scene.[28] The angel of death had enveloped the Peoples Temple followers in an agonizing grip as they gasped for air, their final moments filled with excruciating pain from the toxic effects of cyanide poisoning. Families lay close together, parents with their arms around their children, seemingly soothing their offspring of their greatest fear. It was an eerie sight, one that looked as if everyone were asleep, as one journalist said.

Investigators found a forty-five-minute audio recording of the horrific event, which was later described as a "death tape."[29] On the recording, Jones could be heard urging Peoples Temple members to drink from the poisoned vat. "You can go down in history, saying you chose your own way to go," Jones told his followers, "and in your commitment to refuse capitalism and in support of socialism."[30]

Two men escaped the mass suicide–murder through a combination of luck and deception.[31] Three others were away on an errand to the Soviet Embassy in Georgetown, the capital of Guyana.[32] Eleven Peoples Temple members—including Wilson, who carried her three-year-old son on her back—walked thirty-five miles to the town of Matthew's Ridge on the pretense they were going on a picnic.[33] One elderly African American woman slept inside her cabin throughout the commotion.[34] When she awoke the following morning, she found bodies everywhere, including her sister's.[35]

Jones's two sons, Stephan and Jim Jr., were in Georgetown for a basketball tournament when they received a call from their father asking them to return to Jonestown for the revolutionary suicide.[36] They refused and were spared the terrible death, but their mother, siblings, and Jim Jr.'s pregnant wife all perished.[37]

Jones's body was found in the main pavilion with a bullet wound to the head.[38] He was forty-seven years old. Carter, Jones's aide, identified the body as belonging to Jones. "I remember thinking, the son of a bitch didn't even die the way everybody else died," Carter said.[39]

The Autopsy

Jones's embalmed body, which was rapidly decomposing, was released by the government of Guyana sometime between November 23 and November 26, 1978, and transported to Dover Air Force Base in Delaware.[40] However, the autopsy wasn't performed by medical pathologists of the United States Armed Forces Institute of Pathology until December 15, almost one month after Jones's body was discovered.[41]

"It is difficult to convey to someone who has not had firsthand experience what a week in a tropical climate can do to human remains," D. R. Jones (unrelated to Jim Jones) wrote in an article for the *American Journal of Psychiatry*.[42] "The changes in color and size, the infestation with various insects, and above all the overpowering and unforgettable odor of just one body are beyond recognition."[43]

Fingerprint and dental records were used to identify the body as belonging to Jones.[44] "[It] is that of a Caucasian male with moderate to severe decomposition changes," the medical pathologist wrote in the autopsy report.[45] Measuring sixty-eight inches long, Jones's body weighed 175 pounds and had no scars or tattoos.[46]

According to a team of forensic dentists, the teeth were colored pink, but the discoloration was caused by the very warm and humid environment in Guyana and not by cyanide.[47]

Unfortunately, the autopsy was compromised by the ongoing rapid putrefaction.[48] Nevertheless, an external examination revealed multiple skull fractures and a gunshot wound to the head.[49] The entrance wound was in the left temple, triangular in shape, perforating the underlying temporal parietal skull.[50] The exit wound was in the right temple, about three and a half inches below the top of the head.[51] The path of the wound through the brain could not be identified, owing to the severe decomposition of the brain and its semiliquid state.[52] Nonetheless, no microscopic or grossly anatomical changes were found in the brain.[53]

What I found most puzzling was the absence of gunpowder residue and muzzle imprint around the gunshot entrance wound.[54] Did that mean the wound wasn't self-inflicted and that Jones was shot from a distance by somebody else? Also, since the entrance wound was on the left side of Jones's head, was Jones left-handed? Complicating the forensic analysis further was the fact that Jones's hands were not swabbed for powder residue, on the assumption that the embalming process and the extensive handling of the body would have led to false-positive or false-negative results.[55]

The internal examination was unremarkable. The larynx showed no evidence of obstruction, and the stomach contained no food or pill residues.[56] In addition, the heart was of normal size and shape with no abnormalities, the heart valves were normal, the coronary arteries showed slight to moderate thickening, and the aorta had only a few small plaques, not enough to impede blood flow.[57]

The lungs, liver, spleen, and kidneys were all normal in size and shape, and the pancreas; pituitary gland, thyroid, adrenal glands, and small and large intestines had no abnormality.[58] The prostate was small and without nodules.[59]

It was obvious Jones died from a gunshot wound to the head. However, the lack of forensic evidence that he was shot at close range raised the possibility he was either murdered or possibly shot by someone else to relieve him of the pain that accompanies the agonal phase of cyanide intoxication, a period that can last as long as five minutes, during which there is an abnormal pattern of breathing and brainstem reflexes characterized by gasping and labored breathing. I was anxious to review the toxicology report, hoping it would help explain the mystery surrounding Jones's death.

Cause and Manner of Death

Toxicology testing of Jones's blood was severely limited because of the embalming process, which replaced blood with formaldehyde.[60] In addition, the urinary bladder was empty, so urine could not be tested for the presence of drugs.[61] Nonetheless, using highly specific gas chromatography and ultraviolet and mass spectrometry methodologies, a therapeutic amount of chloroquine, a drug most likely taken as prophylaxis against malaria, was detected in Jones's liver, but its concentration wasn't sufficiently elevated to contribute to Jones's death.[62]

Toxic levels of pentobarbital, a short-acting barbiturate sedative drug, were detected in the lungs, stomach, brain, kidneys, muscle, and liver, with the levels in the liver and kidneys in the lethal range.[63] However, the amount of pentobarbital in the brain, the most important organ for controlling vital functions, was low.[64] The medical pathologist concluded it was unlikely Jones's death was caused by pentobarbital intoxication, since tolerance to barbiturates, including pentobarbital, can develop over a period of time and the lethal level of the drug varies from one person to another.[65] However in my opinion, it is impossible to conclude to what degree, if any, pentobarbital contributed to Jones's death without first measuring its concentration in the blood, something that was impossible to do in this case.

That pentobarbital, a barbiturate drug not present in the poisoned fruit drink, was found in several of Jones's organs is consistent with reports Jones had been a chronic abuser of drugs, including amphetamines and barbiturates.[66] According to Jeff Guinn, author of *The Road to Jonestown: Jim Jones and the Peoples Temple*, Jones started using painkillers as early as the mid-1960s and was abusing amphetamines and tranquilizers on a regular basis by the early 1970s.[67] "I knew drugs were a problem with my father," Stephan, Jones's only biological child, said.[68] "[He] was using drugs to wake up and using drugs to go to sleep."[69]

Cyanide was not detected in any of Jones's organs, which suggests he didn't drink from the poisoned vat.[70] Another possibility is that Jones drank the poisoned fruit drink but the cyanide had rapidly volatilized from his body to undetectable levels by the time the autopsy was done, something that could happen even after death.[71] In my opinion, this is unlikely since diphenhydramine, a drug present in the poisoned fruit drink and which is not depleted from the body after death, was not found in Jones's organs even though it was present in several Peoples Temple members who had ingested the poisoned fruit punch.[72] The absence of both cyanide and diphenhydramine from Jones's system strongly supports the likelihood that Jones did not drink the cyanide-laced fruit drink the day he died.

Some have suggested Jones's death was a homicide, since he had deposited millions of dollars in European bank accounts and would not have committed suicide if he had planned to retrieve the money. This is mere speculation with no confirming evidence.[73] As for whether Jones was left-handed, I did not find any reports describing Jones as either left-handed or right-handed. It is a mystery that, when solved, may help explain whether his gunshot wound was self-inflicted or was caused by somebody else.

Besides Jones, the only other deceased person in the main pavilion with a gunshot wound to the head was Jones's nurse, Annie Moore.[74] Since Moore's muscle tissue contained a lethal level of cyanide, she had obviously ingested the poisoned fruit punch.[75] Her gunshot wound, therefore, was either self-inflicted or she was shot by somebody else.[76] Some people have suggested that Moore shot Jones and then committed suicide; another possibility is that Jones shot Moore and then shot himself.[77] In view of the unanswered questions in Moore's death, it is premature to speculate whether Moore shot Jones until the circumstances of her own death have been satisfactorily determined.

The medical pathologist concluded that the manner of Jones's death was consistent with suicide because of the presence of a hard-contact gunshot wound to the head. He noted that the embalming and extensive handling of the body probably led to loss of important forensic evidence, such as the loss of gunpowder residue and muzzle imprint around the entrance wound.[78] Without additional specific and reliable information, however, he couldn't rule out the possibility that Jones's death was a homicide.[79]

After I reviewed the circumstances surrounding Jones's death, the autopsy findings and results of toxicology testing, published lay articles, and the scientific literature, I was convinced that the cause of Jones's death was a gunshot wound to the head. However, in the absence of a suicide note and information on whether Jones was left-handed, as well as the lack of forensic evidence showing that Jones was shot at close range, and the inability to determine whether Jones committed suicide or was shot by somebody else, I labeled the manner of death undetermined.[80]

Life and Career

Jones was born in 1931 in Crete, a small unincorporated town in Indiana whose population neared fourteen hundred.[81] With one traffic light, one restaurant, five churches, and five coffin makers, the town's economy revolved around religion and funerals.[82]

Jones's father, a disabled World War I veteran, suffered from respiratory ailments and was an alcoholic and a fortune teller; his mother, seventeen years younger than her husband, was a domineering woman who worked as a waitress.[83]

As a child, Jones read books about Joseph Stalin, Karl Marx, Mao Zedong, Mahatma Ghandi, and Adolph Hitler.[84] His exposure to religion began at the age of six when a female neighbor took him to a Church of the Nazarene service.[85] There, Jones took an immediate liking to religion. Surprisingly, Jones was found to have a keen ability to recite sermons and to quote lengthy Biblical verses.[86] The townspeople thought Jones was a "weird kid" because he would deliver sermons to animals and collect roadkill, for whom he provided elaborate funerals.[87] "He was obsessed with religion," recalled Chuck Wilmore, a childhood friend of Jones.[88]

While attending high school, Jones took a job as an orderly at Reid Memorial Hospital, where he met Marceline Baldwin, a nurse at least four years his senior.[89] "Marceline was always for the underdog," her mother recalled, which blended well with Jones's compassion for the poor and for African Americans.[90] On June 12, 1949, shortly before he reached his eighteenth birthday, Jones married Marceline.[91]

Jones enrolled at Indiana University in 1950 with plans to become a doctor, mostly to please his mother. However, his career goals changed in 1952, after he began to serve as an occasional preacher in a fundamentalist congregation in Indianapolis, and then as a student pastor in the Somerset Southside Methodist Church.[92] With his strong passion for racial integration and socialism now fully developed, Jones's dramatic sermons were filled with attacks on "the

Establishment" for its racial discrimination and for ignoring the plight of the poor.[93] Achieving social change through Marxism and mobilizing people through religion became his all-consuming passion.[94]

In 1953, Jones launched his own church, the Peoples Temple Full Gospel Church, which later became the Peoples Temple.[95] It was open to all ethnic groups and was a place where Jones could perform sham "faith healings" and preach messages of socialism, integration, and racial equality while at the same time helping the poor with groceries and clothing, opening a soup kitchen, and establishing nursing homes for the elderly.[96]

To raise money, Jones imported monkeys and sold them door-to-door as pets. Stephan, Jones's son, thought his father's purpose was to "bust down some walls and to create a community where all are welcome, no matter where they came from."[97]

"[Jones] was a changed man in 1957, after he went to see Father Divine," Eugene Cordell of Indianapolis said, referring to Reverend M. J. Divine, an African American preacher in suburban Philadelphia who attracted followers by raising fear of outside enemies and elevating himself to godlike status.[98] "He got a big head and took a different viewpoint to his preaching," agreed Ross E. Case, one of Jones's aides.[99] "He was always talking about sex or Father Divine and Daddy Grace [founder and first bishop of the predominantly African American denomination, the United House of Prayer for All People] and was envious of how they were adored by their people and the absolute loyalty they got," Case said.[100] Jones wanted the same affection and loyalty from his parishioners that Father Divine was receiving from his.[101]

As more people joined the Peoples Temple, the church became a massive voting bloc on social issues. Indianapolis political leaders took notice and began to court Jones, whom they saw as a skilled organizer who could deliver large numbers of people to political campaign rallies.[102] "At that stage of the game," Bishop A. James Armstrong said of Jones, "he appeared to be an idealistic humanitarian. That was many years before he showed what he truly was."[103]

Jones was appointed to the post of director of the Human Rights Commission in 1961, the same year he graduated from Butler University after attending night school and earning a degree in secondary education.[104] "The selection committee thought that, being a pastor, he could pacify businesses that were discriminating, in a calm and unemotional way," remembered Indianapolis Mayor Charles Boswell.[105] After taking office, Jones immediately started to integrate police stations, hospitals, churches, restaurants, amusement parks, the telephone company, and movie theaters.[106] "He was an earnest, idealistic, rather intense young man," Rabbi Maurice Davis said of his time working with Jones on housing issues.[107] "There was no indication that this thing was going to turn into a cult and that he was going to get flaked out with power."[108]

Before Jones and Marceline had their own child in 1959, they adopted several ethnic children—African American, Native American, and Korean American—whom they called their "rainbow family."[109] Between 1963 and 1968, Jones moved his growing family first to Brazil, in part because he was being investigated for shady real estate transfers, and then to Ukiah, in Northern California, to avoid the "cataclysmic thermonuclear war" he claimed would happen on July 15, 1967. While in California, Jones received several humanitarian awards and was appointed chairman of the Mendocino County Grand Jury by Judge Robert Winslow.[110] "He was a very bright, humanistic person," Winslow remembered.[111]

By some accounts, a positive turning point for the Peoples Temple occurred in October 1968. It was then that Tim Stoen, a deputy district attorney and a Stanford University Law School graduate, began to attend services at the Peoples Temple.[112] Influenced by the assassination of Dr. Martin Luther King, Jr., Stoen sold almost all of his possessions and became a full-time aide to Jones.[113] "[Stoen] was a highly respected member of the community," said Thomas E. Martin, a Mendocino County probation officer. "This gave the church instant credence."[114]

After the Peoples Temple relocated to Guyana, Stoen's wife defected back to the United States. A year later, Stoen, who also became disillusioned with the authoritarian practices of the Peoples Temple, followed his wife but left his son in Jonestown, since Jones, claiming to be the boy's father, refused to let the child leave the settlement. Teri Buford O'Shea, a former Peoples Temple member, was adamant when she said in an interview with the *Atlantic*, "There was no way of getting a child out of Jonestown."[115] Once in the United States, the Stoens petitioned the courts and sought out their representative in Congress to help secure the release of their son from Jonestown. Tragically, their young boy was one of the victims of the Jonestown massacre.

In 1971, Jones purchased a church in San Francisco and another in Los Angeles.[116] By then the Peoples Temple ran social and medical programs for the poor, including a free dining room, and drug rehabilitation and legal aid services. In addition, Jones made numerous donations to charitable causes and journalism organizations, and delivered votes for politicians.[117] In return, he was appointed chairman of the Housing Authority by San Francisco Mayor George Moscone.[118]

The decline of the Peoples Temple began in 1973, after eight prominent members defected with stories of financial abuse, mind control, and tax evasion.[119] Sometime thereafter, an article appeared in *New West* magazine alleging that members of the Peoples Temple had been beaten, the church had engaged in financial misdealings, and Jones was nothing more than a charlatan.[120] "He had been paranoid before that," Stoen recalled, "but after the *New West* article, he really became paranoid."[121]

Articles in the *San Francisco Examiner* soon followed, describing Jones as a false messiah who claimed to have resurrected forty-three people from the dead.[122] For Jones, it was too much. He decided to move ahead with his plans to relocate the Peoples Temple to Guyana, in South America.[123]

Conclusions

According to James T. Richardson, professor emeritus of sociology and judicial studies at the University of Nevada, a cult requires a charismatic leader who is viewed as strong and trustworthy, one who has vision and can excite like-minded people to follow him in pursuit of a common goal.[124] Jones was such a leader, offering the vulnerable and the disenfranchised a new way of life free of financial stresses and inequality in pursuit of a shared purpose.[125]

"There was a lot of good in my father," Jones's son, Stephan, observed.[126] "I mean, people were attracted to him for a reason … My father preached tolerance. He preached a lot of truths." But then, ironically, Stephan qualified his remarks. "He didn't live them, but he preached them."[127]

Larissa Piva, a Canadian freelance writer, called Jones "the master of the art of deception."[128] His vision of creating a racially integrated socialist community where everyone was equal was so revolutionary and appealing that highly regarded politicians, mesmerized by Jones's strong personality and oratory, anxiously sought his counsel and support. People willingly gave up their belongings and life savings in exchange for what they believed was the promise of a life-changing experience of security, social justice, and equality, even blindly following Jones and the Peoples Temple wherever the church relocated.[129] "It was all a charade," Mike Cartmell, a former Peoples Temple member, declared.[130]

While Jones preached about communalism, the power of belief, and self-sacrifice, he didn't always practice what he preached.[131] He ate specially prepared steaks, had a color television, and demanded sexual favors from the women members of his church.[132] "All that mattered to my father," Stephan noted, "[were] people's perceptions of him. His entire existence was superficial."[133]

As for Jones's famous "faith healings," it took many years before Stephan realized that his father's so-called ability to extract cancer from a man's body was simply an act using raw chicken giblets.[134] "I think I knew it was just a bunch of junk," Stephan said.[135] "There was nothing spiritual about my father."[136]

As Jones became addicted to drugs and alcohol, his behavior became more bizarre.[137] He manipulated his congregants with blackmail and humiliated them with public beatings.[138] "His message was incredibly violent as time went on, and it was erratic," Stephan observed.[139] Fannie Mobley, a former member of the Peoples Temple, recalled, "He [Jones] turned from a beautiful Christian man to a Jekyll and Hyde monster."[140]

And yet, despite his absolute authoritative power, many members of the Peoples Temple loved Jones, calling him "Father" and respecting his absolute authority.[141] The question was, Why did they do so? Apparently, fear was the underlying factor.

"Like any good demagogue," Stephan explained, speaking of his father, "he would conjure up fear"—fear of an impending nuclear war, fear of being placed in concentration camps, fear of being exterminated by white racists.[142] O'Shea, a Peoples Temple member who survived the massacre, stated, "The first time I met him, I was convinced he could read minds, cast spells, do all kinds of powerful things, both good and evil."[143] But in the long run, "His paranoia got completely out of control. I was afraid of him and stayed afraid of him for seven years."[144]

What kept me wondering as I reviewed the published literature was how Jones could have espoused so many commendable virtues, such as racial equality, integration, and social justice, and then turn into such a horrible human being who could lead his followers to Armageddon. The answer seems to lie in his unrelenting maintenance and pursuit of power. "If you see me as your father, I'll be your father ... If you see me as your savior, I'll be your savior. If you see me as your God, I'll be your God," Jones told his followers.[145] "It was all very sincere to people in the pews," Cartmell, the former Peoples Temple member, explained, "but it was just power. He was a con man."[146]

Antoinette Pick-Jones, writing on behalf of San Diego State University, noted that it was after the Peoples Temple moved to California that Jones's behavior changed from that of compassion to that of control.[147] Peoples Temple members were taught to never question his authority.[148] According to Jose I. Lasaga of the Miami Mental Health Center, Jones used several techniques to hold power over his followers, including control of property and income, weakening of family ties, a sociopolitical caste system, control of the ability to escape, and control of verbal, cognitive, and emotional expression.[149] Deborah Layton, the only person to successfully escape from the Peoples Temple, recalled, "As Father's influence increased, the members became unwitting pawns in his quest for more and more personal power."[150] Without Jones's ability to control his followers, Pick-Jones concluded, the Jonestown massacre would not have happened.[151]

The enormity of the Jonestown massacre is beyond comprehension, but it is important to try to fully understand what led to that horrific event so a similar catastrophe can never happen again. Many scholars believe an appreciation is required of how Peoples Temple members came to a common consciousness in order to arrive at an explanation for the mass suicide in Jonestown, but Albert Black Jr. of the University of Washington disagrees.[152] Black claims there is no reason to assume the massacre was necessarily a homogeneous event.[153] He believes two different types of suicides occurred simultaneously in Jonestown—altruistic suicide, where some Peoples Temple members died because they put the group above themselves, and fatalistic suicide, where the majority of members died because Jonestown became a hopeless, demeaning, and antagonistic environment.[154] While Black's theory may be correct, it doesn't explain why children, who constituted 30 percent of the deaths, do not fit in either of the two categories.

As for the manner of Jones's death, it remains undetermined. In my opinion, there simply isn't enough conclusive evidence to indicate that Jones took his own life. Stephan believes his father must have killed himself and that he wouldn't have left the final act to somebody else. "I think he would be admitting in his own warped mind that … he was a coward, and about nothing," Stephan said.[155] I vehemently disagree.

There is no doubt in my mind that Jones was a coward, whether he shot himself or not. He made his followers drink the poisoned fruit punch and suffer five long, agonizing minutes of the toxic effects of cyanide poisoning, but he, like other mass murderers, chose a relatively quick and painless death from a gunshot wound to the head rather than face the effects of cyanide intoxication or, better yet, the strong arm of the law. If that is not a prime example of cowardice, then nothing is.

CHAPTER 10

David Koresh

Died April 19, 1993

Key Figure in the Waco Siege

ON THE MORNING of February 28, 1993, more than seventy-five agents of the Bureau of Alcohol, Tobacco, and Firearms (ATF) gathered at a staging area near Waco, Texas, prepared to serve a search warrant on the Branch Davidians' rural compound, ten miles east of Waco, and to execute an arrest warrant for David Koresh, the leader of the religious cult.[1] Within hours, the ATF agents unexpectedly found themselves in a war zone that lasted fifty-one days.

Based on interviews of a United Parcel Service driver and former members of the Branch Davidians, as well as a review of documents and records from interstate shippers and arms dealers, federal authorities believed Koresh had been stockpiling weapons at his "Mount Carmel" compound and illegally converting semiautomatic weapons into fully automatic weapons.[2] Dubbed "Operation Trojan Horse," ATF agents had trained to take the Branch Davidian building by force.[3] Dressed in tactical gear, they boarded cattle trailers covered with tarps, hoping to disembark close to the compound and to surprise Koresh.[4]

"That was highly unusual, to say the least," Chuck Hustmyre, an ATF special agent, remembered, "but that part of Texas is just a big, barren, windswept prairie, and there's nothing to hide behind."[5] What the ATF agents did not know at the time was that Koresh had been tipped off about their plans by David Jones, a local mailman who happened to have been his brother-in-law.[6]

"This was going to be a warrant service that would last maybe a day or so for us to complete the search," ATF agent Blake Boteler later said.[7] Instead, as government forces approached the compound, they were met by a barrage of unrelenting gunfire.[8] "We were getting shots from multiple windows and multiple locations with automatic weapon fire," Boteler said.[9] John Risenhoover, another ATF agent, expanded on Boteler's comments. "You have to remember, we were in there with pistols, a couple of MP-5s, and I think a total of four AR-15s," he said, while the Branch Davidians had grenades and automatic weapons.[10] "The biggest problem we had," said Byron Sage, the principal Federal Bureau of

Investigation (FBI) negotiator, "we created a crisis within a crisis."[11]

Inside the complex, "the windows were shot out, and there was glass all over the floor," Catherine Matteson, one of the Branch Davidians who lived in the compound, recalled sometime later.[12] To avoid the broken glass and gunfire, the women took the children to the hall on the second floor and shielded them with their bodies.[13]

As far as his followers were concerned, "[Koresh] had shown us in the Scriptures that it was okay to defend your family and your property," said Clive Doyle, a Branch Davidian who escaped the siege.[14]

Within minutes of the raid, Wayne Martin, one of the Branch Davidians inside the compound, called 911 and pleaded with Larry Lynch, a lieutenant at the McLennan County Sheriff's Office, "Tell them there are women and children in here and to call it off!"[15]

It took Lynch thirty-one minutes to make radio contact with ATF commanders and another hour before he reached the ATF on a secure line before a cease-fire was finally reached.[16] By then, four ATF agents and six Branch Davidians had died.[17] Also, sixteen ATF agents and Koresh had been wounded.[18]

The following day, the ATF officially handed over command of the operation to the FBI.[19] "We quickly realized that this was not a typical hostage situation," said Gary Noesner, the FBI's negotiation coordinator.[20] "No one was being held against their will. The Branch Davidians were very devoted followers of David Koresh, and they didn't want anything from the authorities other than for us to go away."[21]

Considering all the killings, FBI negotiators thought it would be difficult to win Koresh's trust, so in an effort to calm the situation down, they adopted a conciliatory tone, sending Koresh a suture kit for his wounds, cartons of milk for the children, and videotapes of themselves and their families.[22] In return, Koresh agreed to release some of the children if certain passages of Scripture were read over the radio.[23] By the third day, after Koresh's demands were met, eighteen children were let out of the Branch Davidian complex.[24] Three others left in the following days.[25]

Next, Koresh promised to walk out of the compound, along with his followers, as soon as a tape he had prepared was broadcast over the radio.[26] Although his message and his "guarantee" were subsequently played over the Christian Broadcasting Network at nine o'clock in the morning, Koresh did not follow through with his promise, claiming, "God told me to wait."[27]

Meanwhile, two miles away, hundreds of reporters, photographers, and video crews from all over the globe gathered at what became known as "Satellite City."[28]

"David was at the center stage of the world's media, and he ate it up," Sage recalled.[29] James McGee, an FBI special agent, agreed. "He was in no hurry to come out."[30] Sage said, "What the Davidians were doing was stalling for time because David was becoming an international celebrity."[31]

The last child was released on March 5; nearly three weeks later, the last adult came out of the compound.[32] Within a span of two days, nine people had walked out of the Branch Davidian complex, giving hope to the FBI negotiators that their efforts were yielding results.[33] And yet, despite Koresh having released so many of his followers, the commander of the FBI tactical team decided Koresh had not done enough.[34] In retaliation, the commander ordered helicopters to knock down water towers, and he instructed tanks to crush some of the Branch Davidians' automobiles.[35]

Effective negotiations between the federal government and Koresh ended on March 23. By then, thirty-five people had been released, including twenty-one children.[36] Nonetheless, still not satisfied, the tactical unit was pushing for a more aggressive and confrontational approach.[37] After obtaining approval from Attorney General Janet Reno, the commander of the tactical team initiated a "psychological operation."[38]

"They started trying to disrupt our sleep," Doyle, a Branch Davidian, said.[39] "They shone bright lights into the building all night long and blasted…Tibetan monks chanting, Nancy Sinatra singing 'These Boots are made for Walking,' and… Christmas carols."[40]

On April 14, Koresh promised to surrender within two weeks, after he finished writing a manuscript about the Seven Seals.[41] Since he had broken his promises before, FBI negotiators were reluctant to agree to Koresh's terms unless he provided tangible physical proof he was writing the manuscript.[42] Four days later, Koresh still had not produced the first page of his manuscript.[43]

Unwilling to wait any longer, Sage called Koresh shortly before 6:00 a.m. on April 19 and told him to surrender or tear gas would be sprayed into the compound.[44] "It's time to come out with your hands up," Sage announced over the loudspeakers.[45] "The siege is over, David, come on out."[46] In response, Branch Davidians fired as many as two hundred rounds of ammunition at the ATF agents.[47] Four minutes later, the first of the modified tanks started punching holes and firing tear gas into the Branch Davidian main building, hoping to force the cult members out.[48]

"Nothing about April 19 started normal, nothing," said David Thibodeau, a former Branch Davidian who had lived in the Waco compound.[49] "There were no gas masks for the children, so the parents were soaking towels in buckets of water," Doyle said.[50]

Koresh encouraged the mothers to take all the children into the "vault," a concrete bunker in which cult members planned to take refuge when "the end of the world" was near.[51] Later, after the siege ended, remains of nine women, five men, and eighteen children who died from smoke inhalation were found inside the bunker.[52]

Four hours passed, but still no one came out of the Branch Davidian complex.[53] "No one was leaving [because] we didn't trust the FBI," Doyle explained.[54]

"In their view, our actions validated David Koresh's end-of-the-world prophecies that he'd been telling them about," said Noesner, the FBI negotiation coordinator.[55]

At 12:08 p.m., three or more simultaneous fires broke out within the Branch Davidian compound, and flames began to pour out of several second-story windows.[56] After the siege ended, it was determined that the fires had been set by Koresh and his followers.[57] The high winds, blowing at thirty to thirty-five miles per hour, ensured the fires spread quickly, engulfing everything in their paths.[58] "Koresh was manufacturing his own Armageddon," said Lane Akin, a Texas Ranger who assisted with the fire investigation.[59]

As the heavy flames rose skyward, Sage pleaded, "David, *please* don't do this. Don't end it this way. Save your people. Lead them out."[60] Still, no one came out of the inferno. "It was a tinderbox," McGee said.[61]

In total, nine cult members escaped the fire through gaping holes in the burning building and were immediately arrested.[62] Seventy-five others died, twenty-five of whom were children.[63] At least seventeen of the dead had gunshot wounds; one child was stabbed to death.[64]

A 501-page report released by the United States Treasury Department five months after the Waco siege ended concluded, "Despite knowing in advance that the element of surprise was lost, the raid commanders made the decision to go forward."[65] In hindsight, everyone agreed it was a botched operation that should have been called off.

After the embers stopped smoldering, federal agents searched for Koresh's body. It was found in the communication room, on the first floor of the Branch Davidian main building.[66] "Koresh had a bullet wound right in his forehead," said Dr. Nizam Peerwani, the Tarrant County chief medical examiner.[67] Koresh was thirty-three years old.

The Autopsy

The autopsy, which was delayed about two weeks, was conducted by Dr. Peerwani at the Tarrant County Medical Examiner's Morgue on the second and third days of May 1993.[68] Based on the circumstances surrounding Koresh's death, the extensive burning of the flesh, and the mutilation and charring of the body, the autopsy took considerably longer than usual, requiring substantial reconstruction of the skull by forensic anthropologists.[69]

Koresh's body arrived wrapped in a white sheet, dehydrated, significantly reduced in size, and secured in a black body bag that included tissue and bone fragments and construction debris.[70] It was identified using dental records.

Besides the extensive charring and burns, there were heat-related fractures of several bones in the arms and legs.[71] The head sustained massive trauma, with the cranium (skull) fractured into multiple large pieces with several parts missing.[72] Nevertheless, after the skull was reconstructed, two gunshot wounds were identified in the head; a third was found in the left hip.[73]

The gunshot entrance wound was circular, and in the mid-frontal area of the skull, approximately one inch above the glabella, the smooth part of the forehead, above and between the eyebrows.[74] Unlike with Jim Jones, whose body was also incinerated and whose gunshot entrance wound showed no evidence of gunpowder, Koresh's gunshot entrance wound, measuring 1.3 centimeters in diameter, had black powder deposits.[75] When forehead tissue was examined under a microscope, a small greenish particle, identified as gunpowder, was revealed.[76] Chemical analysis of residue from the entrance wound detected significant amounts of barium, antimony, and lead, recognized components of gunpowder that are virtually always deposited in the track of a gunshot wound.[77] Together, these findings confirmed that the wound was a gunshot entrance wound.

The second circular gunshot wound was an exit wound, much larger than the entrance wound.[78] It was located in the occipital bone at the base of the skull at the back of the head.[79]

Both the entrance and the exit gunshot wounds caused considerable radiating fracturing of the skull.[80] There was no charring around the entrance wound.[81] However, the exit wound was "charred around the left superior and right margins of the skull, but not around the inferior border."[82] "This observation clearly establishes that the gunshot wound occurred prior to burning because the bone fragments separated and were exposed differentially to the fire," Peerwani explained.[83]

The skull was totally devoid of brain matter, presumably due to incineration, so the pathway of the projectile through the brain could not be evaluated.[84] With the brain gone, it could not be examined for the presence of anomalies, deformities, or other pathological changes.

The third, partially healing, wound, also caused by a projectile, probably from police, measured 4.3 centimeter in diameter and involved the left innominate bone (the hip bone).[85] Both the entrance and exit hip wounds were obscured by extensive charring.[86]

The internal examination began with the customary Y-shaped incision across the abdomen.[87] Despite the extensive heat damage, the internal organs were essentially well preserved, although they were hardened and dehydrated, with a commensurate loss of weight.[88] There was much destruction of soft tissue due to the fire on the right side of the chest and in the abdominal wall.[89] A heat-related fracture of the tenth right rib was also identified.[90]

As for the cardiovascular system, the heart had the normal shape, although it was reduced in size due to heating.[91] The heart valves were unremarkable, with no evidence of death of heart muscle, as from a heart attack, or any appreciable accumulation of plaque in the coronary arteries and aorta.[92]

The lungs were hyperinflated, presumably because Koresh had been gasping for air after tear gas was introduced into the Branch Davidian compound.[93] In addition, the lungs were severely congested and moderately filled with frothy fluid.[94] Dense deposits of black soot and large amounts of granular aspirated blood were present in the tracheobronchial tree, a system of airways that allows passage of air into the lungs.[95]

Chemical analysis of blood detected a carbon monoxide level at 24 percent saturation, approximately ten times more than the normal level but 50 percent lower than the level reported to cause death.[96] This was consistent with Koresh having inhaled toxic fumes prior to his death.

Most of the esophagus, which had some charring, and the stomach, which was empty and without ulceration, were intact.[97] The appendix had a heat-related injury, the liver had superficial burns, and the gall bladder, spleen, and kidneys were shrunken.[98] The pancreas was absent, presumably because of incineration.[99] The prostate was unremarkable, as was the urinary bladder, which was devoid of urine.[100] The organs of the hormone-producing endocrine system were of normal size and shape.[101]

Based on the autopsy findings, it was apparent Koresh died from a gunshot wound to the head. An entrance wound from close range, complete with gunpowder residue around the wound, was identified in his forehead, with an exit wound located at the back of the head.[102] The question left to investigate was whether Koresh's gunshot wound was self-inflicted or whether it was caused by somebody else.

Cause and Manner of Death

The urinary bladder was empty, so toxicological testing of urine could not be conducted. However, alcohol was detected in blood collected from a blood clot, as well as in bile at one hundred milligrams and one hundred and forty milligrams per one hundred milliliters, respectively.[103] Since the autopsy was performed about two weeks after Koresh died, the elevated alcohol levels most likely were due to putrefaction and postmortem fermentation on the open tissue by microflora deposits, such as bacteria and yeast.[104]

Some people have speculated that Steve Schneider, Koresh's second-in-command, shot Koresh in the head and then shot himself in the mouth, since both bodies and a shotgun were found in the communication room of the Branch Davidian compound.[105] This is certainly a possibility. Since Koresh's gunshot entrance wound was higher than the exit wound, it would have been easier for Schneider to have achieved the downward trajectory if he had shot Koresh while standing and Koresh was sitting than for Koresh to have shot himself in the forehead. If that, in fact, is what happened, then Koresh's death was a homicide.

"Well, it's hard to predict whether he shot Koresh or Koresh shot himself, since the bodies were so badly charred," Peerwani said.[106]

After I reviewed the circumstances surrounding Koresh's death, the autopsy findings and results of toxicology testing, published lay articles, and the scientific literature, I determined that the immediate cause of death was massive head and brain trauma due to a gunshot wound to the head. However, without additional information, I found it impossible to conclude whether Koresh's gunshot wound was self-inflicted or he had been shot by somebody else. I therefore labeled the manner of death undetermined.

Life and Career

Koresh was born in 1959 in Houston, Texas, to an unwed fourteen-year-old mother.[107] His mother went to live with an alcoholic and abusive man who was not Koresh's father, so Koresh spent his early years with his grandparents, who attended the local Seventh-Day Adventist Church.[108]

When Koresh was seven years old, his mother married a carpenter and Koresh went back to live with her.[109] According to Mary Garafolo, a journalist, "[Koresh] claimed that when he was a child, God had spoken to him and said, 'You're the chosen one. You are my messiah.'"[110]

As a teenager, Koresh was lonely, dyslexic, and disruptive. He did not do well academically and was bullied in school.[111] He dropped out of Garland High School in his junior year to become a "rock star," but after moving to Los Angeles and achieving little success, he returned to Texas.[112]

When he was nineteen, Koresh impregnated his fifteen-year-old girlfriend, whom he never married.[113] A short time later, he began to frequent a Southern Baptist church and then a Seventh-Day Adventist church, where he met and fell in love with the pastor's daughter.[114] When Koresh told the pastor that God wanted him to marry his daughter, he was expelled from the congregation.[115]

In 1981, Koresh moved to Waco, Texas, where he joined the Branch Davidians, a splinter group originating from the

Seventh-Day Adventist Church.[116] "He seemed lost," recalled David Bunds, a former member of the Branch Davidians.[117]

The Branch Davidians was founded in 1934 by Victor Houteff.[118] Members of the group strongly believed in Armageddon and were obsessed with their deaths and "the end of the world."[119] In 1978, after Ben Roden, the head of the cult, died, his wife, Lois, took over the leadership of the group.[120] With Lois as his mentor, Koresh soon became an influential member of the Branch Davidians.[121]

When Lois died in 1986, her son, George, assumed he would take over as head of the Branch Davidians, however Koresh had other ideas.[122] A power struggle ensued, at which time Koresh and twenty-five of his followers were forced to leave the Branch Davidian compound at gunpoint.[123] In 1987, Koresh returned with seven heavily armed followers and shot George, who survived the attack with only a minor wound.[124] Although he was tried for attempted murder, Koresh was released in a mistrial.[125]

By the late 1980s, Koresh took total control of the Branch Davidians.[126] According to Garafolo, the journalist, Koresh claimed he had memorized both the New and Old Testaments by the time he was eighteen years old.[127] With his uncanny ability to quote numerous chapters and verses of the Bible from memory, Koresh had his followers convinced of his superior knowledge and understanding, believing he could "unlock the future," and "guarantee" immortality.[128]

"One of the things about being a Branch Davidian," Bunds, the former Branch Davidian, explained, "you're supposed to separate yourself from the world. The world is the sins, the flesh, the desires of the world, and you're supposed to be spiritual."[129] Thibodeau, another former member of the group, agreed. "In many ways, it was a very satisfying life. David's message was incredibly deep, and it rang true with me."[130] Former Branch Davidian Matteson exclaimed, "One time, I sat and listened to him [Koresh] teach a Bible study for eighteen hours. I hated it when he stopped."[131] Sheila Martin, who joined the Branch Davidians with her husband and five children in 1988, had a different view.[132] "It was fun as long as we were being obedient," she said.[133] Bunds observed that Koresh's message kept changing over the years because he was always looking for the next big thing to teach that would shock people into listening to him.[134]

As the group grew, so did Koresh's control over its members.[135] He urged his followers to turn over their possessions and financial holdings to his control.[136] He established rules of behavior and ordered the men separated from the women, with no sexual relations even among married couples.[137] Although he was legally married to Rachel Jones, a Branch Davidian who was only fourteen years old when they married, Koresh nonetheless announced that only he could have sexual relations with women, even with the Branch Davidian married women, who he considered to be his "spiritual wives."[138]

Koresh had a harem of girls as young as ten years old he called the "House of David."[139] "His justification for taking all of the women for himself was theological," Bunds explained, "so yeah, being a member of the House of David was a privilege."[140] Eventually Koresh would "marry" as many as twenty cult women and would father at least twelve of their children.[141]

By the early 1990s, Koresh declared he had cracked the code of the Seven Seals of the Book of Revelation, predicting the events leading up to the Apocalypse.[142] Claiming the compound would someday be attacked by the US government, he began to preach a brand of apocalyptic prophesy while at the same time stockpiling guns and ammunition.[143] The end of the world was coming, he told his followers, but they would survive because they were the chosen people and he was the son of God.[144]

On February 28, 1993, ATF agents stormed the Branch Davidian compound with tanks and tear gas.[145] "Everything that David had been teaching us was actually taking place," Thibodeau said.[146] "It seemed like the prophecy was being fulfilled."[147]

Conclusions

"Who was David Koresh?" asked journalist Muriel Pearson, writing for ABC News.[148] "To his detractors, he was a false prophet, a con man, and a pedophile," Pamella Colloff wrote in the *Texas Monthly*.[149] "To his followers, he was the messiah."[150]

On February 28, 1993, when ATF agents went to execute a search warrant for the Branch Davidian compound, they expected to find a different Koresh than the one Colloff had described, one who preached a doomsday scenario and had stockpiled guns and ammunition. And yet, despite everything ATF knew about Koresh and the Branch Davidians, its agents were not adequately prepared to arrest Koresh—something they had planned to do.

"What do you mean 'They know we're coming?'" thought Bill Buford, the agent in charge at the ATF's Little Rock, Arkansas.[151] "Once we knew the element of surprise had been lost, we should have called it off," he said.[152] Nevertheless, ATF agents marched on, determined to proceed with what turned out to be a deeply flawed plan.

When the shooting started, "I was able to hear specific weapons, like AK-47s and an M60 machine gun," Buford said.[153] It should have been expected. After all, the ATF knew Koresh and the Branch Davidians had weapons and ammunition. That is precisely why the agency deployed its agents to search the compound and to arrest Koresh. Moreover, instead of approaching the compound in a nonthreatening way, more than seventy-five ATF agents appeared in full tactical gear, ready for a confrontation for which they were unprepared and had inappropriate weapons and equipment.[154]

The show of force probably strengthened the resolve of the Branch Davidians and drove them together rather than pulled them apart.[155] Said Sage, the lead FBI negotiator, "We grossly underestimated the control that David exerted over them."[156] The proper approach would have been to avoid being overly threatening and to agree to any reasonable demand.[157] The reason for this, in essence, is that this tactic would have ensured the crisis would not escalate to unreasonable proportions.

The biggest obstacle the ATF agents had to overcome was the significant lack of communication between negotiators and the tactical team.[158] The two teams "absolutely need to be on the same sheet of music," Sage declared.[159] They were not. That was the main takeaway from the subsequent Justice Department and congressional reports.[160]

Communication between ATF and the Branch Davidians wasn't optimal either. "At a certain point we realized that their word meant nothing," said Thibodeau, a Branch Davidian who was inside the compound when the siege began.[161] "The negotiators would tell us one thing, and the guys in the tanks would do the exact opposite."[162]

At the end of the fifty-one-day standoff, the US Department of Justice investigated the events at Waco and issued its final report.[163] While admitting, "The negotiations and tactical components of the FBI's overall approach were not always coordinated and, on occasion, were in conflict with each other," no mention was made of the inadequacy of the overall ATF plan and its execution.[164]

The so-called "Danforth Report," published on November 8, 2000, concluded, "The government of the United States and its agents are not responsible for the April 19, 1993, tragedy at Waco ... Responsibility ... rests with certain of the Branch Davidians and their leader ... David Koresh."[165]

"It was such a waste," declared Peerwani, the coroner who autopsied all the bodies after the siege ended, including those of the children.[166] "So many people died. So many people perished. And I hope we all learned a lesson from this."[167]

So why did otherwise reasonable people, such as the members of the Branch Davidians, at least one of whom was a Harvard graduate, commit such unreasonable and unspeakable acts? "I'll call it a cult, that's what it was," Bunds said.[168] "It's people doing things they wouldn't normally do, like giving up their wives and letting their children have sex with adults, which is crazy. Someone says they have authority and then impose upon you rules and restrictions and it gets down into your soul, it really screws you."[169]

Some former members of the Branch Davidians who had escaped the fire or were released before the siege ended remained in Waco; they occasionally meet for Bible studies.[170] "We are still waiting for the resurrection," Doyle said.[171] "It's not just David who will be resurrected, but all our people who died."[172] They will have a long wait.

CHAPTER 11

Vince Foster

Died July 20, 1993
Deputy White House Counsel

VINCE FOSTER, DEPUTY White House counsel to the president of the United States, was depressed. Things were not going well at the White House ever since Bill Clinton, his childhood friend, was inaugurated president on January 20, 1993. As far as Foster was concerned, it was entirely his fault.

Foster had vetted a number of top appointees during the transition period, but he found the vetting process very stressful. On Friday, July 16, his sister, Sheila, told Foster to seek psychiatric counseling for his depression "off-the-record," but by Monday, he still had not spoken to any of the three doctors she had recommended.[1] Instead Foster saw his physician in Little Rock, Arkansas, who prescribed a low dose of trazodone, an antidepressant medication.[2]

When seven employees of the White House travel office were fired and William Kennedy, one of Foster's former partners at the Rose Law Firm and his associate in the White House Counsel's Office, was reprimanded for what became known as "Travelgate," Foster considered resigning.[3] However, he dreaded the thought of having to face humiliation when he returned to Arkansas.[4] Then, when Zoë Baird withdrew her nomination for attorney general after it was discovered she had failed to pay taxes for her nanny, Foster blamed himself for "Nannygate."[5] Very distraught and clinically depressed, Foster saw his reputation, which he had built over a lifetime, being tarnished with every passing day.[6]

Tuesday, July 20, began as a good day for the Clinton administration. Ruth Bader Ginsburg sailed through her nomination to the Supreme Court, and Louis J. Freeh was nominated to head the FBI.[7] While everyone celebrated these developments, Foster was despondent, and his mood was "markedly understated," according to Special Counsel Robert B. Fiske Jr.[8] Rather than rejoicing with his office mates, Foster ate his lunch in his office and, at about one o'clock, picked up his suit jacket and left.[9] On the way out, he announced, "I'll be back," without saying where he was going.[10]

Three hours later, Foster still had not returned. A search was initiated, and his gray Honda Accord was soon found in a parking lot at Fort Marcy Park in McLean, Virginia.[11] His jacket was neatly folded on the passenger seat.[12]

At about 5:30 p.m., Foster was discovered in the park, his body slumped beside a Civil War cannon, approximately two hundred yards from the parking area.[13] According to police, Foster had taken his .38 caliber Colt handgun from a closet in his home and placed it in an oven mitt, and had then driven to the park, where he shot himself in the mouth.[14] Foster was forty-eight years old; he had been in the Clinton administration for only seven months.

The Autopsy

The autopsy was performed at Virginia's Fairfax Hospital by Dr. James C. Beyer, an assistant chief medical examiner.[15] By 2006, the year he died of a blood disorder, Beyer had conducted more than twenty thousand autopsies.[16]

The internal examination revealed a heart that was of normal size and weight.[17] As for the heart muscle, it was without fibrosis or scarring, free of inflammation, and showed no evidence of a previous heart attack.[18] In addition, the heart valves were without any abnormalities, the coronary arteries were normal with a normal distribution, and the aorta had minimal accumulation of plaque.[19]

The respiratory system—lungs, larynx, trachea, and bronchi—showed no evidence of trauma, inflammation, or obstruction.[20] When lung tissue was examined under a microscope, red blood cells were identified in the alveoli, suggesting Foster had aspirated blood prior to his death.[21]

The endocrine system, including the pancreas and adrenal and thyroid glands, was normal, as were the kidneys and urinary bladder.[22] The stomach contained a considerable amount of digested food material, consistent with Foster having had lunch only hours before he died, but it was free of pill fragments.[23] The liver was unremarkable and without evidence of trauma.[24] The appendix was normal.[25]

The most important anatomical anomaly found in the autopsy related to the cause of Foster's death was the perforating gunshot wound to the mouth and head.[26] The entrance wound was clearly visible in the posterior oropharynx, an area at the back of the throat, approximately seven and a half inches from the top of the head.[27] Some tissue fragments of the palate contained what appeared to be gunpowder debris, which was confirmed when palate tissue was viewed under a microscope.[28] The wound track in the head continued "backward and upward, with an entrance wound just left of the foramen magnum [a large oval opening in the occipital bone at the base of the skull]."[29] The brain stem and the left cerebral hemisphere of the brain were also damaged, with the exit wound through the scalp and skull "near the midline in the occipital region of the brain."[30]

Cause and Manner of Death

Police found Foster lying dead at Fort Marcy Park, covered with gunshot residue–like material, a gun in his right hand.[31] There was no sign of a struggle or evidence of foul play, which precluded the possibility that Foster's death was a homicide.[32]

With the exception of the gunshot wound to the mouth and the back of the head that caused substantial and significant damage to the skull and brain, there were no other anatomical changes to explain Foster's death.[33] However, since Foster's doctor had given him trazodone, a prescription medication for depression, twenty-four to thirty-six hours prior to his death, I wondered whether Foster had taken more pills than he had been prescribed and whether the drug may have affected his state of mind. To answer these questions, I reviewed the toxicology report.

An immunological testing screen did not identify trazodone in Foster's blood, suggesting he had not taken his medication as prescribed.[34] It also meant the drug did not contribute to Foster's death.

Urine and vitreous humor, the clear gel that fills the space between the lens and the retina of the eyeball, were tested for the presence of drugs, but neither alcohol nor ketones were detected.[35] Had there been a high level of ketones, it would have indicated Foster had been suffering from diabetic ketoacidosis at the time of his death, a complication of diabetes that could lead to coma or possibly even death.

A suicide note was not found with Foster's body. However, a draft resignation letter, torn into twenty-seven pieces, was discovered in a briefcase in Foster's office that hinted at Foster's state of mind.[36] It said, in part, "The *Wall Street Journal* editors lie without consequence. I was not meant for the job or the spotlight of public life in Washington. Here, ruining people is considered sport."[37]

After I reviewed the circumstances surrounding Foster's death, the autopsy findings and results of toxicology testing, published lay articles, and the scientific literature, I concluded that the immediate cause of death was a self-inflicted gunshot wound to the mouth and head. The manner of death was suicide.

Life and Career

Born in 1945 in Hope, Arkansas, the county seat of Hempstead County, Foster was the son of a successful real estate developer and a friend of Bill Clinton, the future president of the United States.[38] Foster and Clinton attended the same kindergarten, so their friendship, which began at a very early age, had endured more than forty years.[39]

When Foster was seven years old, Clinton moved to Hot Springs, about seventy miles away from Hope.[40] Nevertheless, Foster and Clinton continued to maintain their friendship, as Clinton often visited his grandparents in Hope during the summers, weekends, and on holidays.[41]

By all accounts, Foster was a high achiever throughout his life. At Hope High School, he was an excellent student, president of the student council, and an athlete.[42] After graduating in 1963, Foster attended Davidson College, where he majored in psychology.[43] Instead of joining the family real estate business as his father had hoped, Foster began pursuing a law degree in 1967 at Vanderbilt University Law School.[44]

Foster married Elizabeth "Lisa" Braden in 1968, the daughter of an insurance broker he met while at Davidson College, after which he transferred to the University of Arkansas Law School, where he was managing editor of the *Arkansas Law Review*.[45] With Foster having joined the Arkansas National Guard, attending law school at the University of Arkansas was more convenient for his guard duties.[46]

In 1971, Foster earned his law degree, graduating first in his class and scoring the highest of his classmates on the Arkansas bar exam.[47] As a newly minted lawyer, he joined the Rose Law Firm in Little Rock as an associate.[48] Three years later, he made partner.[49]

Always extremely well prepared for his cases, Foster quickly built a reputation for being one of the best trial litigators in Arkansas.[50] "Driven to prevail," is the way his wife described Foster, who often stayed up all night to get ready for big cases.[51] Don Moldeo, the writer, described Foster as "a 'can-do' lawyer who worked best when under pressure."[52]

According to the *Washington Post*, Foster had reached the pinnacle of the Arkansas legal establishment by 1992.[53] In June of the following year, he received several awards from the Arkansas Bar Association and was named "Outstanding Lawyer of the Year."[54]

When Bill Clinton won the 1992 presidential election, Foster joined the transition team and became deputy White House counsel in the new administration.[55] Adjusting to Washington DC and a life in politics was difficult for Foster.[56] He had no political experience, and his family was still in Arkansas so his son could finish his senior year in high school.[57]

One of Foster's first official tasks was to vet potential administration appointees.[58] The experience caused him much anxiety, and he became depressed.[59] Foster thought he was responsible for Zoë Baird withdrawing her nomination for attorney general, as well as for the unsuccessful appointments of Kimba Wood, the second nominee for attorney general, and Lanie Guinier, who was to head the Civil Rights Division of the Justice Department.[60] Working twelve-hour days, often seven days a week, Foster started to lose weight.[61]

On May 8, 1993, Foster gave the commencement address at his alma mater, the University of Arkansas Law School.[62] "The reputation you develop for intellectual and ethical integrity will be your greatest asset," Foster told the graduating class.[63] "There is no victory, no advantage, no fee, no favor, which is worth even a blemish on your reputation for intellect and integrity."[64] Four days later, Travelgate erupted in full force.[65]

Stinging editorials critical of Foster appeared in the *Wall Street Journal* in June and July 1993.[66] A congressional hearing potentially was on the horizon, during which Foster would have to testify. Suffering from insomnia and struggling with depression, Foster bade his office coworkers good-bye on Tuesday afternoon in late July 1993 and drove to Fort Marcy Park.

Conclusions

Two law enforcement investigations, one by the United States Park Police and another by the first independent counsel,

Robert B. Fiske Jr., concluded Foster had committed suicide by gunshot at Fort Marcy Park.[67] Two congressional inquiries and a three-year investigation by the second independent counsel, Kenneth W. Starr, reached the same conclusion.[68]

To quell conspiracy theories, Starr's investigation included analysis by experienced FBI criminal investigators and other law enforcement professionals, as well as opinions by Dr. Brian D. Blackbourne, a medical examiner and a forensic pathologist, Dr. Henry C. Lee, one of the world's foremost forensic scientists and an expert in crime scene reconstruction, and Dr. Alan L. Berman, a PhD psychologist, psychotherapist, and suicidologist.[69]

"Vincent Foster committed suicide on July 20, 1993, in Fort Marcy Park by placing a .38 caliber revolver in his mouth and pulling the trigger," Blackbourne concluded.[70] "His death was at his own hand."[71] Lee noted, "The data indicate that the death of Mr. Vincent W. Foster, Jr. is consistent with a suicide. The location where Mr. Foster's body was found is consistent with the primary scene."[72] As for Berman, he reported, "[It is] my opinion and to a one hundred percent degree of medical certainty, the death of Vincent Foster was a suicide."[73]

According to Starr's report, Foster was "a controlled, private, perfectionistic character whose public persona as a man of integrity, honesty and unimpeachable reputation was of utmost importance."[74] Under extreme stress, Foster was overwhelmed with fear and anxiety over real or perceived mistakes, which undoubtedly pushed him over the edge and led to his demise.[75]

"It is not something new to discover that Washington can dash a lot of vision and hope," said Cliff Baker, artistic director of the Arkansas Repertory Theater, where Foster had once served as board chairman, when he heard of Foster's passing.[76] That may be true, but suicide is a tremendously high price to pay for working on behalf of the American people.

CHAPTER 12

John Candy

Died March 4, 1994
Actor-Comedian

ON MARCH 4, 1994, John Candy, a comedian, actor and a former member of Chicago's Second City, was filming *Wagons East*, a Western comedy in which he played a drunken stagecoach driver, in Durango, Mexico.[1] "I don't know if he was excited to work on … [the film] … or wasn't," Chris, Candy's son, said.[2] "Richard Lewis, who worked with him on that movie, told me … when he looked at my dad, he looked so tired."[3]

Shooting in the eighty-degree heat was exhausting, ending at about 10:00 p.m., after which Candy had a spaghetti dinner, took a shower, and went to bed at approximately eleven o'clock.[4] He had completed filming two thirds of his scenes and had only two more left before returning to California.[5]

When Candy did not show up the following morning, his bodyguard, Gustave Populus, telephoned Candy's room.[6] Unable to reach Candy, Populus went to his room and knocked on the door for several minutes.[7] Receiving no response, he entered the bedroom only to find Candy lying dead in bed, wearing a red-and-black-checked nightshirt, half in and half out of the bed.[8]

The medical examiner of the state of Durango arrived at about 1:00 p.m. and pronounced Candy deceased, estimating the time of death at between 5:00 a.m. and 7:00 a.m.[9] Candy had apparently suffered a massive heart attack and died in his sleep, the coroner said.[10] He was forty-three years old.

The Autopsy

It is unclear whether an autopsy or toxicology testing was performed. However, based on published lay articles, Candy, weighing approximately 350 pounds, was obese.[11]

Cause and Manner of Death

"There were no suspicious circumstances" surrounding Candy's death, the coroner who examined Candy's body said.[12] Furthermore, no drugs or alcohol were found in Candy's room.[13]

In the absence of a toxicology report, it was impossible to determine whether cocaine, a drug Candy had been abusing for a long time, contributed to Candy's death.

After I reviewed the circumstances surrounding Candy's death, the death certificate, and published lay articles, I had no reason to disagree with the coroner's conclusion that the immediate cause of death was acute myocardial infarction, or a heart attack.[14] Furthermore, since the coroner concluded the manner of death was natural, it suggests Candy's heart attack was not caused by a drug overdose for if it was, he would have labeled the death an accident.

Life and Career

Candy was born in 1950 in Toronto, Canada.[15] He attended Holy Cross Catholic School up to the eighth grade and then Neil McNeil Catholic High School, where he acted in school plays and played hockey and football.[16]

In 1969, Candy enrolled at Centennial Community College in Toronto, taking journalism and drama courses, after which he landed an acting job as a member of a children's theater group.[17] Soon he appeared in television commercials and in low-budget Canadian feature films before becoming a performer and writer in 1972 for Toronto's Second City, an improvisational comedy troupe.[18] He was later "traded to Chicago, and ... started [his] Second City training there." In 1974, he returned to Toronto's Second City, bringing his skits to Canadian television three years later.[19]

Although Candy had small roles in Steven Spielberg's film *1941*, in *The Blues Brothers*, and in *Stripes*, his big breakthrough was in the 1984 film *Splash*.[20] "The mere sight of the tubby Mr. Candy is funny enough," Janet Maslin of the *New York Times* wrote at the time, "but the spectacle of him playing racquetball really is something to see."[21]

In 1985, Candy co-starred in *The Shmenges: The Last Polka* on HBO; in 1990, he played the leader of a polka band in the film *Home Alone*.[22] In total, in the years between 1981 and 1992, Candy was featured in at least fifteen films, including in the hit movie *Planes, Trains & Automobiles*.[23] While most of his roles were comedic, Candy's dramatic performance in Oliver Stone's political thriller *JFK* was considered by many critics to be his best work.[24] "He worked so hard on that," Candy's daughter, Jen, recalled.[25] "He had a dialect coach, and he worked night and day on that script. He was so worried about it, getting that accent down."[26]

On March 4, 1994, Candy was in Mexico shooting *Wagons East* when he died. Released in August 1994, the film flopped at the box office.[27]

Conclusions

Since Candy's father—who, like Candy, was also obese—died from a heart attack when he was thirty-five years old, Candy always feared he would experience the same fate.[28] "He grew up with heart disease," Candy's son, Chris, said of his dad.[29] "His father had a heart attack, his brother had a heart attack. It was in the family."[30] One report noted that Candy's grandfather had also suffered from heart disease.[31] According to the CDC, genetic factors, which can influence the susceptibility to the underlying etiology of heart failure, the rapidity of disease progression, and the response to pharmaceutical therapy, likely play a role in high blood pressure, heart disease, and other heart-related conditions.[32]

Besides a genetic predisposition for heart failure, Candy had other risk factors for heart disease.[33] "John was obese throughout his adult life," Dr. Michael Hunter, a renowned forensic pathologist, noted.[34] "I've discovered that John was prone to binge eating in response to professional setbacks." Occasionally, Candy had tried to control his weight with different diets, but without success.[35] The American Heart Association reported that not only does obesity contribute to the effects of various cardiovascular risk factors, but it also contributes to the development of cardiovascular disease, particularly heart failure and coronary heart disease, as well as cardiovascular mortality independent of other cardiovascular risk factors.[36]

Unlike Cass Elliot, a member of the singing group the Mamas and the Papas, who was also obese and who died of congestive heart failure, Candy was a heavy smoker.[37] One of his friends said, "When I first met John, he was already smoking. I think he was smoking like a pack a day when he was seventeen [or] nineteen. John never did give up the smokes."[38] Smoking has been linked to heart disease for many years, with smokers two to four times more likely to suffer from heart disease than nonsmokers.[39] Chemicals in tobacco smoke can damage the structure and function of blood vessels and affect the function of the heart.[40] In addition, they can cause an increase in blood pressure and heart rate, reduce the flow of oxygenated blood from the heart to the rest of the body, and increase the risk for blood clots.[41]

Candy had one other significant health risk for heart disease.[42] "John appears to have a history of use of another drug that is also known to have a damaging impact on the heart, and that's cocaine." Hunter said.[43] Chronic cocaine users are more likely to get high blood pressure, thickening of the heart muscle wall, and atherosclerosis, all major risk factors for heart attacks.[44]

Candy's drug problem began when he moved to Chicago to perform at Second City.[45] "The next thing I knew," Candy said, "I was in Chicago, where I learned how to drink, stay up real late, and spell 'd-r-u-g-s.'"[46] When his friend, John Belushi, who was also extremely overweight, tragically died of a drug overdose in 1982, Candy saw it as a message and quit using cocaine, although some reports note he occasionally still used the drug.[47]

Candy's risk for heart disease was greater than the sum of its parts.[48] Although he could have avoided some of the risks, Candy's addiction to drugs, as well as his smoking and obesity, for which surgery might have been helpful, were too much for his heart to bear. "He was an amazing talent, an amazing force," Candy's son remembers.[49] "He was on this planet to do a lot, and he did do a lot."[50] Steve Martin, the comedian, said, "John Candy was a gentleman and a great comic talent."[51] Candy's daughter, Jen, took a more philosophical view of her dad's passing. "As much as he is gone," she said, "he is not gone. He is always there."[52]

CHAPTER 13

Kurt Cobain

Died April 5, 1994

Member of Nirvana

ON MARCH 3, 1994, while Nirvana, the grunge band, was on its In Utero European Tour, Kurt Cobain, the band's left-handed guitarist and lead singer, ingested champagne along with an overdose of flunitrazepam, a benzodiazepine tranquilizer, in an apparent suicide attempt.[1] In a coma, Cobain was rushed to a hospital in Rome, Italy, where, after recovering, his wife, Courtney Love, the lead singer of the band Hole, took Cobain back to their home in Seattle, Washington.[2] Two weeks later, Cobain locked himself in his room with drugs and guns.[3] Fearing he was again trying to kill himself, Love called police.[4]

When police arrived, Cobain denied he was trying to commit suicide, claiming he was simply trying to hide from his wife.[5] Police confiscated four guns, twenty-five boxes of ammunition, and a bottle of pills.[6] Love and some of her friends arranged an "intervention," during which Cobain agreed to enter the Exodus Recovery Center, a drug rehabilitation facility in Marina Del Rey, California.[7] However, after spending just two days in rehab, Cobain climbed over a six-foot fence and fled the facility.[8]

After secretly flying back to Seattle, Cobain roamed the streets for several days while Love reported him missing and frantically searched for his whereabouts.[9] "Kurt hadn't called me," Mark Lanegan, Cobain's close friend, later told *Rolling Stone*.[10] "He hadn't called some other people. He hadn't called his family. He hadn't called anybody ... I had a feeling that something real bad had happened."[11]

On Friday, April 8, an electrician arrived at the Cobain residence to install a security system.[12] As he entered a greenhouse above the garage, he found Cobain dead with a twenty-gauge shotgun in his arms and blood oozing from his ear.[13]

The King County Medical Examiner's office concluded Cobain had died three days earlier, in the afternoon or evening of April 5.[14] He was twenty-seven years old.[15]

The Autopsy

The autopsy was conducted by Dr. Nikolas Hartshorne, an assistant medical examiner at the King County Medical

Examiner's office.[16] The autopsy and toxicology reports were unavailable for review. However, based on published lay articles, Cobain's death was the result of a single gunshot wound to the head, entering the jaw and exiting through the skull.[17] Other autopsy findings included puncture wounds on the insides of the right and left elbows of both arms.[18]

Cause and Manner of Death

Police did not suspect foul play in Cobain's death. "There's nothing suspicious about the scene or the circumstances that bothers me," Hartshorne said.[19]

Toxicology analysis of Cobain's blood detected 1.52 milligrams per liter of morphine, the active metabolite of heroin, a "not insignificant" amount, said Dr. David Bailey, of the University of California at San Diego.[20] Dr. Randall C. Baselt, a forensic toxicologist, was more emphatic.[21] "A high concentration, by any account," Baselt declared.[22] Also present in Cobain's blood was a trace amount of diazepam, a tranquilizer.[23]

A suicide note written in red ink was located at the scene.[24] "We feel confident that this was a self-inflicted gunshot wound to the head," Hartshorne said.[25] The death certificate noted that Cobain died from a self-inflicted "contact perforating gunshot wound to the head ... through the mouth."[26]

Conspiracy theorists claimed that with so much morphine in Cobain's blood, it would have been impossible for him to pull the trigger.[27] They proposed that someone else must have shot Cobain so that his death was a homicide. However, in my view, that is unlikely.[28] Six days before he died, Cobain had his friend, Dylan Carlson, purchase a 20-gauge shotgun and a box of ammunition.[29] In 2014, Mike Ciesynski, a former Seattle Police Department detective, located the receipt for the shotgun shells used to kill Cobain.[30] The date, time, and location of Stan's Gun Shop, where the shells had been purchased, matched the place, date, and time a Seattle cabdriver said he had dropped off a man, most likely Carlson, he had picked up at Cobain's residence.[31]

Since Cobain's body was discovered three days after he died, his blood morphine level may have been subject to postmortem redistribution—changes in the concentrations of drugs in blood that occur after death.[32] Thus, the amount of morphine measured in Cobain's blood at his autopsy could have been 9 to 45 percent higher than on the day he died.[33] As for Cobain being too impaired to pull the trigger, Cobain was a longtime heroin addict, so he undoubtedly was tolerant to many of the drug's effects.[34] Lastly, even if Cobain's blood morphine concentration when he died had been the same as the amount measured at his autopsy, it still would have been 50 percent less than the maximum amount reported in the blood of heroin fatalities.[35]

A study by Sandro Galea and coworkers of firearm deaths in New York City between the years 1990 and 1998 found positive drug use in over half of all firearm deaths, with cocaine, marijuana, opiates, and alcohol accounting for almost all of these deaths.[36] In a separate report, Baselt noted that two highly-tolerant young adults given a single oral 400-milligram heroin dose under laboratory conditions had peak plasma levels of morphine that averaged 1,035 milligrams per liter, which is in the range of the amount detected in Cobain's blood at the time of his death, as corrected for postmortem redistribution.[37]

After I reviewed the circumstances surrounding Cobain's death, the death certificate, the autopsy findings and results of toxicology testing, published lay articles, and the scientific literature, I concluded that the immediate cause of death was a self-inflicted gunshot wound to the head. The manner of death was suicide.

Life and Career

Cobain was born in 1967 in Aberdeen, Washington.[38] His mother was a waitress, and his father, an automobile mechanic.[39] As a young child, Cobain liked art and music, playing the piano by the time he was four years old, and even composing simple songs.[40] "My mother encouraged me to be artistic," Cobain once said, adding sarcastically, "It was written in a contract at an early age that I would be an artist."[41]

When Cobain's parents separated and later divorced, it affected him greatly; he became withdrawn, antisocial, and rebellious.[42] "I had a really good childhood up until I was nine, then a classic case of divorce really affected me," Cobain explained.[43] Splitting his time between his father and seeing his mother on the weekends made Cobain depressed.[44] A therapist recommended that Cobain's parents reconcile for the sake of their son, but they were unable to do so.[45] When they divorced, Cobain's father received full custody of his son, while Cobain's sister went to live with their mother.[46]

When Cobain's father married a woman with two children, Cobain became even more bitter, so much so that he went to live with a family friend.[47] While there, he attended church services for a short while and joined the school's wrestling and baseball teams.[48]

During his second year at Aberdeen High School, Cobain started living with his mother, but when he quit school just prior to graduation, she cast him out of the house.[49]

In 1985, Cobain formed a rock band named Fecal Matter, but it disbanded a year later.[50] His next band, Nirvana, was formed in 1988.[51] Nirvana's first album, *Bleach*, with its punk roots and heavy metal sounds, was released a year later.[52]

In the 1990s, Nirvana signed with Geffen Records, released its second album, *Nevermind*, and toured with the popular rock band Sonic Youth.[53] Their song "Smells Like Teen Spirit" became the band's biggest hit and was voted the third-best pop song of all time by *Rolling Stone*.[54] Recognized as the best songwriter of his generation, Cobain became one of the most influential musicians in alternative rock history.[55]

As Nirvana became more successful, Cobain became unhappy with the band's musical direction. Unable to handle the pressure and professional expectations associated with the growing popularity of the band, Cobain took solace in heroin.[56] "I didn't know how to deal with success," he later said.[57] "If there was a Rock Star 101, I would have liked to take it. It might have helped me."[58]

In February 1992, Cobain married Love, who was already pregnant and, like Cobain, was a heavy heroin user.[59] Their marriage was tumultuous from the start. In 1993, Seattle police broke up a violent domestic dispute at Cobain's house, at which time guns were confiscated and Cobain was arrested for assaulting Love.[60]

Nirvana's third and final album, *In Utero*, released in September 1993, was hugely successful, soaring to number one on the music charts.[61] It included the highly popular song "Radio Friendly Unit Shifter."[62]

In March 1994, while touring Europe with Nirvana, Cobain overdosed on drugs in an apparent failed suicide attempt.[63] A month later, he tried to commit suicide again. This time, he succeeded.

Conclusions

Cobain began using drugs when he was thirteen years old and had become a full-fledged heroin addict within ten years.[64] In his suicide note, Cobain expressed his guilt for not having "felt the excitement of listening to, as well as creating music, along with reading and writing, for too many years now."[65] He ended the note by saying, "I don't have the passion anymore, and so remember, it's better to burn out than to fade away."[66] Could this truly be what Cobain was feeling, or were the words merely a reflection of his heroin addiction?

There is some scientific support for the notion that Cobain's cognitive abilities were affected by his long-term use of heroin. According to the US National Institute on Drug

Abuse, "… repeated heroin use changes the physical structure and physiology of the brain, creating long-term imbalances in neuronal and hormonal systems that are not easily reversed."[67] Some of heroin's effects include deterioration of the brain's white and gray matter, regions of the brain and spinal cord that enable brain cells to quickly send and receive messages up and down the spinal cord. Deterioration of these areas of the brain can affect decision-making, regulation of behavior, and response to stressful situations.[68] In addition, studies have shown that heroin users often show cognitive impairment, an observation that led to scientific exploration of cognitive enhancers as a potential treatment for heroin use disorder and addiction.[69]

It appears likely Cobain was aware of the effects that drug abuse could have on his cognitive abilities. As he said, "Drugs are a waste of time. They destroy your memory and your self-respect and everything that goes along with your self-esteem."[70] And yet, despite knowing the detrimental psychological and physiological effects of heroin addiction, Cobain was unable to overcome the hold heroin had on his health and well-being.

Mounting pressures of fame took a heavy toll on Cobain. "I was tired of pretending that I was someone else just to get along with people, just for the sake of having friendships," Cobain said.[71] "Friends are nothing but a known enemy … I'm so happy because today I found my friends—they're in my head."[72] Cobain also declared, "I would rather be hated for what I am, than loved for what I am not."[73]

Cobain's obtuse yet mind-blowing views on mental illness can be appreciated from his writing. "Just because you're paranoid doesn't mean they aren't after you," Cobain said.[74] He implored people, "If my eyes could show my soul, everyone would cry when they saw me smile."[75]

That Cobain was prepared for death is apparent from some of his quotes. "If you die, you're completely happy and your soul somewhere lives on," he once said.[76] "I'm not afraid of dying. Total peace after death, becoming someone else is the best hope I've got."[77] He also stated, "I'd rather be dead than cool" and "The finest day I ever had was when tomorrow never came."[78]

I would rather remember Cobain for his genius and his captivating insights than for his death. "Wanting to be someone else is a waste of who you are," Cobain said.[79] Such a profound statement from someone so young is startling. "Practice makes perfect, but nobody's perfect, so why practice?"[80] Another priceless quote: "They laugh at me because I'm different; I laugh at them because they're all the same."[81] "I'm worse at what I do best."[82] There are many more such quotable quotes.[83]

Cobain was a strong supporter of the LGBTQ community.[84] "I would like to get rid of the homophobes, racists and sexists in our audience," he told the crowd at one of his concerts.[85] "If any of you in any way hate homosexuals, people of a different color, or women, please do this one favor for us … Don't come to our shows and don't buy our records."[86] That pretty much summarizes who Cobain was—a strong supporter of women, racial equality, and LGBTQ rights, and a man who was willing to put everything on the line for the sake of his principles and beliefs.

In his death, Cobain joined the "Twenty-Seven Club," a group of prominent musicians who died at the age of twenty-seven that includes Brian Jones, Jimi Hendrix, Janis Joplin, Jim Morrison, and Amy Winehouse.[87]

CHAPTER 14

Jerry Garcia

Died August 9, 1995
Member of the Grateful Dead

WHEN I SAY the words, "Jerry Garcia," the image that immediately comes to my mind is of a cherubic face enveloped by lots of long, bushy, graying hair cascading down the back, all the way down to the neckline. A thick, grayish beard, not quite as long as Santa Claus's covers the face, and a full, thick, graying mustache rests squarely above the upper lip. What little of the face remains in view is creased and weathered, looking at least twenty years older that its age. The eyes twinkle behind rounded glasses, the lenses sometimes clear, sometimes darkly tinted, often barely resting on the tip of a

Roman nose. The pot belly, a product of years of abuse by alcohol and junk food, is wrapped in a black T-shirt.

There was much more to Garcia, of course, besides his distinctive appearance. Founder and best-known member of the Grateful Dead, a rock band known for playing psychedelic rock, folk rock, and bluegrass, Garcia may have been too stoned at times to function on stage. He might even have forgotten the words to his songs. But his fans, aptly named "Deadheads," didn't care.[1] Listening to a live performance of the Grateful Dead is a spiritual experience, one not to be missed.[2] "We are like licorice," Garcia once said.[3] "Either people ignore us, or they like us a lot."[4]

What Garcia loved most, besides music, was drugs— heroin and cocaine to be precise. Struggling with his addiction, especially in the last year of his life, Garcia appeared thin, haggard, and very pale.[5]

In July 1995, a couple of weeks after the Grateful Dead's summer tour ended, Garcia checked into the Betty Ford Center, a residential treatment center for people with substance dependence located in Rancho Mirage, California.[6] Having stayed there less than two weeks, he left in good spirits, feeling he had kicked his addiction.[7] But a few days later, Garcia checked himself into the Serenity Knolls Treatment Center, described on its website as "California's best twelve-step drug and alcohol treatment center."[8]

At 4:23 a.m. on August 9, 1995, Garcia was found dead, lying on the floor of his room at Serenity Knolls.[9] A staff nurse attempted to revive Garcia, but she was unsuccessful.[10]

Paramedics were called, and despite heroic efforts, Garcia was pronounced dead at the scene.[11] He was fifty-three years old.[12]

The Autopsy

Garcia "was a fifty-three year old man with hardening of the arteries," said Gary Erickson, a Marin County coroner's investigator.[13] An autopsy revealed an enlarged heart and "multifocal myocardial fibrosis," a condition that can lead to heart failure and death.[14] In addition, Garcia suffered from arteriosclerosis, with an average blockage of 85 percent in two of his coronary arteries and 30 percent blockage in a third artery.[15]

Cause and Manner of Death

Toxicology analysis identified benzoylecgonine, a cocaine metabolite, in the blood and urine, and morphine, a metabolite of heroin, in the urine.[16] No unmetabolized cocaine or heroin was detected in the blood.[17] Most likely, Garcia had ingested the two addictive drugs prior to entering Serenity Knolls, allowing cocaine and heroin sufficient time to be completely metabolized and to be excreted from the body.[18]

Cocaine, a drug associated with a variety of arrhythmias, is especially toxic to the heart in someone with 85 percent blockage of two coronary arteries and an enlarged heart. However, since free, unmetabolized cocaine was not found in

Garcia's blood, it was impossible to determine to what degree, if any, the drug contributed to Garcia's death.

After I reviewed the circumstances surrounding Garcia's death, the autopsy findings and results of toxicology testing, published lay articles, and the scientific literature, I concluded that the immediate cause of death was a heart attack. Without additional information, I had no reason to disagree with the coroner's conclusion that the manner of death was natural.[19]

Life and Career

Garcia was born in San Francisco, California, in 1942.[20] His mother was a nurse, and his father, a jazz musician.[21]

When Garcia was four years old, he lost two thirds of the middle finger of his right hand in a woodcutting accident.[22] A year later, his father drowned while fly fishing in the Trinity River.[23]

After his father died, Garcia and his brother were sent to live with their grandparents while his mother worked full-time in the family's bar.[24] Five years later, after his mother remarried, Garcia and his brother moved back home with their mother and their new stepfather.[25]

As a young boy, Garcia suffered from bouts of asthma.[26] As a teenager, he skipped classes and fought with his classmates.[27] "I was a fuck-up, a juvenile delinquent," Garcia said of his teenage years.[28]

Garcia loved art and music, especially rock 'n' roll, so his mother encouraged him to pursue his passions.[29] In 1957, when he was fifteen years old, Garcia's mother bought him his first electric guitar. Garcia taught himself the basic chords so he could play along with recordings of Chuck Berry, his favorite singer and guitarist.[30] That same year, Garcia discovered marijuana.[31]

After graduating high school, Garcia enlisted in the army, but he was discharged nine months later, after he had been court-martialed twice and had deserted eight times.[32] When his military stint ended, Garcia enrolled in art classes at the San Francisco Art Institute.[33]

In 1961, Garcia survived a serious car accident in which he was a passenger and one of his friends died.[34] He later claimed that surviving the horrific accident gave him a second chance on life. It was then that Garcia decided to become more serious about his music at the expense of art.

Having learned to play the acoustic guitar while in the army, Garcia began to teach himself the five-string banjo, becoming proficient in bluegrass music.[35] Between 1960 and 1964, he spent much of his time practicing the two musical instruments and learning to play the fiddle, bass, and mandolin; he also performed with several local bands.[36]

In 1965, Garcia formed a blues-rock band called Warlocks; a few months later, the band changed its name to the Grateful Dead.[37] With Garcia as the band's main songwriter, the Grateful Dead played improvisational jazz-inspired folk-rock music, gaining a strong reputation and becoming one of the most popular live psychedelic rock bands in history.[38]

Aoxomoxoa, the band's third album, established the Grateful Dead as one of the greatest live bands of all time, averaging eighty concerts per year.[39] "I feel like we've been getting away with something ever since there were more people in the audience than there were on stage," Garcia told one interviewer.[40] "We've been falling uphill for twenty-seven years. I don't know why. I have no idea. All I know is it's endlessly fascinating and incredible luck probably has a lot to do with it."[41]

In the late 1960s through the early 1980s, Garcia was involved in several side projects, including recording five solo albums—*Garcia, Compliments, Reflections, Cats under the Stars*, and *Run for the Roses*.[42] In addition, he was a founding member of the country-rock group the New Riders of the Purple Sage, The Jerry Garcia Band, and the band Old & In the Way, whose record became the biggest-selling bluegrass album of all time.[43]

By the mid-1970s, Garcia had already gotten into hard drugs; by the 1980s, he was a full-fledged heroin and cocaine addict.[44] "We did about all we could possibly do," to encourage Garcia to stop using drugs, said Mickey Hart, drummer for the Grateful Dead, "but the heroin was stronger."[45] Garcia's creativity was affected by his addiction, and his health deteriorated considerably, so much so that by the mid-1980s, he almost died after going into a diabetic coma.[46] By the time he emerged from his coma five days later, Garcia had lost all his musical skills, which he had to relearn over the next several months.[47]

In 1990, Garcia teamed up with David Grisman, a former member of the band Old and In the Way, and together they released several albums, including *Garcia/Grisman*, *Not for Kids Only*, *Shady Grove*, *The Pizza Tapes*, *So What*, and *Been All Around This World*.[48] "The nineties was my least favorite period, because of Jerry's declining health," Hart said.[49] "He was missing so many damn notes!"[50] Looking tired, Garcia was increasingly disoriented during shows.[51] By 1995, he was not only a diabetic and heavily addicted to heroin and cocaine, but he was also significantly overweight as a result of his love of junk food and lack of exercise. He was also a heavy smoker, which affected his breathing.[52] "He was passing out in the middle of the day on his bed, and he was probably high," said Trixie, Garcia's daughter.[53]

On August 7, 1995, Garcia checked into Serenity Knolls Treatment Center in Marin County to try to get healthy.[54] It was too little, too late.

Conclusions

Many remember Garcia as a talented and accomplished musician and the heart and soul of the Grateful Dead, but healthwise, he was a total mess. Suffering from diabetes, Garcia was also significantly overweight, a drug addict, and a chronic heavy smoker of cigarettes, all risk factors for heart disease.

The likelihood of having heart disease is increased when smoking cigarettes is combined with other risk factors.[55] Other musicians have died at a young age with only one or two risk factors for heart disease, such as drug addiction and obesity. That Garcia had four very serious risk factors meant his early demise was almost assured.[56]

Diabetes is a disease in which the level of glucose, a sugar, remains elevated in the blood.[57] Glucose is the main source of energy for cellular activity in the brain, muscles, and other tissues.[58] Insulin, a hormone made by the pancreas that is secreted into the blood, helps glucose leave the blood and enter cells.[59] When the pancreas does not make insulin or insulin levels are too low, glucose levels remain elevated in the blood.[60]

There are several types of diabetes, the most common of which are type 1, which is usually diagnosed in children and young adults; type 2, which occurs mostly in middle-aged and older people (most likely the type of diabetes Garcia had); and gestational, which can develop during pregnancy.[61] About 90 to 95 percent of all cases of diabetes in adults are type 2 diabetes.[62] Some risk factors for type 2 diabetes include obesity and being overweight, inactivity, a family history, age, high blood pressure, and abnormal cholesterol and triglyceride levels in blood.[63] If left untreated, diabetes can lead to various ailments, including cardiovascular disease, a condition with which Garcia had been diagnosed.[64]

Garcia was overweight, mainly because of his unhealthy diet. Being overweight has been linked to high blood pressure (hypertension), elevated levels of cholesterol and triglycerides, heart failure, and an enlarged heart (cardiomegaly).[65] Considering his diet of junk food, it is not surprising Garcia's blood cholesterol and triglyceride levels were elevated and he suffered from high blood pressure.

Researchers have found that being overweight is a risk factor for heart failure even in the absence of other risk factors.[66] In one study, people who were the most obese and had high levels of troponin, an enzyme released from heart muscle when it is injured, were nine times more likely to develop heart failure than those with a normal weight and undetectable troponin levels.[67] Cardiologist Dr. Chiadi Ndumele of Johns Hopkins Hospital said, "Obesity itself can be causing silent damage to your heart muscle."[68] Dr. Jennifer Logue of the University of Glasgow agreed, urging that health-care providers and public officials "need to dedicate far more resources to preventing obesity."[69]

Garcia had another risk factor for heart disease—chronic abuse of cocaine and heroin. Although he did not die from a heroin overdose, Garcia had an enlarged heart and severe atherosclerosis, and he died from a heart attack—all symptoms associated with chronic cocaine use.[70] As cardiologist Dr. Nicole Harkin said, "Long-term users [of cocaine] have an increased risk of heart disease, and cocaine use has been associated with premature blockages in the heart."[71]

Cocaine stimulates the release of endothelin-1, a potent vasoconstrictor, and inhibits the production of nitric oxide, a major vasodilator.[72] It also stimulates the cardiovascular system by increasing heart rate and blood pressure, thereby decreasing myocardial contraction, lessening coronary capacity and blood flow, and depriving heart muscle of oxygen, resulting in cocaine-induced cardiomyopathy and electrical irregularities in the heart.[73]

Garcia's fourth risk factor for heart disease was his chronic heavy smoking. People who smoke cigarettes are two to four times more likely to develop heart disease than nonsmokers.[74] Cigarette smoke causes a rise in blood pressure, an increase in heart rate, and a reduction in oxygenated blood leaving the heart to other parts of the body.[75] Chemicals in cigarette smoke cause cells that line coronary blood vessels to become swollen and inflamed, which can lead to atherosclerosis, a narrowing of coronary arteries due to a buildup of plaque in the arterial walls, a reduction of oxygenated blood to the heart, and death of heart muscle.[76]

Ironically, when Garcia died, he was in a rehab center, trying to get clean. The years of defying the odds had taken their toll, however. "Magic is what we do, music is how we do it," he once said.[77] Apparently it was difficult for Garcia to make music and, at the same time, to take care of his health.

By 1995, the Grateful Dead was no longer merely a band; it was a top-earning touring act that earned over $50 million a year and whose schedule was set years in advance.[78] "We had a payroll and families," said Hart, the band's drummer.[79] "We weren't getting that much money; we were spreading it around. We couldn't stop. We were a snake eating its tail. There was no way for us to take a rest."[80] As for Garcia, he had alimony to pay as well as expenses for illicit drugs.[81] Success for the Grateful Dead came at a price, and the price was making a bargain with the devil. For Garcia, the devil was heroin and cocaine, and the price was his life.

Garcia's death meant the end of the Grateful Dead.[82] "Like everything else, it was too good to last," said Phil Lesh, a founding member of the Grateful Dead who played bass guitar.[83] What did last, however, was the ice cream flavor Cherry Garcia, for which Ben and Jerry's paid Garcia $125,000 for the use of his name.[84] Not bad for someone who couldn't stick to a low-calorie diet.

CHAPTER 15

Mickey Mantle

Died August 13, 1995
Professional Baseball Player

FROM THE 1950S to 1960s, baseball was dominated by the New York Yankees. The team was managed by the colorful and eccentric Casey Stengel.[1] With Yogi Berra as catcher, Whitey Ford as pitcher, Roger Maris in the outfield, and Mickie Mantle in center field, any Yankees game, especially when the team played against the Brooklyn Dodgers or the New York Giants, put the whole city on pause.

Mantle was a nineteen-year-old country boy from Commerce, Oklahoma, when he joined the Yankees.[2] It was also the year he began abusing alcohol. By the time he retired from baseball, his legs and knees were hurting and his career batting average had sunk to 0.298.[3] "I can't play anymore," Mantle said in March 1969, "I don't hit the ball when I need to. I can't steal when I need to. I can't score from second when I need to ... I never wanted to embarrass myself on the field or hurt the club in any way or give the fans anything less than what they are entitled to expect from me."[4] But that wasn't all. By the time he retired, Mantle had also developed a taste for the good life—living high and drinking good liquor—eventually becoming a chronic alcoholic.[5]

By his own admission, drinking was a way of life for Mantle even while he was in the Yankees.[6] "When I was drinking, I thought I was funny—the life of the party," Mantle said, "but as it turned out, nobody could stand to be around me."[7] On January 7, 1994, at the urging of his son Danny and former football player and television broadcaster Pat Summerall, Mantle checked himself into the Betty Ford Center in Rancho Mirage, California, a residential treatment center for people with substance dependence.[8] "Your liver is still working," his doctor told him, "but it has healed itself so many times that before long, you're just going to have one big scab for a liver. Eventually you'll need a new liver. I'm not going to lie to you. The next drink you take may be your last."[9]

In an article entitled "Time in a Bottle" for *Sports Illustrated*, Mantle reflected on his days as an alcoholic.[10] "I began some of my mornings the past ten years with the 'breakfast of champions'—a big glass filled with a shot or more of brandy, and some Kahlúa and cream," Mantle wrote.[11] "Unless I had a business engagement, I'd often keep on drinking until I couldn't drink anymore."[12]

Besides his chronic alcoholism, which undoubtedly caused his liver cirrhosis, Mantle was diagnosed in mid-1995 with hepatitis C, a virus transmitted through contaminated blood and a leading cause of liver cirrhosis and liver cancer.[13] Unlike hepatitis A and B, there is no vaccine against hepatitis C.[14] "It's a silent infection and it's a very clever virus that mutates very fast, so it has been difficult to develop a vaccine," said Dr. Harrys Torres of MD Anderson Cancer Center in Houston, Texas.[15] Having both liver cirrhosis and hepatitis C substantially increases the risk of developing liver cancer, so it was no surprise when Mantle was diagnosed in 1995 with undifferentiated hepatocellular carcinoma, an inoperable liver cancer.[16] "This is the most aggressive cancer that anyone on the medical team has ever seen," said Dr. Goran Klintmalm, medical director of transplant services at Baylor University Medical Center in Dallas, Texas.[17]

On June 8, 1995, Mantle underwent a liver transplant after doctors determined that without it, he would die within two to three weeks.[18] At first the surgery appeared to have been successful, but on July 28, Mantle reentered the hospital after doctors noted his liver cancer had metastasized to his lungs.[19]

At about 2:00 a.m. on August 13, 1995, Mantle died.[20] He was sixty-three years old.[21]

The Autopsy

There is no evidence an autopsy or toxicology testing was done after Mantle died. Based on published lay articles, Mantle had been suffering from cirrhosis of the liver, hepatitis C, and liver cancer that had metastasized to the lungs.

Cause and Manner of Death

After I reviewed the circumstances surrounding Mantle's death, as well as published lay articles and the scientific literature, I concluded that the immediate cause of death was metastatic undifferentiated hepatocellular carcinoma due to chronic cirrhosis of the liver and hepatitis C. The manner of death was natural.

Life and Career

Mantle, the son of a lead and zinc miner, was born in 1931 in Spavinaw, Oklahoma, a small, rural town with a population of only 437.[22] Mantle's father was an avid baseball fan, and he trained Mantle as a young boy to be a switch-hitter.[23] "He and my grandfather, who was left-handed, pitched to me every day after school in the backyard," Mantle said.[24] "I batted lefty against my dad and righty against my granddad."[25]

When Mantle was four years old, his family moved to Commerce, a town near Spavinaw.[26] While at Commerce High School, Mantle played baseball, basketball, and football.[27]

"My mother made every baseball uniform I ever wore till I signed with the Yankees," Mantel recalled.[28]

In his sophomore year, Mantle developed osteomyelitis, a serious bone infection, in his ankle.[29] At first his doctors thought his leg might need to be amputated, but after Mantle was treated with penicillin at the Crippled Children's Hospital in Oklahoma City, the infection was arrested.[30] Within a few weeks, Mantle returned to playing baseball.[31]

In 1949, Tom Greenwade, a New York Yankees scout, saw Mantle hit two homers, one righty and another lefty, while playing for an "under twenty-one" baseball team called the Baxter Springs Whiz Kids.[32] Greenwade wanted to sign Mantle on the spot, but seeing that he was still in high school, he waited until graduation day, at which time he signed Mantle as a shortstop to the Yankees' minor "Class D" team; two years later, at just nineteen years of age, Mantle joined the major league team.[33]

Unfortunately for Mantle, in his first year with the Yankees, he did not perform to everyone's expectations and was sent back to the minor league for additional training.[34] "It's not the end of the world, Mickey," Stengel, the team's manager, told Mantle.[35] "In a couple of weeks you'll start hitting and then we'll bring you right back again. I promise."[36] True to his word, Stengel had Mantle rejoin the Yankees when the 1952 baseball season opened.[37] This time Mantle performed in what became his trademark fashion, hitting a home run against the Washington Senators in 1953 that traveled 565 feet; it is still known as one of the longest hits in the history of Major League Baseball.[38]

The Yankees won all three World Series titles during Mantle's first three years with the team.[39] His golden year, however, was 1956. It was then that he won the "Triple Crown," leading the league in batting average (.353), home runs (52), and runs batted in (130); over that one season, he was also named the league's Most Valuable Player, a title he held the following year and again in 1962.[40]

By the mid-1960s, due in part to the excruciating pain in his knees and legs from several injuries he had sustained throughout his career, Mantle was in a slump.[41] "Hitting the ball was easy," Mantle once said.[42] "Running around the bases was the tough part."[43] On March 1, 1969, Mantle announced his retirement from baseball.[44]

Mantle's illustrious eighteen-year baseball career included 536 home runs and the all-time record for the most home runs in a World Series game—18.[45] During his tenure with the team, the Yankees won seven World Series and twelve American League pennants.[46] "I also broke Babe Ruth's record for strikeouts," Mantle said at his induction into the National Baseball Hall of Fame in 1974.[47] "He struck out only fifteen hundred times. I did it seventeen hundred and ten times."[48]

In retirement, Mantle opened the successful Mickey Mantle's Restaurant on Central Park South in New York City. In addition, he worked as a greeter for the Claridge Hotel and Casino in Atlantic City, appeared in television commercials, and had small roles in films.[49] His early investments in a hotel and a restaurant chain both failed.[50]

After struggling financially for several years, Mantel finally became wealthy in the mid-1980s as a result of the exploding baseball memorabilia industry, as his signature became a hot commodity.[51] At the same time, he continued to grapple with his alcoholism, which only worsened during his retirement.[52] Mantle's drinking got so bad that radio show host Don Imus joked, "If you get to Mickey Mantle's restaurant after midnight, you win a free dinner if you can guess which table Mickey's under."[53]

In his eulogy at Mantle's interment, Bob Costas summed up Mantle best when he said, "In the last years of his life, Mickey Mantle, always so hard on himself, finally came to accept and appreciate the distinction between a role model and a hero. The first, he often was not. The second, he always will be. And, in the end, people got it."[54]

Conclusions

The one constant that plagued Mantle throughout his adult life was the fear of dying young from Hodgkin's lymphoma, formerly known as Hodgkin's disease, a cancer of the lymphatic system, part of the immune system.[55] Mantle's grandfather, father, two uncles, and his son Billy all had Hodgkin's lymphoma, and they all died before the age of forty.[56] Mantle often said, "I'll never get a pension. I won't live long enough."[57] With that kind of an attitude, he decided to make the most of his remaining years. "What the hell, live while you can. I'm not going to be cheated."[58] And so he did, having a good time, laughing and drinking, and then drinking some more. Once, after hitting a home run while under a gray haze of a hangover, Mantle said, "Boy, you'll never know how hard that was."[59]

Although Mantle was at an increased risk of developing Hodgkin's lymphoma because of his genetic predisposition for the disease, scientists are still unsure what causes the cancer. The most that can be said is that males between twenty and forty years old or who are over seventy-five and have had illnesses caused by the Epstein-Barr virus, such as infectious mononucleosis, are more likely to develop Hodgkin's lymphoma than females.[60]

As it turned out, Mantle was never diagnosed with Hodgkin's lymphoma, and neither were his three remaining sons. Moreover, he was sixty-three years old when he died, much older than his male relatives who had died from the cancer.[61] "I always wondered why the disease had skipped me," Mantle said after his son was diagnosed with Hodgkin's.[62] "I had been expecting it all my life. For that matter, why had it spared my brothers, my sister, and their children? Why had it picked Billy?" There is no simple answer.

Mantle eventually developed a different kind of cancer— undifferentiated hepatocellular carcinoma—whose risk is higher in people with long-term liver disease, such as cirrhosis, or whose liver is scarred by infection with hepatitis B or hepatitis C or who drink large quantities of alcohol.[63] All three of these risk factors—alcoholism, hepatitis C, cirrhosis of the liver—are risk factors that Mantle could have avoided acquiring had he chosen to do so.

The risk of contracting hepatitis C increases significantly by having multiple short-term sexual relationships with partners who are infected with hepatitis C.[64] Mantle's promiscuity, which probably contributed to his being infected with hepatitis C, is legendary. As if to cement that notion, Mantle invited both his estranged wife of fifteen years and his mistress to his retirement ceremony in 1969.

As for being an alcoholic, Mantle wrote in his 1994 article "Time in a Bottle," "If alcoholism is hereditary, if it's in the genes, then I think mine came from my mother's side of the family. Her brothers were all alcoholics," thereby suggesting his alcoholism was beyond his control.[65] While it is true that alcoholism is a complex genetic disease, "there is no 'gene for alcoholism,' and both environmental and social factors weigh heavily on the outcome," as stated by Howard J. Edenberg and Tatiana Foroud of Indiana University School of Medicine.[66]

A person's choice of whether to drink alcohol and how much and how often is a strong factor in determining whether he or she becomes an alcoholic. Mantle may have had a genetic predisposition to alcoholism, but he was not genetically destined to become an alcoholic. Had he chosen not to consume so much alcohol over his lifetime, he would not have suffered from cirrhosis of the liver, a recognized risk factor for liver cancer, and probably would have avoided developing undifferentiated hepatocellular carcinoma.

By the time Mantle realized the errors of his ways, it was too late. "If I knew I was going to live this long, I'd have taken better care of myself," Mantle said.[67] Although he was transplanted with a new liver, Mantle's cancer had metastasized to his lungs. "You talk about a role model, this is a role model. Don't be like me," Mantle told his fans four weeks prior to his death.[68] "God gave me the ability to play baseball and I wasted it."[69] It was good advice—advice that he should have heeded himself.

CHAPTER 16

Marshall Applewhite

Died March 26, 1997

Key Figure in the Heaven's Gate Mass Suicide

MARCH 26, 2007 started off like any other day at the San Diego County Sheriff's Office. The phone was ringing off the hook, and people were being brought in for questioning or booked for minor offenses. When the phone rang for the fifth time, a sheriff's deputy picked up the receiver. "I need to report an anonymous tip, who do I talk to?" said the unidentified caller.[1] "This is regarding a mass suicide."[2] Within days, the caller was revealed to be Rio D'Angelo, a former member of Heaven's Gate, a strange and secretive cult of unidentified flying object (UFO) enthusiasts.[3]

The address to which the sheriff's deputies were led was that of a three-story, ninety-two-hundred-square-foot, $2.6 million rented hilltop mansion with seven bedrooms and nine bathrooms that was located in an exclusive suburb thirty miles north of San Diego.[4]

Two days earlier, members of Heaven's Gate started to implement their planned mass suicide so they could leave their bodily "vehicles" or "containers," as they called them, behind and "return their souls to 'a higher level of existence' in a starship" hidden in the tail behind the Hale-Bopp comet, one of the brightest comets known to date.[5] The preparation for their "departure" from Earth began with a group dinner at Marie Callender's, a chain restaurant serving American food.[6]

"They all ordered the exact same thing," a waiter at the restaurant recalled.[7] "They all had iced teas to drink, dinner salads beforehand with tomato vinegar dressing, turkey potpie for the entrée, [and] cheesecake with blueberries on top for dessert."[8]

Later that evening, after the cult members returned to their mansion, Marshall Appelwhite, the leader of Heaven's Gate, provided his followers glasses of vodka and bowls of applesauce or pudding laced with large amounts of barbiturate sedatives, which they enthusiastically and willingly consumed.[9] To make sure they died from the drug overdose, the cult members lay down in their bunk beds or on mattresses and covered their heads with plastic bags to induce asphyxiation.[10]

Death came over three days: fifteen people on March 24, fifteen more on March 25, and nine on March 26.[11] As the days passed, those Heaven's Gate members still living draped purple shrouds over the faces of those who had died.[12]

"These were some dedicated people," said Rick Scully, former lead detective in the San Diego County Sheriff's Office.[13] He then added, "[They were willing] to stand over the person they lived with for twenty years and watch them die."[14]

Calvin Vine, the chief investigator for the medical examiner's office, was one of the first to arrive at the Spanish-style mansion.[15] "The obvious odor of decomposed bodies … hit you as soon as you entered the residence," he remembered.[16] The scene was "like descending into hell," Scully said.[17]

It was only when he entered the bedroom that Vine saw the thirty-nine bodies—eighteen men, some of whom had been castrated, and twenty-one women—all between the ages of twenty-six and seventy-two.[18] The corpses, in various stages of decomposition, were lying on their backs, identically dressed in black shirts and black pants, with customized patches identifying them as the "Heaven's Gate Away Team," and wearing black Nike sneakers.[19] Many had a five-dollar bill and three coins—quarters—in their pockets.[20]

Later, people wondered why the Heaven's Gate members had worn Nike shoes. "They were able to get a good deal on them," said a surviving member.[21] "It was a combination of factors that made the sale happen, not because of a particular model or brand."[22] Nike quickly discontinued that style of shoe due to its association with the mass suicide.[23]

Vine described the scene as follows: "There was no mess. There was nothing out of place. There was no trash in the trash cans. Everything was just immaculate."[24]

"It seemed to be a group decision," Dr. Brian Blackbourne, the medical examiner-coroner of San Diego County, said.[25] "These people all had identification in the front pockets of these big black shirts they were wearing," including driver's licenses and birth certificates. Some even had passports.[26]

Packed luggage, labeled with the name of each cult member, was next to the beds.[27] However, notwithstanding all their careful preparations, while the spirits of the Heaven's Gate members may have gone to the "Next Level," as they called it, their suitcases remained behind.

The body of Applewhite, the only member of Heaven's Gate with a private bedroom, was the last to be found.[28] He was sixty-five years old.

The Autopsy

The autopsy report was unavailable for review. However, based on published lay articles, Applewhite suffered from "constrictive coronary arteriosclerosis," a narrowing of the coronary arteries due to accumulation of plaque.[29] No gross visual or physical evidence of cancer was identified in the liver or in any of Applewhite's other organs.[30]

Cause and Manner of Death

Foul play was not suspected in any of the deaths. Jerry Lipscomb of the San Diego Sheriff's Department said that no blood or signs of trauma were found at the scene; the only weapon was a nine-millimeter handgun packed in one of the suitcases.[31]

Toxicology testing revealed the presence of phenobarbital, a barbiturate sedative, in the blood of all thirty-nine deceased cult members, ranging between 28 micrograms and 164 micrograms per milliliter.[32] Since the average lethal blood level of phenobarbital is 100 micrograms per milliliter, some, but not all, of the Heaven's Gate members ingested a fatal dose of the drug.[33]

Besides phenobarbital, four cult members also had hydrocodone, an opioid medication present in Vicodin, a combination of acetaminophen and hydrocodone, at a blood concentration ranging between 50 nanograms and 1,300 nanograms per milliliter.[34] Since doses of 130 nanograms and 600 nanograms per milliliter are considered fatal, some, but not all, of the cult members ingested a fatal dose of hydrocodone.[35]

One person had butalbital, a short-acting barbiturate sedative, in his system; six others had acetaminophen, most likely also originating from Vicodin.[36]

In addition to the sedative drugs, thirty-three cult members had blood alcohol levels ranging from 0.04 to 0.15

percent.[37] This amount of alcohol was not sufficient to cause death by itself.

"We're not talking about a drug-crazed, party-time situation," Lipscomb said when it was discovered the cult members had taken large amounts of drugs.[38] "The drugs were taken for a very specific purpose and that was to take their own lives. It's our opinion that it was their intent—they planned to do this."[39]

Those cult members who ingested nonlethal amounts of drugs most likely suffocated to death from the plastic bags placed over their heads.[40]

In total, thirty cult members died from the combined effect of phenobarbital intoxication along with probable suffocation by a plastic bag.[41] Nine others died from a combination of phenobarbital, butalbital, hydrocodone, and alcohol.[42]

Death due to a combination of several central nervous-system-depressant drugs, some of which were in the overdose range, is a prime example of polypharmacy. Depression of the central nervous system leads to sedation, progressing to deep coma, followed by respiratory arrest and death. Placement of a plastic bag over the face ensured that respiration was further depressed.

After I reviewed the circumstances surrounding Applewhite's death, the autopsy findings and results of toxicology testing, published lay articles, and the scientific literature, I concluded that the immediate cause of death was respiratory arrest due to drug intoxication and suffocation with a plastic bag. Constrictive coronary arteriosclerosis was a contributing factor. The manner of death was suicide.

Life and Career

Applewhite, the son of a Presbyterian minister, was born in 1931 in Spur, Texas.[43] "He was usually president of everything," Applewhite's sister, Louise Winant, said.[44] "He was always a born leader and very charismatic."[45]

After graduating from Corpus Christi High School in 1948, Applewhite enrolled at Austin College, where he majored in philosophy.[46] He subsequently enrolled at Union Presbyterian Seminary to become a minister, but he dropped out after one year to study music instead.[47] "He was religious, but he was not fanatically religious at all," recalled John Alexander, Applewhite's roommate at Austin College.[48] "He was an extrovert. He was popular. He was very smart. He was not pushy."[49]

Four years later, after getting married, Applewhite was drafted into the US Army, where he served for two years in the Signal Corps.[50]

By 1959, Applewhite had earned a master's degree in music from the University of Colorado.[51] "He was quite a musician and had a beautiful voice," said Edith Warren, a piano accompanist for the children's choir that Applewhite led at the First Presbyterian Church in Gastonia, North Carolina.[52]

In 1962, Applewhite became an assistant professor and choral director at the University of Alabama; he was fired three years later when he was discovered to be having a homosexual relationship with a male student.[53] When his wife learned of the affair, she filed for divorce.[54]

The University of St. Thomas in Houston recruited Applewhite in 1965 to become chairman of its music department.[55] Five years thereafter, he was dismissed from his post when administrators learned he was having sexual relations with a male student.[56]

Ashamed of his sexual tendencies and significantly depressed, Applewhite checked into a psychiatric hospital in 1971; at the time, some psychologists believed it was possible to cure homosexuality.[57] As Applewhite had never spoken to his sister in the past about his sexual preference, he told her he was being admitted to the hospital for a "heart problem."[58] "One of the nurses there told him he had a purpose, that God kept him alive," Applewhite's sister said.[59] "She sort of talked him into the fact that this was the purpose—to lead these people—and he took it from there."[60] That nurse was Bonnie Nettles.[61]

Applewhite and Nettles, an astrologer with a strong interest in metaphysical theologies, immediately took to each other, eventually living together in a sexless, common-law marriage.[62] "The only relationship they shared, certainly having no physical attraction toward each other, was the compulsion to discover what had brought them together," Applewhite wrote in 1988, three years after Nettles died of cancer.[63]

Applewhite claimed he and Nettles came from the "Next Level Above Human," in outer space.[64] He began to preach a "theology" that the human body was merely a vehicle or a container for an asexual soul and that one day a UFO would return him to the next level in outer space.[65]

At its peak, about two hundred members were recruited to Heaven's Gate. "Do and Ti," as Applewhite and Nettles called themselves, required their followers to dress alike, cut their hair to a buzz cut, sever all ties with their families, dispose of all their physical and financial possessions, repress their sexual identities, and follow a unisex lifestyle.[66] Calling it "walking out the door of your life," Applewhite had himself surgically castrated in Mexico City, as did at least six of his followers.[67]

James Lewis of the Institute for the Study of American Religion said "Applewhite was so alienated from his homosexuality ... [that] he would put people of opposite sexes together and force them to learn to become neutral, nonsexual."[68]

In 1975, a group of twenty people from Waldport, Oregon, joined Applewhite and Nettles in eastern Colorado, ready to board a spaceship to take them to the next level.[69] The spaceship never arrived, and the group returned from whence they came.

Over the years, hundreds of followers joined Heaven's Gate; the vast majority eventually left, but some came back.[70] And yet, despite having left the cult, many former members still supported Applewhite's message.[71]

In 1997, thirty-eight followers of Heaven's Gate willingly ingested poisoned applesauce provided by Applewhite. "This is not like Waco or Jonestown," Dick Joslyn, a member of Heaven's Gate for fifteen years, said.[72] "Each one did this of their own volition."[73] Janja Lalich, a sociologist and cult expert, agreed. "Nobody held a gun to their heads."[74]

Conclusions

Is this guy crazy?" Applewhite asked rhetorically in one of his videos, staring directly into the camera, his eyes wide.[75] "Is this a cult?" After a slight pause, he answered, "Yes, it is—it's the cult of cults!"[76]

Alice Maeder, whose daughter, Gail, joined Heaven's Gate in 1993, watched the video with horror.[77] When a news broadcast on March 26, 1997 announced that thirty-nine followers of Heaven's Gate died in a mass suicide, Maeder was sure her daughter was not among them. "[She] has more sense than that," Gail's brother exclaimed.[78]

All hope for Gail's safe return home was dashed when Maeder saw her daughter's farewell video, which had been sent to the media sometime before the mass suicide began. "We are all choosing of our own free will to go to the next level," Gail said, grinning.[79]

"[This is] just the happiest day of my life," a male cult member said on his farewell tape.[80] "I've been looking forward to this for so long."[81] Some Heaven's Gate followers had waited for close to twenty years.

Lalich, the cult expert, explained that by the time members of Heaven's Gate had committed suicide, "They were in a place where they could not imagine existence outside the cult."[82]

People have speculated that the cult members may have been inspired to commit suicide because Applewhite had claimed he was dying of liver cancer and that his body was "disintegrating."[83] "Once he is gone … there is nothing left here on the face of the Earth for me … no reason to stay a moment longer," a female cult member could be heard saying on a tape sent to D'Angelo, the former Heaven's Gate member who alerted the police.[84] However, the autopsy clearly showed that no cancer of any kind was present in Applewhite's body.[85]

According to Louis Jolyon West, a professor of psychiatry at the University of California–Los Angeles School of Medicine, Applewhite's final statements in his videos show him to be delusional, sexually repressed, and suffering from a rare case of clinical paranoia.[86] "We have no hesitation to leave this place, to leave the bodies that we have," Applewhite said on one of his tapes.[87] After all, human bodies are just temporary vessels for the souls.[88]

Nick Cooke, a twenty-three-year "on again, off again" Heaven's Gate member whose fifty-four-year-old wife committed suicide along with Applewhite, explained, "I'm not suicidal … but I have no problem in laying down my shell, or my body as they did that day. I don't consider it suicide."[89]

What made Applewhite's message so appealing to his followers that they were willing to leave their families, all of their earthly possessions, and even give up their lives was his theology and charisma. Applewhite formulated his theology based on the Book of Revelation of the Bible by significantly transforming the original Christian basis to account for transcending from one form to another, "like caterpillars to butterflies," and for traveling into outer space.[90] As one of his male followers proclaimed, "We're going to be moving along to the 'next evolutionary level above humans,' taking on a brand new vehicle that we're going to be using in the next level."[91]

A recent Gallup poll found that one-third of people in the United States believe extraterrestrial spacecraft are visiting Earth from other planets or galaxies.[92] According to a recent survey by the Pew Research Center, 65 percent believe intelligent life exists on other planets.[93] With so many people believing in UFOs and that life exists outside our universe, it is no wonder that, combined with an out-of-this-world message delivered by a charismatic leader, thirty-nine followers of Heaven's Gate enthusiastically embraced their one chance to become extraterrestrial travelers to the "Evolutionary Level Above Human" and to commit suicide together.

"They were rational, lucid, reasonable people," said Alex Papas, a Phoenix, Arizona, film producer who had worked with some of the cult members.[94] Scully agreed. "The Heaven's Gate cultists weren't stupid people," he said.[95] "They were good people, and they had something missing in their lives that they were searching for."[96]

214

About a month after the Heaven's Gate mass suicide, Cooke, the former follower of Heaven's Gate whose wife had died along with Applewhite, sent his daughter a letter and a five-minute audio tape.[97] "I am eager to join my Older Members Ti and Do and my classmates," Cooke wrote.[98] Along with Charles Humphrey of Denver Colorado, another former member of Heaven's Gate, Cooke took a taxi on May 5 to the Holiday Inn Express in Encinitas, California, less than five miles from the mansion in which the mass suicide occurred, and checked into room 222.[99]

The following day, after having been alerted by Cooke's daughter, deputies of the San Diego County Sheriff's Department arrived at the Holiday Inn Express, where they found Cooke's body lying facedown on the floor between two beds; Humphrey, groggy but alive, lay faceup on the floor, between another bed and the window.[100] Both men were dressed in black pants and black tops and had on Nike shoes.[101] Each of them had a five-dollar bill and three quarters in his pockets.[102] Near the beds were purple shrouds and packed suitcases.[103] According to a spokesperson from the Sheriff's Department, the men appeared to have consumed vodka and barbiturates.[104]

Humphrey was transported by ambulance to Scripps Memorial Hospital in Encinitas, where he eventually recovered.[105] About ten months after his suicide attempt, Humphrey's body was discovered in a small tent near Ehrenberg, California.[106] Lt. Don Davis, a spokesperson for the La Paz County Sheriff's Department, said, "His head was sealed in a plastic bag with pipes running to a car's exhaust pipe and a tank marked 'carbon dioxide.'"[107] Wearing black sweatpants and a black T-shirt with a patch on the sleeve reading, "Heaven's Gate Away Team," Humphrey had a five-dollar bill and three quarters in his pocket.[108] Next to his body was a purple shroud.[109] This time, his suicide attempt had been successful.

In his final letter to his daughter, Cooke wrote, "Nothing of this world holds any real promise for me in continuing my growth and service—my teachers and classmates have returned, leaving myself [and] a few other class dropouts, of like mind, to put our houses in order and to follow them."[110] Apparently other members of Heaven's Gate are still out there, monitoring the skies, waiting for the passing of the next comet.

CHAPTER 17

Chris Farley

Died December 18, 1997

Actor-Comedian

ON DECEMBER 11, 1997, after spending a night at the Hazelden Betty Ford addiction treatment center in Minneapolis, Minnesota, Chris Farley, the comedian of *Saturday Night Live* (SNL) fame, returned to his sixtieth-floor condominium apartment in the John Hancock Center, located on a stretch of Chicago's posh Michigan Avenue called "the Magnificent Mile."[1] Over the next three days, he attended mass at St. Michael's Catholic Church, something he often did, baked holiday cookies, bought a Christmas tree, and went to a meeting of Alcoholics Anonymous.[2]

Between Sunday, December 14, and Thursday of that week, Farley went on a drinking and drug binge, consuming large quantities of drugs and alcohol, frequenting several Chicago bars, and mingling with a series of party girls.[3]

Farley's first stop was at the Karma Club, where he stayed until almost two o'clock on Monday morning.[4] That evening, he attended the thirty-eighth anniversary party for Chicago's Second City, an improvisational comedy troupe where he got his start.[5] Later he was spotted drinking at several local pubs.[6]

On Tuesday, December 16, Farley canceled his haircut appointment to spend the afternoon with a call girl smoking pot and drinking screwdrivers.[7] "I don't think he knew what he wanted," the call girl later said.[8] "You could just tell he was on a rampage … He just kept bouncing from room to room."[9]

At about 3:00 a.m. on Friday, December 18, inebriated and stoned, Farley collapsed in his apartment as the call girl with whom he had been using drugs was about to leave.[10] "Don't leave me," he told her.[11] On the way out, the woman momentarily stopped, took a picture of Farley lying on the hallway floor, and then left the premises.[12]

The following afternoon, Farley's body was discovered by his brother, John, lying in the entrance hallway of his apartment, about ten feet from the front door.[13] There was blood-tinged fluid coming from Farley's nose and a white, milky froth coming from his mouth.[14] At about 2:00 p.m., emergency medical services were called.[15] They pronounced Farley dead at the scene.[16] He was thirty-three years old.[17]

The Autopsy

By any measure, Farley was obese, his body weighing 296 pounds and measuring sixty-eight inches long.[18] An examination of the cardiovascular system showed an enlarged heart with severe narrowing of all three coronary arteries due to atherosclerosis.[19] These cardiovascular anomalies put Farley at an increased risk of sudden death from an arrhythmia and a heart attack.[20]

Besides the cardiovascular changes, there was a substantial amount of edema (fluid) and congestion in the lungs. In addition, fatty deposits were identified in the liver. A "fatty liver" can develop when the body produces too much fat or it cannot efficiently metabolize fat.[21] The excess fat is then stored in liver cells, where it accumulates.[22] This is often seen in people who are obese or are chornic abusers of alcohol.[23]

Knowing that Farley was a chronic abuser of illicit drugs, I was anxious to review the findings of the toxicology testing and to determine whether drugs had contributed to his death.

Cause and Manner of Death

Toxicology testing of Farley's blood identified high levels of morphine, a pharmacologically active metabolite of heroin and an opioid analgesic drug in its own right, as well as unmetabolized cocaine.[24] While no alcohol was detected in Farley's blood, therapeutic amounts of an antihistamine and low levels of fluoxetine, an antidepressant drug, were also found.[25] Since Farley had been drinking heavily in the days prior to his death, the lack of alcohol in his system suggested he had probably stopped drinking at least twenty-four hours before he died.

A test of Farley's urine identified a metabolite of marijuana.[26]

The presence of free, unmetabolized cocaine and a large amount of morphine, a pharmacologically active metabolite of heroin, in Farley's blood indicated Farley died from an overdose of a "speedball," a combination of heroin and cocaine.[27] The presence of fluid in the lungs and frothy liquid in the upper airways, well-recognized symptoms of heroin intoxication, confirmed Farley died from opioid intoxication.

Farley had probably taken the heroin and cocaine mixture not long before he died, because insufficient time had passed for the cocaine to be completely metabolized. Undoubtedly, the stimulating effects of the cocaine wore off much sooner than the central-nervous-system-depressant effects of heroin. The delayed effects of heroin depressed the respiratory center in the brain, slowing down the breathing apparatus and leading to death.

Interestingly, John Belushi, a comedian Farley had idolized who was also obese, also died from a speedball overdose— and at the same age as Farley.[28] "Chris loved Belushi," said Charna Halpern, a close friend of Farley and cofounder and director of ImprovOlympic, a Chicago improvisational theater.[29] "He thought Belushi was brilliant."[30]

Belushi wasn't the only celebrity to die after ingesting a speedball. River Phoenix died from a speedball overdose in

1993, and like Farley, he also had a metabolite of marijuana in his urine.[31] Philip Seymour Hoffman, an Oscar-winning actor, had heroin and cocaine in his blood when he died, as well as a benzodiazepine tranquilizer and amphetamine.[32] And just like Farley, the actress Carrie Fisher also had heroin and cocaine metabolites in her system, as well as an antihistamine, diphenhydramine, and the antidepressant drug fluoxetine.[33]

After I reviewed the circumstances surrounding Farley's death, the death certificate, the autopsy findings and results of toxicology testing, published lay articles, and the scientific literature, I concluded that the immediate cause of death was respiratory depression and cardiotoxicity caused by opioid and cocaine intoxication due to a speedball. Coronary atherosclerosis was a contributing factor.[34] The manner of death was accident.[35]

Life and Career

Farley was born in 1964 in Madison, Wisconsin.[36] He attended Edgewood High School of the Sacred Heart and other Catholic schools, where he played football.[37] His first job after graduating from Marquette University in Milwaukee, Wisconsin, in 1986 was at Scotch Oil, a company his father owned.[38]

Having earned a degree in theater and communications, Farley started his professional career by performing at the Ark Improvisational Theater and then at the ImprovOlympic Theater in Chicago before joining the cast of Second City, where he was discovered in 1990 by Lorne Michaels, producer of SNL.[39]

Farley performed in one hundred episodes on SNL in over five years.[40] Playing upon his large size, Farley's self-deprecating style of humor and physical brand of comedy was quickly embraced by the show's viewing audience.[41] Besides his time on SNL, Farley also acted in several films, including *Wayne's World* (1992), *Coneheads* (1993), *Billy Madison* (1995), and *Tommy Boy* (1995).[42] *Black Sheep* (1996) and *Beverly Hills Ninja* (1997), two films with former SNL members David Spade and Chris Rock, soon followed.[43]

According to one reporter, Farley was "a manic cannonball who could appear surprisingly athletic one moment and perilously ungainly the next," able to do perfect cartwheels, but dangerously overweight.[44] "He shouted big, sweated big, laughed big, and fell down big."[45]

Halpern, the director of ImprovOlympic, remembered how Farley called her crying because "They [SNL] were going to make him dance with Patrick Swayze and 'they were making fun of the fat boy.'"[46] The skit became one of the most memorable acts at SNL; another was of Farley as a motivational speaker.[47]

Farley very much wanted to expand his acting range and was afraid he was being typecast. "Sometimes I feel trapped by always having to be the most outrageous guy in the room," he said in a 1996 interview.[48] Halpern thought Farley had the capacity to show more depth in his acting. "He was really trapped in that role of fall-down slapstick comedy," she said.[49] "I felt like people were making him a caricature."[50]

In 1996, Farley left SNL at a time when his substance abuse was already out of control.[51] Production of his next film had to be halted several times so he could go to rehab.[52] By the end of the following year, Farley was dead.

Conclusions

"That's the next Belushi," said Del Close, an improvisational instructor, when he first saw Farley.[53] "The minute [Farley] stepped onstage" at Second City, said Amy Poehler, an alum of the comedy troupe, "the audience fell madly in love with him. I've never seen anyone commit to anything harder than he would."[54]

Farley "was kind of shy," said Molly Shannon, one of Farley's SNL classmates.[55] "Sometimes I'd peek into his dressing room, and he'd always kneel down and pray before he performed."[56] Farley was also extremely kind and generous.[57] He often helped people in need, stopping to give money to homeless people he passed on the street.[58]

Regrettably, Farley also had a dark side—a terrible eating and drinking problem, a history of drug abuse, and regularly hiring prostitutes and call girls.[59] "He loved to drink," Halpern said.[60] "I don't think he felt in control."[61]

Farley's friends saw his drinking and drug use as a battle he had yet to conquer.[62] People close to Farley said he was a very sweet guy—before midnight, that is.[63] "I have a tendency toward the pleasures of the flesh," Farley explained.[64] "I still have to work on my weight and some of my other demons."[65] It was a battle he never won.

No one was surprised when word of Farley's death reached his friends, with one columnist calling it "the least surprising premature death of a celebrity in show business history."[66] Nick Burrows, director of guidance at Edgewood High School of the Sacred Heart, said, "The evils got him. I know he tried to get it under control, but it got the best of him in the end."[67]

Six months before he died, Farley was approached by one of his mates. "Hey, you gotta take it easy," his friend said.[68] Farley replied, "I want to live fast and die young."[69] He got his wish.

CHAPTER 18
Eric Harris and Dylan Klebold
Died April 20, 1999
The Columbine High School Massacre Shooters

COLUMBINE, "ONE OF the best places to live in Colorado," is bordered to the east by Littleton and Columbine Valley and to the west by Ken Caryl. An idyllic town with a population approximating twenty-five thousand, Columbine is filled with parks and is within an easy drive to a beautifully designed eighteen-hole championship golf course.[1]

Columbine High School, which opened in 1973, is located in Littleton and has a student population of about seventeen hundred. It is ranked sixty-ninth in Colorado by *US News & World Report*.[2]

On Tuesday, April 20, 1999, with only seventeen days remaining in the school year, seniors at Columbine were anxiously awaiting their graduation. Unlike their classmates, Eric Harris and Dylan Klebold skipped the morning's bowling class, even though they were both on the bowling team and had arrived at the school on time.[3] Surprisingly, Harris also missed his third-period Chinese philosophy exam, which counted for nearly one third of his grade.[4] And when the fourth-period creative writing class began, neither Harris nor Klebold was in attendance for that class either.[5] Instead the two boys left the school grounds and drove to a field east of Wadsworth Boulevard, where they set two pipe bombs and an aerosol canister to detonate shortly after a quarter past eleven.[6]

At eleven o'clock, Harris and Klebold returned to the school in separate cars, Harris in a gray 1986 Honda Civic and Klebold in his black 1982 BMW.[7] They then headed to the school's cafeteria, each wearing wraparound sunglasses and black leather trench coats, and carrying two duffel bags containing propane bombs.[8] After placing the bags beside two tables and setting the bombs to go off at 11:17 a.m., the time the cafeteria was usually the most crowded, they returned to their vehicles and waited for the explosions to occur.[9]

At 11:19 a.m., the two bombs set as a decoy in a field three miles away from the high school blew up as scheduled.[10] The explosions and subsequent grass fire were enough to divert the attention of the sheriff's office and the Littleton Fire Department away from the high school.[11] However, by 11:20

a.m., the anticipated explosion in the school's cafeteria still had not occurred. Tired of waiting, Harris and Klebold set explosives in their automobiles and, carrying a duffel bag and a backpack containing sawed-off shotguns, a nine-millimeter semiautomatic carbine rifle, and a nine-millimeter TEC-DC9 semiautomatic pistol, they walked to the top of the stairs of the school's west entrance and waited for the bombs to go off.[12] Their plan was to shoot students as they walked up the stairs toward the parking area, trying to escape the explosion in the cafeteria.[13] Fortunately, the bombs failed to detonate.[14]

A witness heard one of the two gunmen shout "Go! Go!"[15] At this time, having pulled out their shotguns, Harris and Klebold immediately began to fire, killing one student on the grassy knoll and seriously injuring another.[16]

"I saw two kids, one in a big black trench coat with a handgun and one on top of the ledge with a huge gun," said Mindy Pollock, a tenth grader.[17] "They were shooting. I saw kids just drop to the ground … I said, 'it's not fake.'"[18]

At some point, Klebold began walking down the steps toward the cafeteria.[19]

Inside the school building, students and faculty, hearing the gunshots, immediately began to run for safety or to hide under tables, in utility closets, and in the bathrooms.[20] Nonetheless, over the next fifty minutes, Harris and Klebold killed thirteen people, including William "Dave" Sanders, a teacher and coach of the girls' basketball and softball teams, and wounded more than twenty others.[21] "Tell my family I love them," Sanders said before he died.[22]

Of the thirteen people who were killed, Harris shot eight and Klebold five.[23] Some were shot outside the school as they tried to flee while others were killed in various areas of the school building, including ten in the library.[24]

"They were laughing about it," said Joshua Lapp, a sophomore, referring to the two shooters.[25] "They'd shoot somebody, they'd laugh, they'd giggle."[26]

Several survivors were left with severe, debilitating lifelong injuries.[27] Witnesses said they heard the killers say, "This is what we always wanted to do. This is awesome!"[28]

Shortly after four o'clock, when the shooting finally stopped and police had secured the school building, Harris and Klebold were found dead in the library from self-inflicted gunshot wounds to the head.[29] It is believed they committed suicide at 12:08 p.m.[30] Harris was eighteen years old, and Klebold, seventeen.

The Autopsy

The two autopsies were performed on April 22 by Dr. Ben Galloway, a forensic pathologist, in the Jefferson County Coroner's Office in Golden, Colorado.[31] Identification of the bodies was made through fingerprint analysis.[32] Besides Galloway and his assistant, Rob Kulbacki, others in attendance included members of the Jefferson County Sheriff's Department.[33]

Harris's body was sixty-eight and a half inches long and weighed approximately 135 to 140 pounds.[34] The hair on top of the head was brown.[35] Interestingly, the right eye was gray but the left was hazel.[36] There were brown whiskers on both sides of the face.[37]

The upper body was clothed in a bloodstained white T-shirt with the inscription "Natural Selection" across the front.[38] A black glove, on which the fingers were cut away, was on the right hand.[39] Other clothing included green plaid jockey shorts, white socks, and black combat boots.[40]

On external examination, the chest had a mild "pectus excavatum," a condition in which a person's breastbone is sunken into the chest.[41] In the sunken area was a curvilinear, horizontally oriented scar.[42]

There was no evidence of external trauma to the neck, chest, abdomen, or back, although a small pigmented nevus, a birthmark, was present on the right lower quadrant of the back.[43] Abrasions (scrapes), lacerations (tears), and cuts were found on the upper arms and right foot, but there was no evidence of recent needle puncture marks or scars.[44]

On internal examination, the cardiovascular system was unremarkable.[45] The heart was without fibrosis or scarring, the heart size was normal and nearly identical in size to Klebold's, and the heart valves were intact.[46] The aorta was without evidence of atherosclerosis.[47]

As for the respiratory system, the lumen of the lower respiratory tract contained a small amount of blood on the right side.[48] The pulmonary arteries, however, were without clots.[49]

A biopsy of the lymph nodes of the lower respiratory tract revealed the presence of "benign reactive lymphoid hyperplasia," a reversible enlargement of lymphoid tissue secondary to an unknown stimulus.[50]

The thyroid, thymus, pancreas, adrenals, spleen, liver, gallbladder, kidneys, and urinary bladder all appeared normal.[51] In addition, the esophagus, stomach, small and large bowel, and appendix were all within normal limits.[52] The stomach contained a brown liquid composed of gastric content.

Of special importance for the identification of cause of death were the findings related to the head. Evidence in the mouth, lower forehead, scalp, bridge of the nose, and orbits of both eyes was consistent with blowout injuries from a high-energy shotgun wound to the roof of the mouth.[53] Blood was present in both ear canals.[54]

The normal contour of the head was distorted by extensive lacerations of the scalp and massive fracturing of the facial bones and cranium, the part of the skull enclosing the brain.[55]

The gunshot entrance wound involved the roof of the mouth and the hard and soft palate.[56] It extended upward, backward, and slightly to the right, involving the nasal pharynx, the part of the nasal cavity above the soft palate, the nasal passages, and the base and back of the skull.[57] The presence of dense powder stain on the surface of the hard palate and black staining on the tongue confirmed the gunshot wound was an entrance wound.[58]

Consistent with a gunshot exit wound was the absence of a large area on the right side of the head, that portion having been blown away by a projectile.[59]

All that remained of the brain was a small portion of the medulla oblongata, one of three regions of the brain stem that plays a critical role in transmitting signals between the spinal cord and the higher parts of the brain, and in controlling autonomic activities, such as heartbeat and respiration.[60] There was no evidence of disease in the brain.[61]

At seventy-four and a half inches long and weighing 143 pounds, Klebold's body was longer than Harris's.[62] The hair on top of the head was brown, and the eyes were bluish-gray.[63] On the upper lip was a blond mustache.[64] The chin had a beard fashioned in a goatee.[65]

The upper body was clothed in a black T-shirt with the inscription "Wrath" across the front.[66] A black glove was on the left hand, consistent with Klebold being left-handed, with the fingers cut away, unlike Harris's glove, which was on his right hand.[67] Other clothing included blue-green plaid boxer shorts, black pants with a black belt, white socks, and black boots on which a red star medallion of a hammer and sickle, similar to the Soviet symbol, was present on the left boot.[68]

On external examination, the neck showed no evidence of injury.[69] In addition, there was no evidence of external trauma to the chest, the abdomen—which had a three-inch horizontal scar in the upper quadrant—or the back.[70]

Small abrasions and contusions (bruises) were found on the left hand involving the thumb and the middle finger, as well as on the index finger of the right hand, the right lower leg, and the left knee.[71] No evidence of recent needle puncture marks or scars was identified on the arms.[72]

Both nasal passages and the oral cavity contained a bloody fluid, as did the lumen of the lower respiratory tract.[73] As for the lungs, there was evidence of aspirated blood, vascular congestion, and early pulmonary edema (fluid).[74]

The cardiovascular system was unremarkable, with a normal heart size, intact heart valves, and no evidence of fibrosis or thickening.[75] The aorta was without plaque.[76]

The thyroid, thymus, pancreas, adrenals, spleen, liver, gallbladder, kidneys, and urinary bladder all appeared normal.[77] As for the gastrointestinal system, the esophagus was normal, as was the stomach, with no evidence of a peptic ulcer or tumor, although fragments of potato skin were identified in the stomach.[78] The small and large bowels and appendix were all unremarkable.[79]

A circular, large-caliber type of gunshot entrance wound from a close range of fire, consistent with nine-millimeter ammunition, was present on the left side of the head, a quarter inch above the left ear, in the region of the temple.[80] Powder stains on the left side of the head confirmed the gunshot wound was an entrance wound.[81] On the right side of the head was a circular type of gunshot exit wound measuring a half inch in diameter.[82]

The projectile traveled left to right through the head, slightly front to back, and slightly downward, in keeping with Klebold being left handed.[83] The wound tracts traveled across the underside of the brain and involved both cerebral hemispheres of the brain in the temporal and frontal regions, the parts of the brain that control muscle functions as well as speech, thought, emotions, reading, writing, and learning.[84]

Numerous fractures of bones within the scalp and substantial injury to the brain, including the presence of more than an ounce of blood overlying the right cerebral hemisphere, were apparent.[85] There was no evidence of an underlying disease in the brain.[86]

Cause and Manner of Death

No alcohol or drugs of abuse were detected in Harris's blood.[87] Also, an immunological drug screen failed to find any pharmaceuticals in his urine.[88]

Using highly specific gas chromatography and mass spectrometry methodology, a therapeutic amount of fluvoxamine, an antidepressant and antianxiety drug, was identified in Harris's blood, confirming Harris was being treated with the drug for anger management since January 1998.[89]

More than five years after the shootings at Columbine High School, the US Food and Drug Administration (FDA) issued a "black box" warning, the most severe warning the FDA can place on a drug short of an outright ban, indicating that the use of certain antidepressant drugs to treat major depressive disorders in adolescents may increase the risk of suicidal ideation.[90] Whether fluvoxamine contributed to Harris's radical behavior on April 20, 1999 is unknown. According to Harris, his goal was to be remembered for having killed more people than Timothy McVeigh, who was responsible for the 1995 Oklahoma City bombing.[91]

After I reviewed the circumstances surrounding Harris's death, the autopsy findings and results of toxicology testing, published lay articles, and the scientific literature, I concluded that the immediate cause of death was a self-inflicted gunshot wound to the mouth and head. The manner of death was suicide.

Neither alcohol nor drugs were detected in Klebold's blood by gas chromatography and mass spectrometry methodology or in urine by an immunological drug screen.[92]

Unlike Harris, Klebold was not being treated with fluvoxamine. Nonetheless, he had been fantasizing about suicide at least since 1997, two years prior to the Columbine massacre.[93] "Thinking of suicide gives me hope that I'll … finally not be at war with myself, the world, and the universe," Klebold wrote in his journal.[94]

After I reviewed the circumstances surrounding Klebold's death, the autopsy findings and results of toxicology testing, published lay articles, and the scientific literature, I concluded that the immediate cause of death was a self-inflicted gunshot wound at close range to the left side of the head.[95] The manner of death was suicide.

Life Experiences

Harris, the son of an Air Force transport pilot and a homemaker, was born in Wichita, Kansas, in April 1981.[96]

When his father retired from the military in 1993, Harris and his family moved to rented accommodations in Littleton, Colorado, before purchasing their own home in 1996.[97]

Harris met Klebold in seventh grade, while they were both attending Ken Caryl Middle School. They soon became close friends.[98] Klebold, who was born in Lakewood, Colorado, was five months younger than Harris.[99] His father was a geophysicist; his mother worked with the handicapped.[100]

As a young boy, Harris was shy, loved baseball, was in Cub Scouts, and was considered highly intelligent, having been in a program for gifted and talented students at his elementary school.[101]

In August 1995, Harris and Klebold enrolled in the ninth grade at Columbine High School.[102] The school had just completed a $15 million renovation, and the two boys were in the first class to see the new makeover.[103] While at Columbine, Harris earned good grades and was on the soccer team.[104] Klebold, although bright, didn't apply himself to his schoolwork, and his grades were mediocre.[105]

Of the various languages offered at Columbine, Harris and Klebold chose to study German, immersing themselves in everything German, even listening to music by German bands.[106] Klebold was also active in the production of school plays as a sound, light, and video operator. As a computer assistant, he helped maintain the school's computer server.[107]

Klebold was friends with Brooks Brown ever since their time together in first grade and in Cub Scouts. Harris, on the other hand, first met Brown as they rode the school bus together to middle school.[108] Soon the three became very good friends.[109] But in late 1997, Harris had a falling out with Brown and, having a mean streak, broke the windshield on Brown's car and terrorized the Brown family by putting firecrackers on the windowsill of their home.[110] Brown's parents filed a complaint with the Douglas County Sheriff's Office, claiming Harris threatened their son on one of his several internet websites, but nothing further came of the complaint.[111]

Another run-in with the law occurred in January 1998. At that time, Harris and Klebold broke into a van and stole electronic equipment, for which they were charged with theft, criminal mischief, and criminal trespassing.[112] Since it was their first offense, they were assigned to a juvenile diversion program that included anger management.[113] Released a month early for good behavior, they received glowing evaluations from their supervisors.[114] Their "good behavior" was all an act.[115]

In late December, Robyn Anderson, who later became Klebold's prom date, purchased two shotguns and a rifle at a gun show on behalf of Klebold and Harris, since they were both underage.[116] A month later, the two boys bought a nine-millimeter TEC-DC9 semiautomatic pistol from Mark Manes.[117] This was the same ammunition the two gunmen later used on students and teachers at Columbine High School.

Three days prior to the Columbine High School shootings, Klebold, dressed in a traditional black tuxedo and bow tie, attended the senior prom with Anderson.[118] "[He] was talking about the future at the University of Arizona and his plans to major in computer science," said Victor Good, a family friend.[119] Harris couldn't get a date for the prom, so he spent the evening at home watching movies.[120] Later, he attended the after-prom party, where he met Klebold.[121]

In the late afternoon of April 19, 1999, the day before the school massacre, Harris and Klebold skipped the last two classes of the day—Creative Writing and Psychology.[122] That night, Klebold outlined in his notebook the schedule for the following day.[123] "About twenty-six and a half hours from now, the judgment will begin," he wrote.[124] "When first bombs go off, attack, have fun!"[125] As for Harris, he had Manes buy him one hundred rounds of ammunition at a local Kmart.[126]

Conclusions

At first everything seemed unreal. The mind just couldn't accept what was happening. Brian Anderson, a student at Columbine, thought the gun Harris was holding was a prop from a film class.[127] Even Patricia Nielson, an art teacher, thought Harris was playing some sort of a prank.[128] "Knock it off," she told him.[129]

Kyle Ross, Harris's former classmate in Plattsburgh, New York, where Harris had lived before he moved to Colorado, was very surprised when he heard Harris was one of the Columbine High School gunmen.[130] "My mouth just dropped," Ross said.[131] "He didn't seem anything like what is portrayed on TV."[132]

That Klebold was one of the shooters was also hard to believe. "You'd better cross [Klebold's] name off," Chris Hooker, an eighteen-year-old senior at Columbine told a reporter at the start of the massacre.[133] "He's not that kind of person. He would never do this."[134] She, too, was wrong.

"It's the horror of all horrors," said Good, the Klebold family friend mentioned above.[135] Speaking of Klebold's parents, Good said, "They knew a different kid than the monster in the school."[136]

It is tempting to think Harris and Klebold had a Jekyll-and-Hyde personality, sometimes friendly and at other times violent, but that may not be accurate, at least not for Harris. Harris readily displayed his rage, for which he had attended anger management classes and was being treated with fluvoxamine.[137] Klebold was quiet and "a nice guy, if you got to know him," according to Jacob Cary, a sixteen-year-old student at Columbine.[138] Tim Kastle, who had been spared being shot by Kelbold, agreed. "He was shy, more than anything else."[139]

There was another side to Klebold that other classmates saw, however. He swore in front of teachers and often lost his temper.[140] Just weeks before the massacre, Klebold had written a paper for one of his classes that was so violent it foreshadowed the events of April 20.[141] A dean of students at the high school who had Harris and Klebold in his office on several occasions said, "[I had seen] the potential for an 'evil side' … that there was a violent, angry streak in these kids."[142]

There is almost universal agreement that of the two shooters, Harris was the instigator and Klebold the follower.[143] "No way he'd do that on his own," Cary said, speaking of Klebold.[144] "He's not a leader in any way."[145]

Terra Oglesbee, who took the creative writing class with both gunmen, described Klebold this way. "He seemed like he had low self-esteem ... He always followed [Harris] around."[146] Although taller than Harris, Klebold lacked self-confidence and always let Harris take the lead.[147]

"I'd say [Harris] had it in him," said Brian Anderson, who was injured in the massacre; Klebold "was kind of influenced and followed."[148]

Dave Cullen, an investigative journalist, summed it up best when he said, Harris was "the callously brutal mastermind" while Klebold was a "quivering depressive who journaled obsessively about love."[149]

Any misconceptions about Harris and Klebold were quickly dispelled when police viewed the threatening, violent, and graphic content on the internet websites Harris had developed.[150] Several journals and videos prepared by the two gunmen at least a year prior to the massacre were also discovered. In these, Klebold and Harris rant about specific people and their plans to kill hundreds of their fellow students and teachers on what they referred to as "Judgment Day."[151]

Three months after the massacre, the FBI sponsored a workshop of highly regarded mental health experts to try to analyze the two shooters and to discern their motivation for committing such an atrocity.[152] The group of psychiatrists and psychologists concluded that Harris and Klebold most likely were not motivated by revenge against any particular person or group. Instead they were looking for "devastating infamy," according to FBI special agent and clinical psychologist Dwayne Fuselier.[153]

Harris and Klebold had significantly different mental conditions, the mental experts concluded. Harris was cold, calculating, and homicidal, a real psychopath, while Klebold was manic depressive and suicidal, blaming himself for his problems.[154] "Harris wanted to hurt people" while "Klebold was hurting inside," Fuselier said.[155]

Robert Hare, author of *Without Conscience*, described psychopaths as lacking empathy, guilt or remorse.[156] "[They] are rational and aware of what they are doing and why. Their behavior is the result of choice, freely exercised."[157]

Frank Ochberg, a Michigan State University psychiatrist, noted that Harris was a brilliant killer without a conscience whereas Klebold would never have carried out the Columbine High School shootings without Harris.[158]

In my view, Harris's and Klebold's motives for committing the massacre were best expressed by the two killers themselves in their final farewell video, shot in the early morning of April 20, 1999.[159] "Hey Mom," Klebold began. "It's about a half an hour till Judgment Day ... Just know I'm going to a better place. I didn't like life too much, and I know I'll be happy wherever the *** I go."[160] Not to be outdone, Harris faced the camera and added his own final thoughts. "I know my mom and dad will be just like ... just *** shocked beyond belief.

I'm sorry, all right. I can't help it."[161] As if for good measure, Klebold, standing behind the camera, then interrupted Harris and said, "It's what we had to do."[162]

The massacre at Columbine High School may not have been the first mass shooting in a public school in the United States, but it was not the last one either. On December 14, 2012, after killing his mother, twenty-year-old Adam Lanza went to Sandy Hook Elementary School in Newtown, Connecticut, wearing black fatigues and a military vest and carrying a semiautomatic assault rifle and two pistols.[163] He then shot and killed twenty students, six- and seven-year-olds, and six adults before committing suicide with a gunshot to the head.[164]

Since the shootings at Columbine, at least eleven more mass school shootings occurred—six in colleges and five in grade schools, each with four or more victims.[165] A more recent shooting in which a gunman killed nineteen elementary schoolchildren and two teachers and injured seventeen others occurred on May 24, 2022 at Robb Elementary School in Uvalde, Texas. At least ten other school shootings at various elementary schools did not qualify as "mass shootings."[166] According to John Cohen, a former Department of Homeland Security official, "The people who conduct school shootings … go online, they look at past attacks, and in a perverse way, they connect with not only past incidents, but also past attackers. The story of the Columbine shooters is a story that resonates with a group of kids that are experiencing similar situations."[167]

CHAPTER 19

Timothy McVeigh

Died June 11, 2001

The Oklahoma City Bomber

TIMOTHY MCVEIGH WAS a twenty-seven-year-old former US Army soldier.[1] At about eight thirty on the morning of April 19, 1995, wearing a T-shirt with a drawing of Abraham Lincoln and the words "Sic Semper Tyrannis" (thus ever to tyrants) printed on the front, McVeigh drove his rented Ryder truck south toward Oklahoma City.[2] Ten minutes later, after he stopped at a tire store to ask for directions, a video camera captured McVeigh's truck as it headed downtown.[3]

Shortly before nine o'clock, McVeigh parked his rented truck in the handicapped zone beside the Alfred P. Murrah Federal Building.[4] In the truck was a five-thousand-pound bomb made of ammonium nitrate, a common ingredient in fertilizer, and dynamite.[5] McVeigh lit the fuse, locked the vehicle, and then walked away toward a nearby YMCA building where his getaway car was parked.[6] At two minutes past nine, the bomb in the Ryder truck exploded, toppling the north side of the nine-story federal building and killing 168 people, including nineteen children in the building's day care center, and injuring over five hundred more.[7]

Approximately seventy-five minutes after the explosion, Oklahoma Highway Patrol officer Charles Hanger pulled over a Mercury Marquis automobile on Interstate 35, about twenty miles from the Kansas border.[8] The car, which was driven by McVeigh, had no license plates.[9] McVeigh, who did not have his driver's license or the vehicle's registration, was carrying a concealed weapon without a permit.[10] He was immediately arrested, booked, and placed in the county jail in Perry, Oklahoma.[11]

Within hours of the bombing, federal agents found the vehicle identification number (VIN) of the Ryder truck with the bomb and located where it was rented—Elliot's Body Shop in Junction City, Oklahoma.[12] The man who rented the truck, described as "a white male with a brush cut and a strong nose," was quickly identified as McVeigh.[13]

A computer search in Washington, DC, located McVeigh in a Noble County jail, arrested on an unrelated misdemeanor charge.[14] "Yes, I did the bombing," McVeigh told his two court-appointed attorneys before his arraignment for the Oklahoma City bombing.[15]

McVeigh's trial was held in a Denver, Colorado, courtroom in late May 1977. On June second, after twenty-three hours of deliberation, the jury found McVeigh guilty on all counts.[16] Eleven days later, US district judge Richard Matsch imposed the sentence—death by lethal injection.[17] After appealing his verdict several times, McVeigh decided to drop all further appeals in January 2001.[18] At first his execution was scheduled for May 16; however, it was postponed to June 11 to allow McVeigh's defense team time to review forty-five hundred pages of newly discovered documents previously withheld by the FBI.[19]

The execution was held at the US Penitentiary in Terre Haute, Indiana.[20] Approximately two dozen people viewed the execution in person, while more than 250 others watched it on closed-circuit television in Oklahoma City.[21] Per McVeigh's wishes, none of his family members was present.[22]

Dressed in a white T-shirt, khaki pants, and sneakers, his head almost completely shaved, McVeigh was led at seven o'clock in the morning to a green-tiled execution chamber, where he was strapped onto a padded gurney.[23] In lieu of a final statement, McVeigh left a handwritten copy of the poem *Invictus*, in which the concluding lines are "I am the master of my fate / I am the captain of my soul."[24] He was pronounced dead at 7:14 a.m. by Warden Harley Lappin.[25]

The Autopsy

An autopsy is usually conducted on inmates executed at federal prisons. However, prior to his execution, McVeigh's attorneys and Susan Amos, the coroner of Vigo County, Indiana, reached an informal agreement to dispense with an autopsy or other invasive procedures following McVeigh's execution.[26] In exchange, McVeigh, who opposed "the planned mutilation of my corpse," agreed to sign a statement saying he had not been abused while in custody.[27]

Judge Matsch, who had presided over McVeigh's trial, did not object to the informal agreement, saying, "My jurisdiction ends when Timothy McVeigh ends."[28]

Cause and Manner of Death

McVeigh's was the first execution in a federal prison in nearly forty years.[29] According to eyewitness accounts, he was tight-lipped as he entered the execution chamber.[30] After he was strapped onto a gurney, a white sheet covering him up to midchest, McVeigh stared at the ceiling, where a camera transmitted a video of his execution to viewers in Oklahoma City.[31]

A series of three ten-second injections, spaced one minute apart, flowed through intravenous tubing directly into a vein in McVeigh's right leg.[32] The first injection was sodium thiopental, a barbiturate drug with general anesthetic properties.[33] The drug had a rapid onset but a short duration, thereby putting McVeigh into a deep sleep for only five minutes.[34] A minute later, pancuronium bromide, a muscle relaxant, was injected to block nerve impulses from reaching muscles responsible for movement.[35] The third and final drug was potassium chloride to stop McVeigh's heart.[36]

"We were standing at a glass window about eighteen inches from his [McVeigh's] feet," said Shepard Smith from Fox News Channel.[37] "When we were told that the first drug was administered [at 7:10 a.m.], his lips relaxed … his eyes seemed to roll back only slightly, his body seemed to relax, his feet shifted just a bit."[38] Linda Cavanaugh, a reporter from KFOR-TV agreed. "His lips began turning a little bit paler, his skin became pale," she said.[39]

"After they administered the next drug [at 7:11 a.m.], it appeared that [McVeigh] was breathing through his mouth for the first time," Cavanaugh reported.[40] "He took two or three [heavy] breaths … and then from that point on, for the next several minutes, when the final drug was administered [at 7:13 a.m.] until he was pronounced dead [at 7:14 a.m.], there was no additional movement from Timothy McVeigh."[41]

"His skin began to turn a very strange shade of yellow toward the end," said Susan Carlson of WLS radio, "and he remained extremely rigid."[42]

"Timothy James McVeigh died with his eyes open," declared Byron Pitts of CBS News.[43]

"It was a very orchestrated, clinical procedure," Cavanaugh noted.[44] "I think it went very much as they planned it."[45]

After I reviewed the circumstances surrounding McVeigh's death, the death certificate, published lay articles, and the scientific literature, I concluded that the immediate cause of death was respiratory depression and cardiotoxicity due to a court-mandated series of three lethal injections. The manner of death was judicial execution.

Life and Career

McVeigh was born in 1968 in Lockport, New York, outside of Buffalo, but he grew up in nearby Pendleton.[46] When he was a young adolescent, his parents separated, eventually divorcing in 1986, after which McVeigh went to live with his father, while his two sisters lived in Florida with their mother.[47]

McVeigh developed an interest in guns after his grandfather began taking him to target practice.[48] This is similar to Charles Whitman, the University of Texas shooter, whose father, a gun enthusiast, taught him how to handle firearms at an early age.

As a teenager, McVeigh was tall and lanky, and he was often bullied.[49] In 1986, he graduated from high school, earning a partial scholarship to any state university in New York.[50] However, after briefly attending Bryant & Stratton College, he dropped out of school and took a job at a Burger King, and then as an armored car driver for security companies.[51]

In 1988, McVeigh enlisted in the US Army. After completing basic training at Fort Benning, Georgia, he was promoted to sergeant.[52] Almost three years later, he was deployed under Operation Desert Storm to the Persian Gulf War, where he served with distinction. Driving a Bradley Fighting Vehicle, McVeigh earned several awards, including a Combat Infantry Badge and a Bronze Star for bravery.[53] He was discharged from the military in 1991.[54]

Already filled with anger against the US federal government and its policies on gun control, McVeigh was further radicalized in the 1990s by two specific events.[55] The first occurred in August 1992. It was then that, during an attempt to arrest the white separatist Randy Weaver, an FBI sniper killed Weaver's wife and his fourteen-month-old son during a standoff at their cabin in Ruby Ridge, Idaho.[56] The second occurred the following year when a fifty-one-day standoff in Waco, Texas, between ATF agents and the Branch Davidians, a religious cult headed by David Koresh, ended in a firestorm as the Branch Davidian compound was engulfed in flames, killing seventy-four men, women, and children.[57] As McVeigh watched the inferno in Waco on television, he decided to avenge what he considered was the government's assault on individual liberty.[58] "What is this?" he asked Terry Nichols, his army buddy.[59] "What has America become?"[60]

On the second anniversary of the burning of the Branch Davidians' compound, McVeigh conducted "an act of terror, violence, intended to serve selfish political purposes," according to prosecutor Joseph Hartzler.[61] "They [the nineteen children who died] were in a building owned by a government that Timothy McVeigh so hated that ... he chose to take their innocent lives to serve his twisted purpose," Hartzler said.[62] McVeigh, however, believed the children were simply in the wrong place at the wrong time, calling them "collateral damage."[63]

Conclusions

The life and death of Timothy McVeigh raise two issues of national importance, namely domestic terrorism and execution by lethal injection.

Domestic terrorism, as defined by federal law, is "activities that involve acts dangerous to human life that are a violation of the criminal law of the United States ... intended to intimidate or coerce ... or ... affect the conduct of a government by mass destruction, assassination, or kidnapping, and occur primarily within the territorial jurisdiction of the United States."[64] According to the White House National Security Council, domestic terrorism and domestic violent extremists pose a serious and evolving threat to the United States.[65]

The Center for Strategic and International Studies (CSIS) categorized domestic terrorism into five groups: "religious terrorism," which supports a faith-based belief system, such as Islam; "ethnonationalist terrorism," which supports ethnic or nationalist goals; "far-right extremist terrorism," whose goals may include racial or ethnic supremacy, opposition to government authority, anger against women, belief in certain conspiracy theories, or outrage against certain policies, such as abortion; "far-left extremist terrorism," which opposes capitalism, imperialism, and colonialism, and advocates black nationalism, pursues environment or animal rights issues, espouses procommunist beliefs, or supports anarchism; and "other."[66]

Of the sixty-one incidents of domestic terrorist attacks or plots identified by CSIS occurring in the first eight months of 2020, 67 percent were committed by white supremacists and far-right extremists, 20 percent by far-left extremists, and 7 percent by jihadists or "other."[67] And yet, according to CSIS, the total number of deaths (five) resulting from domestic terrorism during that time period was small compared to the 168 deaths in the 1995 Oklahoma City bombing, the nearly 3,000 deaths on 9/11, and the 49 deaths in the 2016 gay nightclub shooting in Orlando, Florida.[68]

The likelihood that the incidents and severity of domestic terrorism may escalate in the coming years is of major concern to law enforcement and security agencies. In August 2017, a white nationalist rally in Charlottesville, Virginia, resulted in numerous injuries and the death of a thirty-two-year-old woman.[69] President Donald Trump downplayed the danger posed by the extremist groups involved, saying there were "very fine people on both sides."[70]

In October 2020, the FBI arrested several people in a plot to kidnap and potentially execute the governor of Michigan, Gretchen Whitmer.[71] And on January 6, 2021, a violent and heavily armed mob of supporters of outgoing president Donald Trump stormed the US Capitol.[72] A National Terrorism Advisory System bulletin issued on January 27, 2021, described the seriousness of the matter as follows: "The Department of Homeland Security is concerned … some domestic violent extremists may be emboldened by the January 6, 2021 breach of the U.S. Capitol Building in

Washington D.C. to target elected officials and government facilities."[73]

"The problem of domestic terrorism has been metastasizing across the country for a number of years now, and it's not going away any time soon," said Christopher Wray, director of the FBI, at a Senate judiciary hearing following the January 6, 2021, attack on the Capitol.[74]

On April 29, 2021, Jill Sanborn, executive assistant director at the National Security Branch, FBI, said at a hearing of the House Appropriations Committee, "Homegrown violent extremists are the greatest, most immediate international terrorism threat to the United States."[75]   Speaking to the House Judiciary Committee on June 10, 2021, Wray said, "The top threat we face from domestic violent extremists continue to be from … racially or ethnically motivated violent extremists, largely those who advocate for the superiority of the white race."[76]

"We cannot ignore this threat [domestic terrorism] or wish it away," President Joe Biden wrote in the preamble to the *National Strategy for Countering Domestic Terrorism* published by the White House National Security Council in June 2020.[77] "Together we must affirm that domestic terrorism has no place in our society."[78]

Of the fifty states in the nation, Texas conducted the most executions since it reinstated the death penalty in 1976, while Virginia is second, with 108 executions during the same time period.[79] In the 110 years between 1900 and 2010, there were

8,776 executions in the United States, either by hanging, electric chair, gas chamber, lethal injection, or firing squad.[80]

In a seven-to-two decision, the US Supreme Court decided in 2008 that since the death penalty is constitutional, execution by lethal injection was also constitutional.[81] The Supreme Court further noted that it was important that the first drug, sodium thiopental, in the three-drug lethal injection protocol used at the time rendered the inmate unconscious so as to avoid an unacceptable risk that the inmate would be aware of being suffocated.[82]

Since August 2009, Hospira, Inc., the manufacturer of sodium thiopental stopped providing the drug in America for lethal injections.[83] The company did not want to expose itself to liability in Europe, where export of sodium thiopental, which is prescribed at much lower doses for therapeutic purposes, would not be permitted if it might be used for executions.[84] This has led to a significant shortage of the medication and a scramble for alternative pharmaceuticals that will not violate the Eighth Amendment prohibition of "cruel and unusual punishment."[85] One such drug is pentobarbital.

Pentobarbital is a powerful barbiturate drug that is longer acting than sodium thiopental.[86] On December 16, 2010, Oklahoma became the first state in the nation to use pentobarbital as the first drug in the three-drug injection protocol when it executed John David Duty.[87] Three months later, Ohio became the first state to use pentobarbital alone to execute Johnnie Baston.[88]

In total, fourteen states have used pentobarbital to execute inmates on death row.[89] On July 25, 2019, after a hiatus of more than fifteen years, the federal government resumed executions by lethal injection with a protocol that utilized only pentobarbital.[90]

Nebraska was the first state to use fentanyl, a powerful opioid drug, along with diazepam, cisatracurium, and potassium chloride, to execute Carey Dean Moore on August 14, 2018.[91]

Seven states have used midazolam, a benzodiazepine-type sedative drug, in their lethal injection protocols, but the drug has proven to be controversial.[92] On April 29, 2014, the execution of Clayton D. Lockett in Oklahoma was one of the most publicized botched executions with midazolam.[93]

There were 1,054 executions by lethal injection between 1900 and 2010, seventy-five (7.12 percent) of which were "botched" and involved "unanticipated problems or delays that caused … unnecessary agony for the prisoner or that reflect gross incompetence of the executioner."[94] This is almost four times as many botched executions as with the electric chair.[95] In many cases, botched executions occurred because executioners had a difficult time finding a vein, with the search sometimes taking as long as sixty minutes, since inmates often are significantly obese or are former drug users with collapsed veins.[96] In a February 22, 2018, capital punishment in Alabama, the executioner tried to find a vein for two and a half hours before the execution was finally called off.[97]

According to Austin Sarat of Amherst College, other reasons for botched executions include "an adverse reaction, such as convulsions … [and the fact that] the [intravenous tubes] that carry the drugs can get clogged," as well as equipment failure or a kink in the tubing.[98]

Joel Zivot, an anesthesiologist at Emory University Hospital in Atlanta, Georgia, and Mark Edgar, a professor of pathology at Emory University School of Medicine, reviewed twenty-seven autopsies of inmates who had undergone lethal injection executions using midazolam.[99] They found that about 75 percent of the cases showed heavy lungs, many of which held bloody froth and foam, with evidence of pulmonary edema, an accumulation of fluid in the lungs.[100] "When [pulmonary edema] is this severe, you can experience panic and terror," said Edgar.[101] The two academics claimed that an inmate with pulmonary edema caused by a lethal injection experiences a feeling akin to drowning.[102]

Following his review of Zivot's and Edgar's findings, Judge Michael Mertz ruled that pulmonary edema caused by midazolam was "painful … inducing a sense of drowning and the attendant panic and terror, much as would occur with the torture tactic known as waterboarding."[103]

National Public Radio (NPR) conducted an investigation that expanded on Zivot's and Edgar's findings.[104] In its review of 216 autopsies of inmates executed by lethal injection, NPR found signs of pulmonary edema in 84 percent of all autopsies across different drug protocols, with sodium thiopental showing the most cases, 45 percent, pentobarbital about 23 percent, and midazolam approximately 14 percent.[105]

Attorneys have now used Zivot's and Edgar's findings to argue in front of the US Supreme Court that executions with lethal injection protocols constitute "cruel and unusual punishment" under the Eighth Amendment.[106]

CHAPTER 20

George Harrison

Died November 29, 2001
Member of the Beatles

DESPITE THE PUBLIC adulation and good fortune that former member of the Beatles, George Harrison, had as a musician, he unfortunately had very little good luck with his health. "It reminds you that anything can happen," Harrison said after his first health scare.[1]

In 1997, when he was fifty-four years old, Harrison discovered a lump on his neck.[2] A biopsy of his enlarged lymph node revealed it to be a malignant form of "oropharyngeal cancer," a throat cancer located in the oropharynx, an area just behind the oral cavity.[3] In August 1998, doctors at Princess Margaret Hospital in Windsor, England, successfully removed the cancer, after which Harrison underwent two series of radiation therapy at the Royal Marsden Hospital in London.[4] "Luckily for me," Harrison said after his surgery and radiotherapy, "they found this nodule; was more of a warning than anything else."[5]

Then, at three o'clock on one early morning in December 1999, a knife-wielding deranged man broke into Harrison's 120 room Victorian neo-Gothic mansion in Henley-on-Thames in Oxfordshire, England, and stabbed Harrison several times.[6] While he fought off the intruder, Harrison's wife, Olivia, hit the man on the head with an iron poker and a lamp.[7] Harrison suffered a punctured lung and minor stab wounds, while his wife had several cuts and bruises.[8] "Aren't you glad you married a Mexican girl?" The singer-songwriter, Tom Petty, wrote Harrison after the incident.[9]

As if that wasn't enough, in March 2001, on one of Harrison's regular visits to the Mayo Clinic in Rochester, Minnesota, doctors found a large cancerous growth on one of his lungs, described as "non-small cell lung cancer."[10] Harrison underwent an operation in May of that year in which half a lung was removed.[11] A statement released after the surgery noted, "He is in the best of spirits and in top form."[12] Pictures showed Harrison on holiday with his wife, enjoying their time in Tuscany, Italy.[13] In true gentlemanly fashion, Harrison told his fans, "I am feeling fine and I am really sorry for the unnecessary worry which has been caused by the reports appearing in today's press."[14]

By July 2001, Harrison's lung cancer had metastasized to his brain.[15] His treatment, which included conventional cobalt radiotherapy by Dr. Franco Cavalli, was performed at Saint Giovanni Hospital in Bellinzona, Switzerland.[16] A week later, Harrison went to convalesce at his secluded sixty-three-acre estate in Hana, on the northern coast of East Maui, Hawaii.[17]

In late October of the same year, Harrison, now extremely thin and in great pain, decided to try one last treatment for his cancer—Dr. Gil Lederman's "stereostatic radiosurgery" at the Staten Island University Hospital in New York.[18] The innovative radiotherapy is often administered to patients considered untreatable and is designed to specifically target the cancer, allowing for fewer doses of radiation, with each at a much greater intensity.[19]

After three weeks, Harrison was ready to return to California, but on the night prior to leaving New York, Lederman and his three children appeared at Harrison's home.[20] According to a lawsuit filed more than two years later by Harrison's wife, Lederman "coerced Mr. Harrison [that night] into autographing a guitar [for Lederman's son] and cards [for Lederman's daughters] in order to create valuable memorabilia."[21] The lawsuit further claimed that Lederman, who had provided personal anecdotes about his treatment of Harrison on several television shows and to *US Weekly*, *Newsweek*, the *New York Post*, and the *National Enquirer*, had "abused Mr. Harrison's trust by leaking confidential information about his treatment and [had] traded upon his fame to promote [his] cancer treatment techniques."[22]

Within ten days of the filing of the lawsuit, a settlement was reached.[23] In a joint statement read aloud in federal court, both parties agreed that the guitar Harrison signed would be returned to the Harrison estate; it "[would] be disposed of privately," and the Harrison estate would give Lederman's son a new guitar.[24] Lederman also agreed not to speak any further about Harrison or the case.[25] Later that week, the Staten Island University Hospital announced it had replaced Lederman as director of its radiation oncology department.[26]

Harrison entered hospice care upon his return to Los Angeles.[27] His wife said he was "getting up early, going to bed early, taking care of himself and having some sort of spiritual quality to his life."[28] Sadly, Harrison died at 1:20 p.m. on November 29, 2001. He was fifty-eight years old. "[He] was at peace and ready," Harrison's wife said. "There was a great light in the room when he passed."[29]

The Autopsy

Per the family's request, no autopsy or toxicology testing was performed on Harrison's body, which was cremated within ten hours of his death.[30] Harrison's ashes were taken to the family home in Hawaii and then to India, where they were scattered in a private ceremony in the River Ganges.[31]

Cause and Manner of Death

After I reviewed the circumstances surrounding Harrison's death, the death certificate, published lay articles, and the

260

scientific literature, I concluded that the immediate cause of death was metastatic non–small cell lung cancer. The manner of death was natural.

Life and Career

Harrison was born in Liverpool, England, in 1943 to a stay-at-home mom and a father who was a school bus driver.[32] He attended Dovedale Primary School, where John Lennon, later of the Beatles, had also been a student.[33]

In 1954, Harrison was admitted to the prestigious Liverpool Institute High School for Boys, where he met Paul McCartney.[34] As Harrison often admitted, he wasn't much of a student.[35]

When he was thirteen years old, Harrison purchased his first guitar.[36] After teaching himself to play a few chords, he and his brother, Peter, along with a friend, formed a band they called Rebel.[37] A year later, McCartney, who had joined Lennon's band, the Quarrymen, encouraged Harrison to audition for their band.[38] Impressed with Harrison's talent, Lennon invited him to join the Quarrymen.[39]

In 1960, Lennon renamed his band the Silver Beetles and then the Beatles.[40] With Harrison as lead guitarist, the Beatles played at small clubs and bars in Liverpool, including at the Cavern, and at the Kaiserkeller in Hamburg, Germany.[41]

By 1962, the Beatles had a new drummer, Ringo Starr, and a new manager, Brian Epstein.[42] Their first single, "Love Me Do," was a huge hit in England, as was "Please Please Me" the following year.[43] "She Loves You" and "I Want to

Hold Your Hand," songs written by Lennon and McCartney, ensured that "Beatlemania" was in full swing in England. Within two years, after an American tour and appearances on *The Ed Sullivan Show*, Beatlemania crossed the Atlantic and swept the United States.[44]

Although often referred to as the "quiet Beatle," Harrison could be quick-witted. Once, when a reporter asked him what he called his hairstyle, he responded, "Arthur."[45] In no time, Sybil Christopher, ex-wife of the actor Richard Burton, founded a very successful nightclub she named Arthur that attracted top-named celebrities from film, dance, and the visual arts.[46]

"I always really enjoyed it in our early years, before we got too famous," Harrison once said.[47] "We used to play clubs and that kind of stuff all the time. And it was fun, it was fun. It was good, because you get to play and you get to get quite good on the instrument. But then we got famous, and it spoiled all that, because we'd just go round and round the world singing the same ten dopey tunes."[48] The other band members agreed, and soon, the "Fab Four," as the Beatles were sometimes called, stopped touring and spent their time in the recording studio instead.[49]

Over the eight years the Beatles were together, Harrison contributed twenty-one memorable songs to the band's repertoire, including "Don't Bother Me," "While My Guitar Gently Weeps," "Here Comes the Sun," and "Something."[50] Often written in minor keys, Harrison's songs provided a sharp contrast to Lennon and McCartney's uptempo tunes.[51]

By 1965, with his interest in Indian music developing, Harrison played the sitar on "Norwegian Wood."[52] In 1968, in large measure because of Harrison's urging, the Beatles traveled to India to study transcendental meditation under the Maharishi Mahesh Yogi.[53]

The Beatles disbanded in 1970; feeling stifled, Harrison was ready to go solo.[54] "There was never anything in any of the Beatles experiences really, that good," Harrison wrote in his 1979 autobiographical book, *I, Me, Mine*. "Even the best thrill soon got tiring."[55] When asked how it felt to be part of the Beatles and now to be on his own, Harrison replied, "My first big break was getting in the Beatles. My second big break was getting out of them."[56]

Harrison didn't waste any time after the Beatles split up. He immediately recruited drummer Ringo Starr, guitarist Eric Clapton, keyboardist Billy Preston, and several others to help him record the songs he had amassed over the years but had never recorded.[57] The result was a three-disc album, *All Things Must Pass*, that included Harrison's signature song, "My Sweet Lord."[58] Other projects soon followed, including the Concert for Bangladesh, several more albums, some more successful than others, and a movie production company, HandMade Films.[59]

In the mid-1980s, Harrison teamed up with Jeff Lynne, Roy Orbison, Tom Petty, and Bob Dylan to form the band the Traveling Wilburys.[60] Together the group produced two commercially successful studio albums.[61]

By the 1990s, Harrison had retreated to his home in Henley-on-Thames, claiming, "I'm really quite simple. I don't want to be in the business full-time, because I'm a gardener. I plant flowers and watch them grow. I don't want to go out to clubs and partying. I stay at home and watch the river flow."[62]

In 1988, the Beatles were inducted into the Rock and Roll Hall of Fame.[63] Ten years later, Harrison had his first health scare.[64]

Conclusions

In 1997, Harrison was diagnosed with oropharyngeal cancer, a "head and neck cancer" of the middle part of the throat.[65] Of the several head and neck cancers, oropharyngeal cancer is much more common than cancer of the salivary glands or cancer of the sinuses and nasal cavity.[66] In 90 percent of patients with oropharyngeal cancer, the malignancy begins in squamous cells in the outermost layer of mucosal surfaces of the throat.[67] When the oropharyngeal cancer metastasizes, it almost always does so locally or to the lymph nodes in the neck.[68] Harrison's cancer was detected when he felt a lump in his neck.[69]

Infection with the human papillomavirus (HPV) is believed to cause about 70 percent of all cases of oropharyngeal cancer in the United States.[70] Patients with HPV-positive oropharyngeal cancer have a much better prognosis as opposed to patients with HPV-negative tumors.[71] Harrison's oropharyngeal cancer was probably HPV-negative, since he admitted after his diagnosis, "I got it purely from smoking."[72]

The two most important risk factors for patients with HPV-negative oropharyngeal cancer are alcohol and tobacco use, as well as secondhand smoke.[73] People who use both tobacco and alcohol in excess are at a much greater risk of developing oropharyngeal cancer than people who use only tobacco or alcohol.[74] Harrison had smoked cigarettes most of his life.

According to the American Cancer Society, the five-year relative survival rate for people with oropharyngeal cancer is 70 percent.[75] By the time Harrison died in 2001, nearly four years after his diagnosis, his cancer had still not reappeared. Nonetheless, since people who have been treated for oropharyngeal cancer have an increased risk of developing a new primary cancer, usually in the lungs or in the head, Harrison's diagnosis in March 2001 with non–small cell lung cancer wasn't a surprise.[76] By July, the lung cancer had metastasized to Harrison's brain.[77]

Lung cancer is the second most common cancer in the United States, about 85 percent of which is non–small cell lung cancer.[78] Smoking cigarettes is the major risk factor for developing the disease.[79] The five-year survival rate for people with non–small cell carcinoma that has not spread beyond the lungs is about 63 percent.[80] If the cancer has metastasized to a distant site, as it did in Harrison, the five-year survival rate drops precipitously to 7 percent.[81] Harrison lived only eight months after he was diagnosed with lung cancer.[82]

Harrison's lung cancer was treated with conventional cobalt radiotherapy followed by stereostatic radiosurgery, but according to his wife, Harrison wanted to embrace his dying and not run away from it at the end of his life.[83] A statement issued by the Harrison family upon his death said, "He left this world as he lived in it, conscious of God, fearless of death, and at peace, surrounded by family and friends. He often said, 'Everything else can wait but the search for God cannot wait, and love one another.'"[84]

Now that Harrison has died, his guitar gently weeps, but his spirit and music will live forever.

CHAPTER 21

Dee Dee Ramone

Died June 5, 2002
Member of the Ramones

DEE DEE RAMONE played bass guitar and was a founding member of the pioneering punk rock band the Ramones.[1] At the band's induction ceremony into the Rock and Roll Hall of Fame on March 18, 2002, each member spoke on behalf of the band. "I'll never forget Dee Dee's classic acceptance speech," said Gary Kurfirst, manager of the Ramones.[2] "I'd like to congratulate myself, and thank myself, and give myself a big pat on the back. Thank you, Dee Dee, you're very wonderful," Ramone joked.[3] Said Kurfirst, "That was Dee Dee, direct and to the point."[4]

Ramone had been booked to perform at the Majestic Ventura Theater in downtown Ventura, California.[5] At about 2:00 p.m. on June 5, 2002, Ramone's wife, Barbara, left their Hollywood home to do some errands. When she returned at 8:25 p.m., she found Ramone collapsed with his face down over the arm of the couch; he was unresponsive.[6] Pulling Ramone off the couch, she lay him down on his back on the carpeted floor and called 911.[7]

When police arrived, they noted vomit on a couch cushion on which Ramone's head lay.[8] A spoon with possible drug residue, five balloons with possible drug contents, and one broken balloon were found on a table in front of the couch.[9] "The investigator noted drug paraphernalia, including a single syringe on the kitchen counter. "We are handling it as a possible accidental overdose," said Craig Harvey, operations chief for the coroner's office.[10]

Paramedics pronounced Ramone dead at 8:40 p.m.[11] He was fifty years old.[12]

The Autopsy

The autopsy was conducted at nine in the morning on June 6, 2002, by Dr. Solomon L. Riley, deputy medical examiner of the County of Los Angeles, California.[13] Six feet long and weighing one hundred and seventy-nine pounds, the body was well-nourished and well-developed with no evidence of trauma.[14]

Multiple tattoos were present on the chest, the abdomen and the arms.[15] With the exception of a horizontal surgical scar at the right lower quadrant of the abdomen and a needle puncture wound in the left "antecubital fossa," an area located in a depression on the anterior surface of the elbow joint, the body was unremarkable.[16] A one-inch abrasion on the left side of the forehead had probably occurred when Ramone slumped over the arm of his couch.[17]

The cardiovascular system was within normal limits, with the heart weight in the normal range, the heart valves unremarkable, the coronary arteries without plaque, and the aorta showing only a slight amount of atherosclerosis.[18]

The right and left lung weights were significantly over the normal range, at 790 grams and 720 grams, respectively, as a result of severe edema and congestion, which, in the absence of any indication of drowning, was a clear sign of an opioid overdose.[19]

The liver had no evidence of cirrhosis, the spleen was congested but otherwise unremarkable, and the endocrine system—pituitary, thyroid, and adrenal glands—was normal.[20]

The kidneys, each weighing 170 grams, were congested but otherwise normal and unremarkable in appearance.[21] The prostate was without nodules.[22]

The appendix was absent, which explains the presence of the abdominal surgical scar.[23] As for the digestive system, the esophagus was unremarkable, and the stomach contained digested food but was otherwise normal, as were the small and large intestines and pancreas.[24]

No evidence of hemorrhage was apparent in the head, below the scalp; the brain was normal and unremarkable.[25]

While the autopsy revealed a normal heart and other organs, the circumstances surrounding Ramone's death and the lung congestion strongly suggested Ramone died from an opioid overdose. I was anxious to review the toxicology testing results, wondering whether it would confirm my suspicion.

Cause and Manner of Death

No foul play was suspected in Ramone's death.

According to David Campbell, a coroner's spokesperson, toxicology tests determined Ramone had a lethal amount of morphine in his system as the result of a heroin overdose.[26] Invariably, after heroin entered Ramone's bloodstream, it was rapidly metabolized by the liver to morphine. The morphine, in turn, bound to areas in the brain responsible for respiration, with death following from respiratory depression. While it was a painless way to die, it possibly could have been prevented had Ramone been treated with naloxone, a recognized antidote for an opioid overdose had paramedics arrived at the Ramone house early enough.

After I reviewed the circumstances surrounding Ramone's death, the autopsy findings and results of toxicology testing, published lay articles, and the scientific literature, I concluded that the immediate cause of death was respiratory depression due to a heroin overdose. The manner of death was accident.

Life and Career

Ramone, whose mother was German, was born in 1951 in Fort Lee, Virginia.[27] Since his father was in the army, Ramone moved often, spending most of his childhood in Berlin, Germany.[28]

"I got exposed to Rock and Roll real early cause my mother always liked it," Ramone told Legs McNeil in an interview for *Vice*.[29] He started to play the guitar when he was twelve years old, the same age he started to use drugs.[30]

"I don't know how I got turned on to morphine—I was just in the wrong place at the wrong time," Ramone told McNeil.[31] "I started getting high on morphine—they didn't have pot or heroin or anything like that in Germany."[32]

Ramone's parents separated when he was in his early teens. They eventually divorced, in part because of his father's alcoholism.[33] When he was fifteen years old, Ramone's mother took him and his sister to Forest Hills, New York, a middle-class neighborhood in Queens, where Ramone attended Forest Hills High School, the same school from which I, as well as Paul Simon, Art Garfunkel, Burt Bacharach, Jerry Springer, and other famous people, had also graduated.[34] It was only then that Ramone began to smoke pot.[35]

In the early 1970s, Ramone, who by then was addicted to heroin, worked as a printer's helper at the Bureau of Advertising in Manhattan, spending much of his time in the art department.[36] His other jobs included working as a barber, in a post office, and in construction. To earn enough money to maintain his drug habit, Ramone became a drug dealer and a male prostitute, and even turned to armed robbery.[37] It was while working at a construction site that Ramone met John Cummings, a member of a band named Tangerine Puppets.[38] Together, Ramone and Cummings, who became known professionally as Johnny Ramone, formed their own band in 1974 they called the Ramones, recruiting Jeffrey Hyman, later known as Joey Ramone, as its lead singer and Thomas Erdelyi, known as Tommy Ramone, who was also in Tangerine Puppets, to play the drums.[39] "I can see now how it was only natural that I would gravitate to Tommy, Joey, and Johnny," Ramone recalled in his autobiography.[40] "They were the obvious creeps of the neighborhood ... No one would have ever pegged any of us as candidates for any kind of success in life."[41]

Besides playing the bass guitar, Ramone wrote or cowrote many of the best-known songs for the Ramones, including "Fifty-Third and Third," "Glad to See You Go," "It's a Long Way Back," "Wart Hog," and "Chinese Rock."[42]

At their live performances, the Ramones always wore black leather jackets, ripped jeans, and tight T-shirts.[43] Their songs were short, seldom lasting more than three minutes, and fast, utilizing only three or four chords.[44] In time, the band's music became the inspiration for punk, indie, grunge, and heavy metal rock, as well as for the bands the Sex Pistols and the Clash.[45] "They're the daddy punk group of all time," said Joe Strummer, lead singer of the Clash.[46]

In 1987, Ramone had a brief career as a rapper with little success.[47] Matt Carlson, a music critic, said Ramone's rap album *Standing in the Spotlight* "will go down in the annals of pop culture as one of the worst recordings of all time."[48] Although he left the Ramones in 1989 because "he needed to find himself and grow," Ramone continued to write songs for the group until the Ramones disbanded in 1996.[49] "We could go on forever, but you want to go out great," Johnny Ramone said.[50]

"One thing that's always been important to me is to be myself," Ramone told McNeil in an interview.[51] "I don't write music according to a certain style that I'm noted for or familiar with. I write how I feel at the moment. I write current. I don't try to recreate the past, and that was the Ramones' thing. That was hard to deal with."[52]

In the 1990s, Ramone formed the bands Dee Dee Ramone and the Chinese Dragons, Dee Dee Ramone I.C.L.C. (Inter-Celestial Light Commune), and a tribute band called the Remainz; he also recorded several solo albums, all of which achieved moderate success.[53] In 2002, he tried acting, appearing in the low-budget film *Bikini Bandits*.[54] And in 2009, he wrote an autobiography entitled *Poison Heart: Surviving the Ramones*, which was republished in 2016 as *Lobotomy: Surviving the Ramones*.[55] Ramone also wrote a novel, *Chelsea Horror Hotel*, and a travelogue of his 2001 European tour, *Legend of a Rock Star*.[56]

Ramone's final career move was to become a painter, selling his paintings for a few hundred dollars each.[57]

Conclusions

Ramone's drug use began at a very young age, and he could never shake off his addiction to heroin, which ultimately led to his demise. "I'm really lucky I'm still around," he said in late 2000.[58] "Everybody expected me to die next ... It was sad when Sid Vicious died ... I was freaked out when Phil Lynott died from [the band] Thin Lizzy ... It was always someone else instead of me."[59]

Ramone was always the wildest member of the Ramones, partaking in legendary drug binges and fighting with the other members of the band.[60] Nonetheless, his publisher, Neil Ortenberg, said of Ramone, "He was an amazing person. He could be so otherworldly that people would disregard him and then he'd suddenly say something that would make you realize what kind of genius he was."[61]

Deborah Harry, of the band Blondie, described Ramone this way.[62] "He was sort of a wacky guy who wrote great songs. He was a really good songwriter, though a little self-destructive ... He had this sort of manic energy. I always thought that the Ramones were this tactical force, like the Marines jumping out of a plane or something. They had this focus and energy that I really admired."[63]

When he heard of Ramone's passing, his brother said, "For me, he was one of the greatest rock and roll songwriters alive. Sadly, another life becomes legend."[64] Guitarist Johnny Ramone declared, "He was a star and the most influential punk rock bassist. I believe he has influenced every kid playing bass that saw him perform."[65]

In the introduction to Ramone's autobiographical book *Lobotomy: Surviving the Ramones*, McNeil summed it up best when he wrote, "Dee Dee was the archetypical f--k-up whose life was a living disaster. He was a male prostitute, a would-be mugger, a heroin user and dealer, an accomplice to armed robbery and a genius poet who was headed for an early grave, but was sidetracked by Rock and Roll."[66]

Despite never reaching commercial success, the Ramones managed to "reinvent Rock and Roll," wrote Jim Greer in *Spin* magazine.[67] "No group in the last eighteen years has been more important or influential."[68] David Fricke of *Rolling Stone* wrote that they "torched the sluggish Seventies with their debut album, *Ramones*, the punk-rock blast that shook the world."[69] A *New York Times* poll voted the band's debut album one of the twenty most influential albums of the twentieth century.[70]

"I think Rock and Roll should be three words and a chorus," Ramone once said in an interview, "and the three words should be good enough to say it all."[71] He was probably right.

CHAPTER 22

Maurice Gibb

Died January 12, 2003
Member of the Bee Gees

ON WEDNESDAY, JANUARY 8, 2003, Maurice Gibb, one of the three brothers of the popular singing group the Bee Gees, was at his 13,447-square-foot thirteen-bedroom home off La Gorce Circle in Miami Beach, Florida, when he began to experience severe stomach pain.[1] He was immediately rushed to Mount Sinai Medical Center, but before he could undergo emergency abdominal surgery, he suffered cardiac arrest.[2]

Successfully resuscitated, Gibb was nevertheless significantly weakened.[3] Due to the grave nature of his medical condition, Gibb underwent an abdominal operation early Thursday morning at the conclusion of which he was placed in intensive care and was listed in critical but stable condition.[4]

"Maurice has undergone surgery for an intestinal blockage," a spokesperson for the Gibb family announced. "We are awaiting a full medical prognosis later today, but everyone is very, very worried."[5]

Robin, Maurice Gibb's twin brother, flew in from London when he heard of the seriousness of his brother's unexpected medical situation.[6] Echoing the sentiments expressed by the family spokesperson, Robin noted, "The latest update is that all his vital organs are A1 and he's recovering. Obviously, it's been very bad but every hour is a bonus."[7]

After the surgery, Gibb appeared to show signs of recovery.[8] On Saturday, he opened his eyes and squeezed his daughter's hand, but as the day progressed, his condition rapidly deteriorated.[9]

Gibb died at one o'clock on Sunday morning.[10] He was fifty-three years old.

"We're both devastated," Robin said, speaking on behalf of his remaining brother, Barry.[11] "It's like a nightmare that you wake up to every day. It's going to take a long time even just for it to sink in."[12]

The Autopsy

"This is the body of a five foot, eight inches, one hundred and forty-nine pound, embalmed adult white male who appears of the reported age," Dr. Bruce A. Hyma wrote in the autopsy report.[13] The chief medical examiner of Miami-Dade County, Florida, Hyma made no mention the deceased was a member of the Bee Gees or that he was a famous musician and record producer.

Around Gibb's right wrist was an identification band bearing the name "Ted Dugal," presumably because Gibb had been admitted to the hospital under an assumed name.[14] A second band noted that Gibb was allergic to penicillin and strawberries.[15] Around the left ankle was an identification tag with Gibb's correct name, date of birth, and the date of his death.[16]

On external examination, the face, neck, chest, back, arms, and legs were all free of visible scars and tattoos.[17] A flat gray-white "verrucous nodule" measuring 1.1 centimeters was identified on the foreskin of the penis.[18] While the lesion may have been a penile wart or even penile verrucous carcinoma (cancer), it is impossible to provide an accurate diagnosis without a microscopic examination of the tissue.

Doctors had diagnosed Gibb with "congenital malrotation of the small intestine," a birth defect in which there is a misalignment of the bowels during fetal development, and "volvulus," a twisting of the bowels.[19] This, in turn, caused ischemic enteropathy, a condition in which there is substantial reduction of blood flow to the intestines and death of intestinal tissue.[20] It was a medical emergency that, had it not been surgically treated, could have led to Gibb's imminent death.

Evidence of a recent surgical operation was readily apparent. The abdomen had a thirty-centimeter midline vertical laparotomy incision that had been closed with twenty-seven metal staples.[21] A sutured gastrostomy site, an opening through the abdominal wall into the stomach for the introduction of food and medication, was also present.[22]

Large portions of dead sections of the small intestine were missing, including the distal part, called the jejunum, and the entire ileum, the final section of the intestine.[23] The fundus, the upper part of the stomach, was sutured to the abdominal wall and to the gastrostomy site.[24] The appendix was absent, and various surgical procedures had been performed on the cecum, a pouch connected to the junction of the small and large intestines, the ascending colon, and the remaining jejunum.[25]

Since Gibb had suffered cardiac arrest prior to his operation, I was especially interested to examine the autopsy findings related to the cardiovascular system.

The heart weight was in the normal range.[26] There was mild accumulation of plaque in the aorta, and 60 percent narrowing of the left anterior descending coronary artery, which put Gibb at an increased risk for a heart attack. However, it remains a mystery why Gibb's heart stopped beating prior to his surgery.[27]

Other significant anomalies identified on internal examination, none of which contributed to Gibb's death, included cerebral edema; emphysema in both lungs, a condition that causes shortness of breath; edematous vocal chords; and tracheobronchitis. Gray-white exudate was present in the epiglottis and larynx, with mucus and pus-containing gray-brown secretions in the trachea.[28]

Interestingly, since Gibb had a history of alcohol abuse, I expected to find evidence of cirrhosis, a chronic liver disease typically caused by alcoholism; however, this was not the case; Gibb's liver was normal both in weight and in appearance.[29] As for the esophagus, gallbladder, spleen, prostate, kidneys, pineal gland, and endocrine system, they were all normal.[30]

Cause and Manner of Death

While Gibb had 60 percent narrowing of one of his coronary arteries, a risk factor for a heart attack, and his heart had stopped beating, it was restarted prior to his operation. He also suffered from emphysema. Had Gibb lived, he may have eventually died from heart disease or emphysema.

After I reviewed the circumstances surrounding Gibb's death, the autopsy findings, published lay articles, and the scientific literature, I concluded that the immediate cause of death was ischemic enteropathy due to volvulus resulting from intestinal malrotation.[31] The manner of death was natural.

Life and Career

Gibb was born in 1949 on the Isle of Man in the United Kingdom, within half an hour of his fraternal twin brother, Robin.[32] His father was a bandleader and an accomplished drummer, so music was always an important part of the Gibb family.[33] The twin boys and their older brother, Barry, often accompanied their father in family jam sessions, harmonizing at a very young age, with Maurice singing the higher notes.[34]

When Gibb was eight years old, he and his two brothers got a few of their friends together, and they formed a band they named Rattlesnakes.[35] In December 1957, Rattlesnakes made its first public appearance at Manchester's Gaumont Theater, singing "Wake Up Little Suzie" by the Everly Brothers; they were a huge hit.[36]

The following year, Gibb and his family moved to Australia, eventually settling in Redcliffe.[37] The Redcliffe Speedway, where Barry worked selling soda during races, invited the three brothers to sing over the public address system.[38] On one such occasion, Bill Gates, a popular DJ, heard the trio sing and took on the role of their promoter, playing the group's recordings at his station and renaming them the Bee Gees.[39] Soon, the Bee Gees were performing at outdoor exhibitions, appearing on television shows such as *Anything Goes* and *Cottie's Happy Hour*, and even hosting their own television show, *The BG Half Hour*. In 1963, the Bee Gees released their first single, "The Battle of the Blue and the Grey."[40]

By the early 1960s, Maurice Gibb was providing his vocals to many of the Bee Gees' songs and had become the group's lead bass guitarist, as well as its keyboard and percussion player.[41]

The three brothers moved back to London in the late 1960s, where they released their first studio album, *Bee Gees*

First. It quickly reached the top ten on music charts, both in the United Kingdom and the United States.[42] "Massachusetts," one of the ballads on the album, became the number-one single on the UK charts, where it stayed for several weeks.[43]

As the Bee Gees' popularity increased and the group became commercially successful, Gibb enjoyed the rock 'n' roll lifestyle and overindulged in alcohol.[44] By the time he was twenty-one years old, he owned six Rolls Royce automobiles and eight Aston Martins and had become an alcoholic.[45]

In 1969, Gibb married pop singer Lulu, but four years later, the marriage ended because of Gibb's alcoholism and his extravagant "high-life."[46] "No one knew me until I met my wife Lulu," Gibb said.[47]

The Bee Gees had several commercial hits, including "How Can You Mend a Broken Heart" (1971), "Jive Talkin'," (1975), and the bestselling soundtrack ever for the film *Saturday Night Fever* (1977), with more than 40 million copies sold.[48] Nevertheless, years later, Gibb recounted, "We've been up and down like yo-yos," during the 1970s.[49]

In 1977, after he attended rehab, Gibb told a reporter, "I used to be a real terror [but] I just enjoy life to the fullest now. There's two days a week I don't worry about now, and that's today and yesterday."[50]

Despite having refrained from alcohol for nearly ten years, Gibb suffered a relapse in 1988 after his younger brother, Andy, died.[51] "When [Andy] died, I just drank to numb my mind," Gibb said.[52] In 1991, Gibb even threatened his second wife, Yvonne, and their two children with a gun; that led him to increase his resolve to being sober.[53]

After Gibb bought his waterfront home in Miami Beach in 2002, all three Gibb brothers lived on the same street in Miami.[54] Following Gibb's death, his wife put their two houses in Miami Beach up for sale, as well as their two houses in England, a house in Spain, and another in the Bahamas.[55]

Conclusions

The incidence of congenital intestinal malrotation has been reported to be as high as one percent.[56] It is generally formed during the fourth through twelfth weeks of gestation, with approximately 90 percent of all cases exhibiting symptoms in the first year of life.[57] The condition, which is usually detected in early childhood, is caused by incomplete rotation and fixation of the intestines, often leading to life-threatening volvulus of the midgut.[58]

While a malformed small intestine can develop kinks, causing blockage and backup of fluid and waste materials, it can also form crimps in blood vessels.[59] Without an adequate blood supply, intestinal tissue can die, rupture, and spill its toxic contents into the abdominal cavity, leading to a fatal infection and death.[60]

Cases of intestinal malrotation in adults are rare and can have life-threatening consequences if they are not detected early.[61] Symptoms are nonspecific, which makes diagnosis very difficult; these may include chronic abdominal symptoms, such as intermittent abdominal pain and vomiting, bloating, malabsorption, and alternating constipation and diarrhea.[62]

"People can live to middle age [with a malformed, twisted intestine] with no symptoms," said Dr. Jeffrey Raskin, interim chief of gastroenterology at the University of Miami Memorial Medical Center, "or they can present on the first time with a catastrophic event," as apparently happened with Gibb.[63] Unfortunately, there is no way to predict which patients will proceed to potentially fatal midgut volvulus or bowel ischemia.[64]

According to Dr. Jacob C. Langer, "The most important goal of clinicians is to determine whether the patient has midgut volvulus with intestinal ischemia, in which case an emergency laparotomy should be done."[65] This is precisely the protocol that was followed with Gibb. While Gibb's surgery was successful, the outcome was tragic, mainly because Gibb was older at the time of his diagnosis than most intestinal malrotation patients and his intestines may have already burst, spilling their contents of toxins and wastes into the abdominal cavity.

Almost as soon as Gibb died, his two remaining brothers threatened to take legal action against the hospital, claiming it was negligent in its treatment of Gibb.[66] However, Gibb's wife, who was originally from England, would not hear of it.[67] "[It's] so American to sue," she declared. Instead she negotiated an amicable settlement.[68]

After Maurice Gibb's death, Robin and Barry equivocated as to whether to retire the Bee Gees name.[69] "In the beginning,

Barry and I couldn't decide if we were going to go forward with the name of the Bee Gees or just Barry and Robin," Robin told a British newspaper.[70] "Now, we've decided to continue as the Bee Gees because we feel we can and Maurice would have wanted it."[71]

On August 14, 2010, seven years after Maurice Gibb's death, Robin began to feel abdominal pain while performing in Belgium. Four days later, he underwent emergency surgery at an Oxford hospital for a blocked intestine.[72] Over the following months, he continued to experience severe abdominal pain, cancelling a tour in Brazil in April 2011 and two concerts in October of that year, one in Paris and another in London.

In November 2011, Robin was diagnosed with colorectal cancer that had metastasized to his liver.[73] In March 2012, he underwent surgery to remove a blood clot in his colon; in mid-April, he contracted pneumonia and fell into a coma.[74] He died in May 2012 from liver and kidney failure brought on by his colorectal cancer.[75]

Only one member of the Bee Gees remained—Barry Gibb.

CHAPTER 23

John Ritter

Died September 11, 2003

Actor in *Three's Company*

UNLIKE OTHER WELL-KNOWN comedians who became sitcom stars and late-night television hosts, John Ritter never did stand-up comedy. And yet he was a lovable, popular comic actor whose star rose to great heights after he landed the role of Jack Tripper in the television sitcom *Three's Company*.[1]

On Thursday, September 11, 2003, while rehearsing on the set of his latest show, *8 Simple Rules ... For Dating My Teenage Daughter*, Ritter suddenly began experiencing nausea and vomiting.[2] At 6:00 p.m., feeling faint and complaining of chest pain, he was rushed to the emergency room at Providence St. Joseph Medical Center in Burbank, California, where a doctor prescribed aspirin and antinausea medication and ordered medical tests, including a chest X-ray; for some unknown reason, the X-ray was never done.[3] A "code AMI"—acute myocardial infarction or heart attack—was activated sometime around 7:15 p.m. after one of the test results came back showing abnormalities consistent with a heart attack.[4]

Dr. Joseph Lee, a cardiologist, arrived at Ritter's bedside at 7:25 p.m.[5] Lee planned to order an angiogram, a medical imaging procedure used to visualize the inside of coronary blood vessels. When Ritter asked whether he could get a second opinion before agreeing to the procedure, Lee replied, "No, there's no time. You're in the middle of a heart attack."[6] Seeing that Ritter was anxious, Ritter's wife leaned down and whispered in her husband's ear, "I know you're scared but you have to be brave and do this because these guys know what they're doing."[7]

After ordering anticoagulants to be administered to Ritter, a standard treatment for a heart attack, Lee placed a catheter into a vein in Ritter's groin, threading it through the blood vessel and into the heart.[8] But sometime during the catheterization procedure, a large aortic dissection was found—a tear in the inner layer of the body's main artery that carries oxygenated blood away from the heart to the rest of the body—and Ritter's condition worsened.[9] Surgeons attempted to repair the aortic dissection, but they couldn't.[10] Despite heroic measures, Ritter, who was fifty-four years old, was pronounced dead at 10:48 p.m., the same day his daughter, Stella, celebrated her fifth birthday.[11]

The Autopsy

Per the family's request, no autopsy was performed.[12] However, based on published lay articles, Ritter had an undiagnosed aortic dissection.[13]

Cause and Manner of Death

After I reviewed the circumstances surrounding Ritter's death, as well as published lay articles and the scientific literature, I concluded that the immediate cause of death was internal bleeding due to aortic dissection. The manner of death was natural.

Life and Career

Ritter was born in 1948 in Burbank, California. His mother was an actress, and his father, a well-known country singer and Western film star.[14]

Ritter attended Walter Reed Junior High School and Hollywood High School, where he was student body president.[15] After graduating, he enrolled at the University of Southern California (USC), majoring in psychology with a minor in architecture.[16] It was while at USC that Ritter joined a drama class and changed his major to theater arts. He graduated in 1971 with a degree in drama.[17]

While still in college, Ritter appeared in several stage performances in Europe. After returning to the United States, he made guest appearances on *The Mary Tyler Moore Show*, *The Waltons*, *Hawaii-Five-O*, and *M*A*S*H*.[18]

Ritter's big professional break came in 1977, when he was cast in *Three's Company*.[19] The popular sitcom ran for 172 episodes until 1984, earning Ritter a Golden Globe and an Emmy.[20] "I always wanted to be a liar," Ritter said, "and if you're in television, you're lying because you're just pretending to be yourself."[21]

Over the following eighteen years, Ritter appeared in several television shows and specials, including *Hooperman* and *Hearts Afire*, as well as in films, such as *Real Men, Problem Child*, and *The Dinner Party*.[22] In 2002, Ritter was again cast in a television sitcom, *8 Simple Rules ... for Dating My Teenage Daughter*, and it quickly became a huge hit.[23]

On Thursday, September 11, 2003, while rehearsing for his television show, Ritter fell ill and was quickly rushed to the emergency room of a nearby hospital. He never returned to finish rehearsing.

Conclusions

Two years prior to his death, Ritter had a whole-body computed tomography (CT) scan.[24] The images showed a normal-size aorta with no indication of dissection.[25] Nevertheless, the radiologist, Dr. Matthew Lotysch, seeing that Ritter had blocked coronary arteries that put him at an increased risk for heart disease, urged Ritter to consult a cardiologist or an internist, but he failed to do so.[26] "He implied to me that he was reassured he was okay," Ritter's wife said after Ritter came back from his radiological appointment.[27]

The aorta is made up of three layers—an inner, a middle, and an outer layer.[28] The three layers are made up of connective tissue and elastic fibers, allowing the aorta to stretch from pressure produced by the flow of blood.[29] Aortic dissection is a slow, ongoing breakdown over many years of cells that make up the wall of the aorta, leading to an abrupt, abnormal separation or tear in the inner layer of the aorta.[30] When that happens, blood surges through the tear, allowing the blood to be diverted between the inner and middle layers, slowing or stopping the flow of blood to vital organs and potentially leading to rupture of the aorta or formation of an aneurysm, a balloon-like expansion of the aorta.[31]

The average age for aortic dissection is in the sixties, with two thirds of dissections occurring in men.[32] Some risk factors for developing aortic dissection include chronic high blood pressure; certain medical conditions, such as pregnancy, lupus, and Cushing's syndrome; chest injury, as that which can be sustained in a car crash; and a family history of aortic dissection.[33] One of the most significant and easily preventable risk factors for aortic dissection is drug abuse, specifically that of cocaine and stimulants, neither one of which was a factor in Ritter's death.[34]

Aortic dissections are uncommon, but they are life-threatening.[35] If surgical treatment is not immediate, death will quickly follow from internal bleeding and loss of blood.[36]

About 40 percent of patients immediately die from complete aortic rupture and internal bleeding.[37]

The most common sign of aortic dissection is sudden and abrupt severe sharp pain in the chest or upper back.[38] Other symptoms include shortness of breath, heavy sweating, weakness, and fainting.[39] Ritter had all of these symptoms the day he died.[40]

Diagnosing aortic dissection requires specialized equipment. While a complete physical examination to detect a heart murmur, an electrocardiogram (ECG), and chest X-rays may provide clues, the results of the tests are often completely normal.[41] The most frequently performed and highly accurate tests to diagnose aortic dissections, all of which are expensive, include a CT scan, transesophageal echocardiogram, and magnetic imaging (MRI). Of these, MRI takes longer than the other two tests and is usually not the first choice.[42]

After Ritter died, his older brother was also diagnosed with aortic dissection. He had his operation, and "he is here for Stella and John's kids," Ritter's wife said.[43]

Ritter died at an early age, but he was loved and appreciated by many, as evidenced by the number of accolades that poured in upon his death. Don Knotts, a famous American comedic actor, called Ritter the "greatest physical comedian on the planet."[44] Neil Simon, the playwright, expressed it best when he said, "He was more than a comic. He was a real actor with a genius for comedy."[45]

CHAPTER 24

Bobby Hatfield

Died November 5, 2003

Member of the Righteous Brothers

THE RIGHTEOUS BROTHERS, of which Bobby Hatfield was a member along with Bill Medley, who was not his brother, had been nominated twice for a Grammy, but they had never won the coveted award.[1] The duo had been singing together on and off since 1962 and were extremely popular, but it took forty-one years for them to finally be recognized by their peers in 2003 and to be inducted into the Rock and Roll Hall of Fame at the eighteenth annual induction ceremony at the Waldorf-Astoria Hotel in New York.[2]

Sporting a goatee and reading from his notes, Billy Joel, a 1999 inductee, made colorful introductory remarks before calling Hatfield and Medley up to the podium.[3] "Sometimes, people with blue eyes transcend the limitations of what their color and the culture is supposed to be," Joel said.[4] "Sometimes white people can actually be soulful!"

The Righteous Brothers were often told they sounded like African American gospel singers.[5] In 1966, *Life* magazine wrote, "Right now, the big new sound is blue-eyed soul, a white man's version of Negro soul music, invented by an inventive dynamic duo called the Righteous Brothers."[6]

When Hatfield and Medley approached the podium to accept their award and to sing their biggest hit, "You've Lost That Lovin' Feelin'," ranked by BMI as the most-played radio song of all time, they were cheered on by an enthusiastic audience that had looked forward to what many had considered an overdue occasion.[7] "I had pretty much given up hope," Hatfield told the attendees. "I'm just thrilled that I'm still around to accept it in person. I really didn't want to have to send a videotaped acceptance speech after I was gone."[8] I wondered whether he knew something the rest of us didn't. At that moment, no one suspected that within eight months, Hatfield would be dead.

On November 5, 2003, the Righteous Brothers were in Kalamazoo, Michigan, ready to begin a Midwestern tour through Michigan and Ohio, their first stop being Western Michigan University.[9] Hatfield was staying downtown, at the Radisson Plaza Hotel, but thirty minutes before he was to take the stage at the Miller Auditorium, he still had not shown up.[10] Anxious to begin on time, Medley and Dusty

Hanvey, the Righteous Brothers' road manager, went to the Radisson to investigate.[11] At about 7:00 p.m., a security guard let Medley and Hanvey into Hatfield's hotel room, where they found Hatfield lying dead in his bed.[12] He was sixty-three years old.[13]

The Autopsy

The autopsy was conducted at Sparrow Hospital in Lansing, Michigan.[14] The body was normally developed, weighing one hundred and eighty pounds and measuring seventy-eight and a half inches long.[15] An old, illegible tattoo was identified on the left bicep.[16]

An examination of the cardiovascular system identified 95 percent blockage of a coronary artery.[17]

As for the digestive system, the stomach contained fragments of potatoes, Hatfield's last meal.[18]

Cause and Manner of Death

According to Dan Weston, chief of the Kalamazoo Department of Public Safety, no illegal substances or drug paraphernalia were found in Hatfield's hotel room at the time of his death.[19]

Toxicology testing revealed the presence of cocaine in Hatfield's blood at a concentration of 143 nanograms per milliliter.[20] Cocaine is a stimulant and taken long-term, it is toxic to the heart. Tom Nasser, assistant director of forensic science services for the Orange County Sheriff's Department, said lethal levels of cocaine are closer to 900 nanograms per milliliter, so the amount of cocaine in Hatfield's blood was not an overdose.[21] Other drugs identified in Hartfield's blood included traces of two cocaine metabolites, norcocaine and benzoylecgonine, as well as caffeine and verapamil, a medication used to treat an irregular heart rate.[22]

Cocaine alone may not have been enough to cause Hatfield's death from an overdose, but as a stimulant, along with advanced heart disease, it proved a deadly combination.[23] "In this case, there was already a significant amount of blockage in the coronary arteries," said Richard Tooker, the chief medical examiner for Kalamazoo County.[24] "The blockage was not allowing enough blood to flow to the heart muscle tissue to keep up with the demand the cocaine was placing on the heart."[25]

After I reviewed the circumstances surrounding Hatfield's death, the death certificate, the autopsy findings and results of toxicology testing, published lay articles, and the scientific literature, I concluded that the immediate cause of death was a heart attack, most likely in combination with an arrhythmia caused by acute cocaine intoxication.[26] The manner of death was accident.[27]

Life and Career

Hatfield was born in Beaver Dam, Wisconsin, in 1940, but when he was four years old, his family moved to Anaheim, California.[28] In third grade, Hatfield sang "Shortnin' Bread" on a local radio show.[29] It was his first experience in show business.

At Anaheim High School, Hatfield played football and baseball, was cocaptain of the basketball team, and sang in the school's choir.[30] In his senior year, he was elected student body president.[31]

In 1958, after graduating high school, Hatfield attended Fullerton Junior College, a community college, and then California State University–Long Beach.[32]

Hatfield formed his own singing group, the Variations, and was performing at coffee houses and high school proms when a mutual friend introduced him to Bill Medley, leader of the Paramours, another singing group.[33] In 1962, Hatfield joined Medley as a co–lead singer of the Paramours, along with three other members.[34] It was a perfect combination of Hatfield's soaring tenor and falsetto and Medley's low, contrasting baritone.[35] The group's first performance was at a club called John's Black Derby in Santa Ana, California.[36]

In 1969, discussing his early singing experiences in an interview, Hatfield recalled, "We [were] working in a little club in Orange County, California [when] on this one particular evening there were several black Marines in there, and when Bill and I finished doing a duet, one of them yelled out, 'That's righteous brothers'."[37] It was then that Hatfield and Medley decided to leave the Paramours and form their own group, which they named "the Righteous Brothers."[38]

The Righteous Brothers released their first record, *Little Latin Lupe Lu*, in 1963, with Hatfield screaming at the end of the song like Little Richard.[39] The record was stuck at number forty-nine on the US music charts, mainly because radio stations assumed Hatfield and Medley were African American and refused to play their song.[40]

In 1964, record producer Phil Spector saw the Righteous Brothers perform at the Cow Palace near San Francisco and thought the group's approach to a song was perfect for his "Wall of Sound" style.[41] Spector signed Hatfield and Medley to his record label and invited Barry Mann and Cynthia Weil to write a ballad for the duo.[42] When they finished writing "You've Lost That Lovin' Feelin'," they played the song for Hatfield, who was not happy with it because Medley had the whole first verse.[43] "What am I supposed to do while the big guy's singing?" Hatfield asked, to which Spector replied, "You can go to the bank!"[44] The tune was released in 1964 and became the song most played on the radio in the twentieth century.[45]

In time, Hatfield became disillusioned that Medley was always taking the lead vocals, so in 1965, he recorded a solo performance of "Unchained Melody" that quickly climbed to number four on the US charts.[46] "(You're My) Soul and Inspiration" soon followed, becoming number one on the US charts under the Verve record label.[47]

By 1968, Medley was interested in pursuing a solo career, so the Righteous Brothers parted ways with Hatfield, retaining the group's name and replacing Medley with Jimmy Walker.[48] Six years later, Medley and Hatfield reunited to record "Rock and Roll Heaven," a successful tribute to deceased rock 'n' roll stars.[49] They reunited several more times—in 1982, on the thirtieth anniversary of *American Bandstand*; in 1986, when "You've Lost That Lovin' Feelin'" was included on the soundtrack of the film *Top Gun*; and in 1990, when "Unchained Melody" was featured in the hit film *Ghost*.[50] Since 1990, Medley and Hatfield continued to perform on the "oldies circuit," at county fairs and in colleges.[51]

In 2003, the Righteous Brothers were inducted into the Rock and Roll Hall of Fame.[52] It was a glorious black-tie affair at an upscale hotel in New York City. None of the invited guests thought it would be the last time Hatfield and Medley would sing together.

Conclusions

In 2007, 2.1 million Americans reported recent cocaine use, 1.6 million of whom met the criteria for cocaine dependence or abuse.[53] According to the American Heart Association, chronic cocaine users are more likely to suffer from high blood pressure, heart muscle wall thickening, and stiff arteries—all major risk factors for a heart attack.[54] Cardiologist Dr. Nicole Harkin observed, "Long-term users ... have an increased risk of heart disease, and cocaine use has been associated with premature blockages in the heart. Cocaine-related chest pain or heart attacks can occur the first time a person uses it or the one hundredth — there's really no way of knowing or predicting when it will happen."[55]

Clinically, cocaine increases the oxygen demand of heart muscle by increasing both heart rate and blood pressure.[56] At the same time, it decreases oxygen supply as a result of coronary vasoconstriction, which is much more pronounced in atherosclerotic coronary arteries.[57] When cocaine use is combined with smoking, there is an additive effect on coronary vasoconstriction, resulting in heart dysfunction, arrhythmias, atherosclerosis, and hypertrophy of the left ventricle of the heart.[58]

At the molecular level, cocaine stimulates the sympathetic nervous system, especially at low doses, by inhibiting the reuptake of the neurotransmitter catecholamine and increasing the sensitivity of adrenergic nerve endings to epinephrine, a neurotransmitter known as adrenaline.[59] The drug also acts like a local anesthetic, especially at higher doses. It stimulates the release of a potent vasoconstrictor, inhibits the production of a vasodilator, and promotes thrombosis (blood clots) by activating platelets and increasing their aggregation, leading to calcification and aneurysm, an excessive localized enlargement of an artery caused by a weakening of the arterial wall, more frequently seen in coronary arteries.[60] Often, aneurysms have no symptoms, but when they rupture, they can result in internal bleeding and stroke and could be fatal.

Cocaine can adversely affect every organ in the body, but its most lethal effects are on the cardiovascular system, which explains why cocaine use is the leading cause of drug-abuse-related visits to the emergency room, accounting for 31 percent of all visits.[61] In one study of 233 emergency room visits by cocaine abusers, 56 percent were for cardiovascular complaints.[62]

Most cocaine-related deaths occur after prolonged drug use and not because of a cocaine overdose.[63] In one study in which the pathology of the heart was compared among deaths due to cocaine toxicity and deaths due to opioid toxicity or hanging, neither of which had exposure to cocaine, the cocaine group had significantly greater proportions of hypertrophy (enlargement) of the heart's left ventricle; ischemic heart disease, a condition caused by narrowed coronary arteries; and coronary artery atherosclerosis than either of the other two groups.[64]

At the time of his death, Hatfield's heart was very fragile, having significant blockage and narrowing of a major coronary artery, thereby putting his heart muscle under extreme stress due to an insufficient supply of oxygen. In addition, large amounts of cocaine were detected in his blood.[65] While Hatfield did not die from a cocaine overdose, the drug undoubtedly increased his heart rate to accommodate for the need for more oxygen, leading to an arrhythmia and a heart attack, from which Hatfield ultimately died.

CHAPTER 25

Johnny Carson

Died January 25, 2005

Host of *The Tonight Show*

"AND NOW, HEEEEERE'S Johnny!"

The resounding baritone voice of Ed McMahon, Johnny Carson's announcer, introducing the host of *The Tonight Show* reverberated off the walls of NBC Studio 6B at New York's Rockefeller Center. With the spotlight focused on the multicolored curtain, Carson emerged, taking center stage. Smiling and performing his trademark imaginary golf swing, he appeared to be holding back a full, throated laugh.[1] After a quick glance toward the band and doing a double take upon seeing Doc Severinsen's wildly colorful jacket, Carson began his opening monologue. "I know a man who gave up smoking, drinking, sex, and rich food," he said.[2] "He was healthy right up to the day he killed himself."[3] The audience went wild with hoots, hollers, and applause.

Carson became host of *The Tonight Show*, the most popular late-night talk show in the United States, in 1962, but before him there had been Jack Paar and Steve Allen.[4] Of the three hosts, Carson held the job the longest—thirty years.[5] The question remains, What made him such a great host?

Born in Iowa and raised in Nebraska, Carson had just the right mix of Midwestern charm and East Coast sophistication that appealed to a vast audience. Comedian Jerry Lewis said, "I think that Johnny, no matter how long he lived in Hollywood and no matter how much money he made, he still had a piece of straw stuck in his ear."[6] Writing for the *New York Post*, the journalist Nora Ephron noted that Carson was "just sophisticated enough to talk to sophisticates, just hayseed enough to seem astounded by what they [told] him."[7]

Carson projected a quick-witted personality, a boyish grin, and a steady, nonthreatening presence that put his guests and the viewers at home completely at ease. "The nervousness never lasted more than a second because he was so congenial and comfortable," said comedian Jackie Mason of his time on *The Tonight Show*.[8] Actress and singer Bette Midler said of Carson, "He had it all. A little bit of devil, a whole lot of angel, wit, charm, good looks, superb timing and great, great class."[9]

After he finished delivering his nightly monologue, Carson sat down behind his desk and, nonchalantly holding a cigarette between his second and middle fingers, began introducing his guests.[10] Arnold Schwarzenegger, the thirty-eighth governor of California and a former bodybuilder, said of Carson, "He welcomed me on his show when no one knew who I was and helped me promote the image of bodybuilding."[11] Comedian Joan Rivers, whom Carson featured on his show numerous times, said, "Every solid comedian today really got their break on the Carson show."[12] David Letterman, another comedian who later became a late-night television host himself, agreed. "He gave me a shot on his show and in doing so gave me a career."[13]

Carson did not limit his guests to the entertainment industry. American animal and environmental advocate Joan Embery brought a marmoset from the San Diego Zoo to *The Tonight Show*. It immediately climbed on Carson's head and urinated.[14] Carson deadpanned, "I'm glad you didn't bring a baby elephant."[15] And when Miss Piggy of The Muppets appeared on the show and asked, "Can you stand there in your rented tuxedo and honestly say that I am not Oscar material?" Carson replied, "Oscar Mayer, maybe."[16]

American psychologist Dr. Joyce Brothers, who appeared on *The Tonight Show* about ninety times, said Carson "never said a cutting remark in all of the years that I watched the show, and I watched it for years and years ... He was kindness personified."[17]

Carson smoked cigarettes throughout his years on *The Tonight Show*, reportedly going through four packs of Pall Mall cigarettes a day.[18] In the 1960s, smoking "was the sign of being an intellectual," said Ron Simon, television and radio curator at the Paley Center for Media in New York.[19] "Edward R. Murrow smoked [on *Person to Person*], Leonard Bernstein [the conductor] smoked."[20] In a 1979 interview on *60 Minutes*, Carson told Mike Wallace, "I feel guilty … it's compulsive."[21]

At an NBC dinner party in 1982, Carson announced he quit smoking.[22] "I smoked for forty-six years and finally quit the habit. I've been off thirty-one days, and I have to thank my wife, Alex, who has stood by me closely."[23] Yet despite his announcement, Carson remained a heavy smoker for many years, hiding the ashtray and cigarettes under his desk during taping of *The Tonight Show.*[24]

In May 1992, after hosting *The Tonight Show* for thirty years, Carson announced his retirement.[25] "I am one of the lucky people in the world," he told the 50 million viewers that night.[26] "I found something that I always wanted to do and I have enjoyed every single minute of it. I bid you a very heartfelt good night."[27] Just like that, Carson was gone, never to be seen on television again—well, almost. When he heard that Carson retired, the comedian Bob Hope remarked that it was like "a head falling off Mt. Rushmore. He's had a profound impact on millions of lives. He changed people's sleeping habits, sex habits and their midnight eating habits."[28]

On May 13, 1994, Carson briefly appeared in a cameo performance on *The Late Show with David Letterman.*[29] After receiving a standing ovation, he sat for a few minutes behind Letterman's desk and then left without speaking to the audience.[30] This time, it definitely was his final good bye.

At 3:30 a.m. on March 19, 1999, Carson suffered a massive heart attack at his beachfront home in Malibu, California.[31] Hospitalized at Saint John's Health Center in Santa Monica, California, he underwent quadruple-bypass surgery.[32] "The operation went very well and his heart is functioning normally," said Lindi Funston, a spokeswoman for the hospital.[33] It was Carson's first health scare, undoubtedly contributed to by his chronic heavy smoking.

In 2002, Carson announced he was suffering from emphysema, a chronic obstructive pulmonary disease (COPD).[34] On January 5, 2005, he was hospitalized at Cedars Sinai Medical Center in Los Angeles, California, for breathing difficulties; after he was stabilized, he insisted he wanted to go home.[35] On January 16, Carson was back in the hospital; on January 21, he was transferred to the intensive care unit.[36]

At 6:50 a.m. on January 23, 2005, Carson died.[37] He was seventy-nine years old.[38] His younger brother, Dick, recalled that during their last conversation, Carson kept saying, "Those damn cigarettes, those damn cigarettes."[39]

The Autopsy

No autopsy or toxicology testing was performed after Carson died.[40]

Cause and Manner of Death

After I reviewed the circumstances surrounding Carson's death, the death certificate, published lay articles, and the scientific literature, I concluded that the immediate cause of death was emphysema.[41] The manner of death was natural.

Life and Career

Carson was born in Corning, Iowa, in 1925.[42] His mother was a homemaker, and his father was a manager of the Iowa-Nebraska Light & Power Company.[43] When he was eight years old, Carson's family moved to Norfolk, Nebraska.[44]

Carson purchased a magician's kit when he was twelve years old; at fourteen, he began performing magic tricks as "The Great Carsoni" for his family and friends, and later at county fairs, for the local Rotary and Kiwanis Clubs, and at Methodist Church socials.[45]

After graduating high school in 1943, Carson joined the US Navy, serving as an ensign aboard the *USS Pennsylvania*.[46] Upon his discharge from the navy in 1945, Carson attended the University of Nebraska, where he studied journalism with the intention of becoming a comedy writer, eventually switching majors and receiving a bachelor's degree in radio and speech.[47]

Carson's broadcasting career began at WOW radio station in Omaha, Nebraska.[48] Soon thereafter, he started hosting television shows, including *The Squirrel's Nest*, a local early-afternoon show, *Carson's Cellar*, in which he performed comedy routines and chatted with celebrities, and *Earn Your Vacation*, his first national television appearance, as host of a game show.[49]

When *The Red Skelton Show* hired Carson as a comedy writer, he got the opportunity to substitute for an injured Skelton, delivering his first monologue in front of a national audience.[50] A year later, he had his own half-hour variety show on CBS called *The Johnny Carson Show*.[51]

In 1957, Carson went to New York City, where he hosted the television show *Who Do You Trust?*[52] The show became so successful that in 1958, Carson was asked to temporarily substitute for Paar on *The Tonight Show*.[53] Four years later, when Paar decided to leave *The Tonight Show*, Carson became his replacement.[54]

The Tonight Show, which initially ran for ninety minutes, was later shortened to an hour, becoming hugely popular. Over his fifteen years with the show, Carson earned a total of six Emmys, a Peabody Award, and the Presidential Medal of Freedom.[55] In 1987, he was inducted into the Television Academy Hall of Fame; in 1993, he was a recipient of a Kennedy Center Honors.[56]

The audience loved it when Carson declared, "We have certain high standards for this show and some day we hope to live up to them."[57] In 1969, he made headlines when he featured the wedding of "Tiny Tim" and "Miss Vicki," winning the biggest ratings ever for *The Tonight Show*—58 million viewers.[58]

Carson's opening monologue was his chance to poke fun at the latest newsworthy stories. No politician was immune from being on the receiving end of one of Carson's jibes. When a joke failed, as they sometimes did, Carson simply pulled down the boom mike and announced, "Attention K-Mart shoppers, clean up in aisle four!" or broke into a soft-shoe dance.[59]

When Mayor John Lindsay described New York as "Fun City," Carson noted, "New York is an exciting town where something is happening all the time, most of it unsolved."[60] In 1974, when President Richard Nixon visited the Middle East, Carson remarked, "Egyptian President Sadat had a belly dancer entertain President Nixon at a state dinner. Mr. Nixon was really impressed. He hadn't seen contortions like that since Rose Mary Woods."[61] And in May 1991, Carson said of President George H. W. Bush, "I know what it feels like having a young guy waiting around for you to keel over."[62] Of Ronald Reagan, Carson declared, "The President has asked for severe cuts in aid to the arts and humanities. It's Reagan's strongest attack on the arts since he signed with Warner Brothers."[63]

Some of Carson's more memorable characters on *The Tonight Show* included Carnac the Magnificent, Aunt Blabby, and Art Fern.[64] One of the best moments on the show was when Ed Ames, who was regularly cast as a Native American on Broadway, demonstrated his tomahawk-throwing technique, striking a cowboy sketched on a prop wall squarely in the crotch, to which Carson exclaimed, "I didn't even know you were Jewish!"[65]

Carson had his detractors. Las Vegas entertainer Wayne Newton called Carson "a very mean spirited human being."[66] Novelist Jacqueline Susann called Carson "unbearably rude," to which he replied, "You're not that great a comedian." Her rebuttal was to fling her alcoholic drink directly into Carson's face.[67]

Despite being very well known, Carson was shy off-camera.[68] "Nobody got to know him," Rivers said. "He was very private."[69] Peter Jones, a documentary filmmaker, said, "Johnny Carson did not really exist anywhere else except in front of the camera. Privately, he was John William Carson."[70] Dick Cavett, the talk show host, called Carson "the most private public man who ever lived."[71]

After he retired from *The Tonight Show*, Carson stayed away from the limelight, spending his time in his $81 million one-bedroom Malibu home, content in his privacy and happy to "let the work speak for itself."[72] Enjoying his retirement, he sailed on his 130-foot yacht, the *Serengeti*, traveled frequently; and played tennis until 2002, when he started experiencing shortness of breath and was diagnosed with emphysema.[73]

Conclusions

Emphysema destructs the walls of the alveoli in the lungs.[74] This causes the alveoli to lose their ability to stretch and shrink with each inhalation and exhalation, the walls between the alveoli to become thick and inflamed, and the airways to make more mucus than usual, thereby clogging the airways and blocking airflow.[75] As a result, oxygen and carbon dioxide exchange between the lungs and the blood is substantially decreased, leading to progressive development of respiratory symptoms, including shortness of breath, chronic cough, wheezing, tightness in the chest, and death.[76]

Approximately 80 to 90 percent of deaths due to emphysema are caused by smoking cigarettes.[77] Other causes of emphysema include occupational exposure to chemical dust and lung irritants, such as air pollution; rarely, it is due to a genetic abnormality called alpha-1-antitrypsin deficiency.[78]

Damage to the alveoli occurs slowly over time, so it typically takes many years of smoking to gradually develop symptoms of emphysema.[79] However, once the damage has begun, it is irreversible.[80] Quitting smoking slows down the progression of emphysema, but it does not reverse it.[81] The best way to prevent emphysema is to never start smoking cigarettes.[82]

Since smoking has also been linked to heart disease, Carson, who was a longtime heavy smoker, not only had emphysema but also had a heart attack and quadruple bypass surgery in 1999.[83]

"We will not see the likes of him again," Letterman said of Carson.[84] "He was the best, a star and a gentleman."[85] Jay Leno, who took over *The Tonight Show* after Carson retired, agreed. "No single individual has had as great an impact on television as Johnny. [He was] the gold standard [for late-night talk show hosts]."[86]

CHAPTER 26

Ken Lay

Died July 5, 2006

Former CEO of Enron

ON JULY 5, 2006, Ken Lay, the disgraced founder and former chairman and chief executive officer (CEO) of the Enron Corporation, an energy company based in Houston, Texas, and his wife, Linda, were vacationing in Snowmass, Colorado.[1] Snowmass is a small resort town located in the valley of the Roaring Fork River, between Aspen and Basalt. Only six weeks earlier, on May 25, Lay was found guilty of six counts of fraud and conspiracy and four counts of bank fraud.[2] Free on $5 million bond, he was scheduled to be sentenced on September 11 at a Houston courthouse.[3]

At about one o'clock in the morning, Lay awoke, and after speaking with his wife, he went into the bathroom.[4] Minutes later, his wife heard a loud thump. When she went to investigate, she found Lay on the bathroom floor; he was unresponsive.[5]

Lay had collapsed while sitting on the commode, after he vomited and had a brief seizure-like episode.[6] Emergency medical services were called, and life-support measures were initiated.[7]

Lay was transported to the Aspen Valley Hospital in Aspen, Colorado, where he was pronounced dead at 3:11 a.m. by Eric Hansen, Deputy Coroner of Pitkin County.[8]

"His heart simply gave out," said Lay's pastor, Reverend Stephen Wende of First United Methodist Church in Houston.[9] Lay was sixty-four years old.

The Autopsy

Dr. Robert A. Kurtzman, an osteopathic physician, a forensic pathologist, and the coroner of Mesa County in Colorado, conducted the autopsy at eleven in the morning, less than eight hours after Lay died.[10] He was assisted by Jill Johnson-Dare.[11] The autopsy was performed at Community Hospital in Grand Junction, Colorado.[12]

"The body is that of a normally developed, well-nourished male who appears appropriate for the reported age," Kurtzman wrote in the autopsy report.[13] Sixty-eight inches long, it weighed 173 pounds and had no tattoos.[14]

314

The scalp, which was balding, had slightly wavy gray hair up to four inches in length.[15] The eyes were brown, and the cornea was clear and without petechia (bleeding) on the conjunctiva or on the sclera, the white outer layer of the eyeball.[16] In addition, the nose was intact, the teeth were natural, and the neck, chest, and abdomen had no deformities.[17]

Besides chest and vocal cord injuries due to attempts at intubation and cardiopulmonary resuscitation, there were superficial injuries typical of a fall, including abrasions on the left side of the forehead and the left knee.[18] These were consistent with reports of the circumstances surrounding Lay's death.[19] No skull fractures or brain injuries were identified.[20]

All in all, the external examination found nothing unusual about Lay's body or its injuries.

The internal examination identified a fracture of the second rib, probably from a fall, but otherwise the contents of the abdomen and chest were all in their normal anatomical location.[21] The lungs, liver, bile ducts, gallbladder, pancreas, spleen, thymus, kidneys, and urinary bladder were all normal in appearance, as were the adrenals, thyroid, parathyroid, and pituitary glands.[22] While the prostate was enlarged and nodular, microscopic examination of prostate tissue identified only chronic inflammatory changes that were not cancerous.[23]

The brain was normally formed, with no evidence of swelling.[24] When brain tissue was examined under a microscope, only age-related changes were identified.[25]

I was especially interested to review the autopsy findings related to the gastrointestinal system, since prior to his death, Lay had complained of upper gastrointestinal symptoms, for which he had been taking medication.[26] However, when I reviewed the autopsy findings related to the esophagus and stomach, they were completely normal.[27] The stomach was not ulcerated, although it contained a half a liter of a turbid, light brown liquid with fragments of tomatoes, bacon, and a yellowish-white pasty substance, most likely cheese.[28] Besides digested food, the stomach also contained four partially dissolved capsules of drugs, the composition of which was never identified.[29] As for the small and large intestine and appendix, they were all unremarkable.[30]

Since so far none of the autopsy findings was abnormal, there was only one other physiological system that potentially could have been responsible for Lay's death—the cardiovascular system. I reviewed those findings next.

At 440 grams, the weight of Lay's heart was 33 percent more than the average weight of a normal heart.[31] Also, the aorta had marked atherosclerosis with accumulation of plaque and calcium in its distal end, which undoubtedly impeded the flow of oxygenated blood, especially to the heart and brain.[32] The presence of dead cardiac tissue in the left ventricle of the heart was clear evidence that Lay had suffered a heart attack.[33] Lastly, not only were two stents present in coronary arteries, one in the right coronary artery and another in the left anterior descending coronary artery, but there was also between 75 to over 90 percent occlusion of three major coronary arteries—the left circumflex coronary artery, the left anterior descending artery, and the right coronary artery—as well as diffuse calcification of all three arteries.[34] This undoubtedly put undue strain on Lay's heart and was a ticking time bomb, ready to explode with a massive heart attack.

Since Lay's esophagus, stomach, and the rest of his digestive system were normal, I wondered whether his esophageal symptoms may not have been caused by gastroesophageal reflux disease (GERD) at all.[35] A report published by the Mayo Clinic in Cleveland, Ohio, notes that symptoms of heartburn, angina (heart pain), and a heart attack can all feel very much alike.[36] Even experienced doctors cannot always tell the difference.[37] Considering Lay had two stents in his coronary arteries, three severely occluded coronary arteries, and evidence of a previous heart attack, it would not be surprising if his symptoms of chest pain had been due to heart disease and not heartburn.

Cause and Manner of Death

According to his wife, Lay did not complain of chest pain, nausea, or shortness of breath before he collapsed on the bathroom floor.[38] However, since he had vomited before he died, and since vomiting, as well as constipation, can be a potential side effect of an opioid overdose, I wondered whether Lay had been taking morphine-like drugs.[39] While the toxicology report was not available for review, Kurtzman reported that "analysis of bodily fluids did not reveal any significant toxicology findings."[40]

The circumstances surrounding Lay's death are very similar to the way Elvis Presley died.[41] Like Lay, Presley was also found unresponsive on the bathroom floor after falling from the commode.[42] And like Lay, Presley was pronounced dead sometime after three o'clock, although Presley's death was at three o'clock in the afternoon whereas Lay was pronounced deceased at three in the morning.[43] In addition, both Presley and Lay died from similar heart-related events, Presley "from hypertensive cardiovascular disease with arteriosclerotic heart disease as a contributing factor" and Lay from "arteriosclerotic cardiovascular disease."[44]

Both Presley and Lay had an enlarged heart, a risk factor for sudden death from an arrhythmia.[45] That they both fell from the commode before they died suggests they may have both been constipated and had pressed hard on their diaphragm as they defecated, thereby putting significant pressure on their heart and initiating an arrhythmia.[46] For Presley this is very likely, since he was known to be severely constipated.[47] As for Lay, while there is no mention in the autopsy report that he suffered from constipation, considering that he had an enlarged heart and from 75 to over 90 percent blockage of three major coronary arteries, it wouldn't have taken much pressure on his heart to cause an arrhythmia.[48]

After I reviewed the circumstances surrounding Lay's death, the autopsy findings and results of toxicology testing, published lay articles, and the scientific literature, I concluded that the immediate cause of death was a heart attack due to severe atherosclerotic cardiovascular disease, possibly in combination with an arrhythmia. The manner of death was natural.

Life and Career

Lay was born in 1942 in Tyrone, Missouri, an unincorporated community in southern Texas County.[49] Unlike his mother, who was a farmer, and his father, a Baptist minister who held several jobs to make ends meet, Lay dreamed of becoming rich.[50] "I was enamored with business and industry," Lay remembered.[51]

When Lay's family was taken in by relatives to live on a farm, Lay "spent a lot of time on a tractor and had a lot of time to think," he told the *Houston Chronicle*.[52] It wasn't until he was eleven years old that Lay lived in a house with indoor plumbing.[53]

In 1964, Lay graduated with a degree in economics from the University of Missouri.[54] A year later, he earned a master's degree in economics from the same university and became a senior economist at the Humble Oil and Refining Company, now known as Exxon.[55] While there, Lay took part-time courses toward his doctorate at the University of Houston, from which he graduated in 1970.[56]

Lay joined the navy in 1967 and was assigned to the Pentagon, where he studied the effect of defense spending on the economy.[57] After his military discharge in 1971, and while teaching night school at George Washington University in Washington, DC, Lay was recruited to become an assistant at the Federal Power Commission to his mentor and former professor of economics at the University of Missouri, Pinkney Walker.[58] In October 1972, Lay was appointed deputy undersecretary for energy.[59]

Between 1973 and 1984, Lay held positions at two pipeline companies—Florida Gas in Winter Park, Florida, and Transco Energy in Houston; he also became CEO of Houston Natural Gas Corporation.[60] In 1985, InterNorth of Omaha, Nebraska, purchased Houston Natural Gas Corporation for $2.4 billion and renamed the company Enron Corporation, with Lay as its new CEO.[61]

When Congress deregulated the sale of natural gas in 1989, Lay saw it as a business opportunity.[62] He hired Jeffrey Skilling as chief operating officer (COO) and transformed Enron into a company that traded energy derivative contracts.[63] In essence, Enron bought natural gas from a network of suppliers and then sold it to a network of consumers.[64] By signing contracts with Enron for a fee, it allowed natural gas producers to mitigate the risk posed by fluctuating energy prices.[65] In time, Enron became the world's largest energy trading company with more than $68 billion in market value.[66]

As COO, Skilling instituted the practice of "market-to-market accounting," a system in which Enron's outstanding derivative contracts on its balance sheet at any particular quarter were adjusted to the fair market value.[67] At the time, there were no quoted prices upon which to base valuations for derivative contracts, so Enron was free to develop its own discretionary valuation models, which often overstated the company's earnings.[68] This gave investors the false impression that Enron was achieving higher-than-actual profits.[69] Other shady accounting practices soon followed, including formation of "special purpose entities" and sham companies to hide Enron's losing assets.[70]

John Clifford Baxter, vice chairman of the board, warned Lay about accounting irregularities in May 2001.[71] On August 15, Sherron Watkins, an accountant and vice president at Enron, informed Lay of her concerns about the company's murky finance and accounting practices.[72] Enron might "implode under a series of accounting scandals," Watkins told Lay.[73]   After hearing from Baxter and Watkins, Lay immediately began to sell about $100 million worth of his own Enron stock while at the same time assuring his employees that Enron's future was secure and urging them to buy more stock.[74]

The Securities and Exchange Commission began to investigate Enron on October 22, 2001.[75] As details of the company's accounting fraud began to emerge, Enron's stock price plummeted from its high of ninety dollars per share to an astonishing twenty-six cents a share by November 30, 2001.[76] Two days later, Enron filed for Chapter 11 bankruptcy protection.[77] As for the company's employees, many lost their life savings, which in many cases were tied up in Enron shares, as well as their 401(k) pensions.[78]

On January 28, 2002, Lay's wife appeared on the *Today* show and declared that she and Lay were broke.[79] In the same month, Baxter was found dead in his locked automobile with a gunshot wound to the head—an apparent suicide.[80] A month later, Lay put his numerous houses and estates up for sale.[81] Soon thereafter, his wife opened a shop in Houston where she sold furnishings and knickknacks she had accumulated over the years and with which she had decorated her several homes.[82]

Despite his wrongdoings and accounting trickery, Lay remained a member of Houston's social elite until July 2004.[83] It was then that he was indicted by a federal grand jury on eleven counts "for his role in a wide-ranging scheme to defraud by falsifying Enron's publicly reported financial results and making false and misleading public representations about Enron's business performance and financial condition."[84]

Twenty-two people were convicted for their actions related to Enron's fraud, including nearly all of the company's executive management team, according to Michael E. Anderson, assistant special agent in charge of the FBI's Houston Division.[85] Lay continued to maintain his innocence even after he was convicted on May 15, 2006.[86]

"Certainly, we're surprised," Lay said outside of the courtroom after he heard the jury's verdict.[87] "I firmly believe I'm innocent of the charges against me."[88] To the end, Lay claimed that business failure was not the same as a crime.[89] "As CEO of the company, I accept responsibility for Enron's collapse," Lay told reporters.[90] "However, I firmly reject any notion that I engaged in any wrongful or criminal activity."[91]

Lay's thoughts on the subject did not matter. Within six weeks, he was dead.

Conclusions

"I always thought of Ken … as a very decent, good human being," said John Olson, a Houston energy analyst at the Sanders Morris Harris Group.[92] Lay had a winning personality that made people love to be around him.[93]

"Ken Lay was a charming fellow and always presented himself as such," said Curtis L. Hébert Jr., chairman of the Federal Energy Regulatory Commission.[94]

The question remains, How could Lay, a man who came from such modest beginnings, who was revered as a visionary, and who, by the late 1990s, enjoyed a lavish, luxurious lifestyle and great popularity, have fallen so low?[95] The answer, according to Gordon Gekko, the fictionalized financial tycoon in the movie *Wall Street*, is "greed."[96] "The thing with money, it makes you do things you don't want to do," said Lou Mannheim, the fictionalized character with a conscience in the film.[97]

"The Enron and Ken Lay stories are best told in an English literature or a classics class, where you are trying to explain what hubris is all about," said Bill Burton, a Texas lawyer who by 2002 had known Lay for more than ten years.[98] Kathleen Magruder, a former Enron regulatory lawyer, still sympathizes with Lay, despite having lost $1.3 million in savings and investments when Enron went bankrupt. "Ken

Lay was a good man," she said.[99] "It is a shame people won't remember the good things he did for this city."[100]

"I wanted very badly to believe what they were saying," Wendy Vaughan, a juror in the Enron case said after the verdicts were announced.[101] "[However,] there were places in the testimony I felt their character was questionable."[102]

After Lay died, Judge Simeon T. Lake III vacated Lay's fraud and conspiracy conviction because Lay wasn't able to pursue an appeal of his guilty verdict.[103] The judge's ruling had no impact on any of the many pending civil claims made against the Lay estate.[104]

CHAPTER 27

Alexander Litvinenko

Died November 23, 2006

Former Officer of the Russian Federal Security Service

NOVEMBER 1, 2006, was a very special day for Alexander Litvinenko, a vocal critic of the Kremlin and a former officer in the Russian Federal Security Service (FSB) of the Russian Federation.[1] It was the sixth anniversary of his arrival in the United Kingdom and the first time he and his wife, Marina, celebrated the momentous event after becoming British citizens.[2] To commemorate the occasion, Marina, a former dance instructor, cooked a special meal, which she and Litvinenko ate together later that night.[3]

Litvinenko had spent the morning of November 1 at his home on Osier Crescent in Muswell Hill, making arrangements for his meetings later in the day, but at about 12:30 p.m., he left the house and traveled by bus and Tube into central London, arriving at Oxford Circus at about one thirty.[4] After a short two o'clock meeting at the office of Dean Attew, director of Titon International, Litvinenko walked to Piccadilly Circus, arriving at 3:00 p.m., just in time to meet Mario Scaramella, an Italian academic nuclear expert who was attending the annual conference of the International Maritime Organization.[5] Scaramella wanted to pass along information he had received from Yevgeny Limarev, a former employee of SVR, the Foreign Intelligence Service of the Russian Federation, about a list of "enemies of Russia" who were to be "eliminated," possibly by poisoning with radioactive thallium; the list included Litvinenko's name.[6]

When they reached the Itsu sushi restaurant, Scaramella showed Litvinenko the threatening emails from Limarev, but Litvinenko brushed them off, saying, "It doesn't matter, if it's from Evgeni, it means not credible … it's shit if it's from Evgeni."[7] Unlike Litvinenko, Scaramella took Limarev's warnings very seriously, especially since his name also was on the list.[8]

At 3:38 p.m., Litvinenko received a phone call from Andrei Lugovoy, a former Russian KGB intelligence officer, who was at the Millennium Hotel on London's Grosvenor Square, along with Dmitry Kovtun, a former officer in the Russian army.[9] The three men had planned to meet at five o'clock at the Pine Bar on the ground level of the hotel, next to the reception area.[10] "Come quicker, I am waiting for you,"

Lugovoy told Litvinenko.[11] It took Litvinenko only a couple of minutes to end his conversation with Scaramella and walk to the Millennium Hotel, which he arrived at just before four o'clock.[12]

When Litvinenko entered the hotel's lobby, Lugovoy was already sitting alone at the bar.[13] As he later recounted, "There was nobody else there ... There were a few mugs on the table and there was also a tea pot."[14] The waiter approached the two men and asked whether they wanted anything else, to which Litvinenko replied he did not.[15] Addressing Litvinenko, Lugovoy said, "Okay, well, we're going to leave now anyway. There is still some tea left here, if you want you can have some," at which time Litvinenko poured himself tea into a clean cup.[16] "Although there was only little left on the bottom and it made just half a cup ... It was green tea with no sugar and it was already cold," Litvinenko later recalled.[17] "I don't drink alcohol generally."[18] Soon Kovtun joined them, and after talking for about twenty minutes, they ended the meeting at about 4:40 p.m.[19]

According to his wife, Litvinenko was "absolutely fine" when he returned from central London later that evening.[20] But sometime in the middle of the night, during the early hours of November 2, Litvinenko became sick with severe vomiting.[21] By daybreak, he looked "very exhausted," could not keep his food or drink down, and was vomiting "again and again."[22] When his condition worsened, Litvinenko's wife called Dr. Yuri Prikazchikov, a well-known doctor in the local Russian community, who suggested Litvinenko take salt and a mineral solution.[23] Litvinenko did as the doctor suggested, but he was unable to keep the solution down.[24]

By the early hours of November 3, with Litvinenko not getting any better, his wife called for an ambulance.[25] Paramedics arrived and concluded that Litvinenko was probably suffering from "the flu" and advised him to stay home.[26] But by morning, Litvinenko felt worse, experiencing bloody diarrhea and complaining of abdominal pain. Prikazchikov, the Russian doctor, was summoned, and he diagnosed Litvinenko with food poisoning, or possibly some sort of infection.[27] Prikazchikov arranged to have Litvinenko admitted to Barnet Hospital, where he was diagnosed with gastroenteritis and mild dehydration and treated with a regimen of ciprofloxacin, a broad-spectrum antibiotic.[28]

Over the following days, Litvinenko began to lose his hair.[29] Blood tests showed a decreasing platelet count, an elevated hemoglobin level, and a significant drop in red and white blood cell count.[30]

On or around November 9, Litvinenko's wife, knowing that Russian FSB agents had poisoned other defectors in the past, raised the possibility her husband had been poisoned, but Dr. Dean Creer, a consulting physician at Barnet Hospital, told her Litvinenko's symptoms were unlikely the result of intentional poisoning or an infection.[31]

On November 13, Dr. Andres Virchis, a consulting hematologist, took over Litvinenko's care.[32] Virchis soon realized Litvinenko's symptoms were not consistent with a diagnosis of gastroenteritis or with ciprofloxacin toxicity.[33]

Based on his experience with cancer patients, he felt the symptoms were more similar to those of a patient suffering from acute leukemia who had been treated with chemotherapy and irradiation prior to a bone marrow transplant.[34] However, when he examined Litvinenko with a Geiger counter on November 15, he did not detect any radioactivity.[35]

The following day, the hospital's poison unit informed Virchis that despite a low thallium level, Litvinenko's condition should be considered as "suspicious thallium poisoning" and that he should begin treating Litvinenko with Prussian blue, a recognized treatment for thallium poisoning.[36]

Thallium, one of the most toxic heavy metals, is in a group that includes mercury, cadmium, arsenic, chromium, and lead.[37] It can cause adverse health effects in many organs, most severely in the nervous system.[38] Although thallium had previously been used as an insecticide and rodenticide against rats and squirrels, that was no longer the case due to its severe toxicity and occasional use in suicide and homicide.[39] Currently, thallium use is increasing in emerging new technologies and in the high-tech industry.[40]

Virchis was concerned that blood tests showed that Litvinenko's blood-forming elements were no longer identifiable in his bone marrow.[41] On November 17, he transferred Litvinenko to the University College Hospital for a possible bone marrow transplant.[42]

Despite some improvement due to his treatment with Prussian blue, Litvinenko soon began vomiting blood and having abdominal pain.[43] His temperature became elevated, he experienced an irregular heartbeat, and his kidney and liver functions were rapidly deteriorating.[44] Dr. Amit Nathwani, a consulting hematologist at the hospital, described Litvinenko's condition as "uncharted territory."[45] On November 20, he transferred Litvinenko to the intensive care unit, where he was given a blood transfusion and underwent dialysis to remove toxins from his blood.[46]

A consensus soon emerged among Litvinenko's treating physicians that his symptoms were not consistent with thallium poisoning, mainly because of the low thallium blood levels, the absence of neurotoxicity—peripheral neuropathy, pain, or numbness in the fingers and feet—and the lower-than-normal number of platelets and red and white blood cells in the blood ("pancytopenia").[47] The hospital's poisons unit advised Nathwani to consider the possibility Litvinenko's symptoms were not caused by thallium at all but instead were caused by an unidentified radioisotope.[48]

In two separate instances during the night of November 21, Litvinenko underwent cardiac arrest, for which he was resuscitated.[49] The following day, his treatment with Prussian blue was discontinued and samples of his blood and urine were sent to the Atomic Weapons Establishment for testing.[50] The test results, which arrived sometime on November 23, revealed that Litvinenko had been poisoned with radioactive polonium-210, an "extremely rare" radioisotope.[51] The results were subsequently confirmed with a second urine test.

At 8:51 p.m. on November 23, 2006, Litvinenko suffered a third cardiac arrest.[52] A half hour later, he was pronounced dead after further attempts at resuscitation were terminated.[53] He was forty-three years old.[54]

The Autopsy

I reviewed medical records of November 3 to 23, 2006, which showed bone marrow and multiorgan failure, as well as the development of alopecia (hair loss)—symptoms consistent with acute radiation exposure—and inflammation of the back of the throat and esophagus consistent with ingestion of the radioisotope.[55] Other factors noted in the hospital records included sepsis, fungal infection, arrhythmias, and cardiorespiratory arrest due to bone marrow failure and its metabolic consequences.[56]

The autopsy was conducted on December 1, 2006, at the Royal London Hospital by two forensic pathologists—Drs. Nathaniel Cary and Benjamin Swift.[57] Special safety precautions were taken because of the radioactivity present in Litvinenko's body.[58] These precautions included the wearing of white safety suits, protective gloves taped at the sleeves, and specialized hoods into which air was piped through a filter.[59] Cary described the autopsy as "one of the most dangerous postmortem examinations ever undertaken in the Western world," an observation with which Swift concurred.[60]

The external examination did not reveal any evidence of underlying natural disease that could have caused Litvinenko's death.[61]

The internal examination identified "changes in the internal organs ... typical of those seen at the end stage of multi-organ failure in an intensive care setting."[62]

Cause and Manner of Death

Prior to November 1, 2006, Litvinenko was "an extremely healthy man."[63] He exercised regularly and did not drink alcoholic beverages or smoke cigarettes.[64]

Routine microscopic pathological examination could not be done owing to the hazardous nature of the tissue samples taken from Litvinenko's body.[65]

Radiological testing of Litvinenko's urine on November 20, 2006, identified extremely high levels (4.4 Gbq) of polonium-210, a radioactive material that emits alpha particles.[66] Of the various bodily organs, the highest level of radioactivity was in the kidneys, and the lowest in the lungs.[67] Low levels of polonium-210 were detected in the mesentery, a fold in the peritoneum; testicles; muscle; brain; bile; heart; and blood.[68] "The calculated amount [of radioactivity] absorbed was far in excess of known survivability limits," Carey concluded.[69]

Analysis of samples of Litvinenko's hair indicated he had been exposed to polonium-210 on two separate occassions.[70] Based on extensive evidence collected in support of "The Litvinenko Inquiry," as well as closed-circuit television footage, it was determined that the fatal second exposure to polonium-210 occurred on November 1, 2006.[71] Because of uncertainties over the rate of hair growth and the potential effects that radiation may have on hair growth, it was estimated that the first exposure had taken place sometime between October 14 and 23.[72]

Dr. John Harrison, director of the Public Health England Center for Radiation, Chemical, and Environmental Hazards, explained that while alpha particles emitted by polonium-210 are too weak to penetrate the skin, they are lethal if ingested.[73] "Ionizing radiation, including gamma rays and alpha particles, can kill cells by damaging biological molecules within them, including DNA," Harrison said.[74] "Enough alpha particles will kill enough cells to cause gross tissue damage, organ failure and death."[75] Harrison further concluded, "Death is the inevitable outcome of the radiation doses estimated to have been received by Mr. Litvinenko's red bone marrow, kidneys and liver. Bone marrow failure is likely to be an important contributory cause of death occurring within a few weeks of intake, as a component of multiple organ failure."[76]

Some people have suggested Litvinenko accidentally poisoned himself while handling polonium-210, but that is mere speculation.[77] Litvinenko had never been involved in dealing with radioactive materials, and the radioactive contamination in his home was consistent with low-level incidental contamination.[78] Furthermore, since Litvinenko's exposure to polonium-210 was by ingestion, it would seem highly unlikely he could have accidentally drunk a solution containing the radioactive material.[79]

Another theory proposed for Litvinenko's poisoning with polonium-210 is that he intentionally ingested this radioactive substance when he attempted to commit suicide, but there is no evidence to support this claim either.[80] Litvinenko had not been depressed prior to November 1.[81] On the contrary, he was busy and active.[82] According to his family and friends, Litvinenko had "everything to live for, a happy marriage, very fond of his son, British citizenship, he'd made the leap from [Russia]. Opportunities ahead of him."[83] And while Litvinenko left a written statement two days prior to his death, the note was far from a suicide note. In it Litvinenko not only thanked his wife, the British public, and the hospital staff who took care of him but also addressed the president of Russia, writing, "You may succeed in silencing one man, but the howl of protest from around the world will reverberate, Mr. Putin, in your ears for the rest of your life."[84]

After I reviewed the circumstances surrounding Litvinenko's death, the autopsy findings and results of toxicology testing, published lay articles, and the scientific literature, I concluded that the immediate cause of death was multiple organ failure, including progressive heart failure, due to radiation syndrome caused by oral exposure to high levels of radioactive polonium-210.[85] The manner of death was homicide.

Life and Career

Litvinenko was born in 1962 in the Russian city of Voronezh.[86] His parents divorced when he was very young.[87] Thereafter, he shuttled between living with his father and grandparents in Nalchik, in the North Caucasus, and living with his mother in Moscow, or an aunt in Morzovsk.[88]

In 1980, when he was twelve years old, Litvinenko began living full-time with his grandparents in Nalchik, in the foothills of the Caucasus Mountains, near the Chechnya border.[89]   Litvinenko finished school when he was seventeen years old.[90] Not having been accepted into a university, he went to a military college instead.[91] Located about eighty miles from Nalchik in the city of Ordzhonikidze in North Ossetia, the college was a training center for Ministry of Internal Affairs of the USSR (Interior Ministry) forces.[92] After graduating as a lieutenant in 1985, he served for three years as a platoon commander in the Dzerzhinsky Division of the forces of the Interior Ministry.[93]

In 1988, Litvinenko was recruited by the KGB into its counterintelligence section as an informant.[94] He studied for a year at the Novosibirsk Military Counter Intelligence School in Siberia, after which he was detailed to the Third Chief Directorate, Military Counterintelligence, at the KGB headquarters in Moscow, where he became an operational officer.[95] Assigned to the Economic Security and Organized Crime Unit in 1991, Litvinenko was transferred three years thereafter to the Anti-Terrorism Department, which later became the Federal Counterintelligence Service (FSK), where he specialized in counterterrorism activities and infiltration into organized crime.[96] It was while working at the FSK, investigating the activities of criminal groups, that he became convinced there was widespread collusion between various criminal groups and KGB senior officials, including Vladimir Putin and Nikolai Patrushev, the director of the FSB.[97]

In June 1994, Boris Berezovsky, an "oligarch" with considerable wealth and political influence, narrowly escaped an assassination attempt.[98] Asked by the FSB to "maintain regular contact" with the oligarch, Litvinenko soon developed a close relationship with Berezovsky that further flourished in March 1995 when he prevented the police from arresting Berezovsky for the murder of Vlad Listyev, who at the time was the most popular television presenter in Russia.[99] "After that, Boris Berezovsky said many times Sasha [Litvinenko] saved his life, and he was very grateful," Litvinenko's wife later said.[100]

In 1994, Litvinenko became actively involved in the first Chechen War, doing "analytical work" and planting FSB agents in Nalchik, near Chechnya.[101] There is also evidence he participated in combat operations inside Chechnya.[102]

In the summer of 1997, Litvinenko was promoted to senior operational officer and deputy head of the "Seventh Section" at the Department for the Investigation and Prevention of Organized Crime (URPO).[103] The role of this "top secret department" was "killing political and high business men … without verdict," Litvinenko said.[104] By the end of the year, Litvinenko was asked to conduct several operations he regarded as unlawful, including "to physically exterminate Berezovsky … I disobeyed the order only because it was an illegal order."[105]

Litvinenko's frustration with corruption in the FSB came to a head in November 1998 when he and four other FSB officers appeared in a press conference and publically accused their superiors of ordering the assassination of Berezovsky.[106] "Never in the history of the Russian security services has the FSB experienced such a public exposure," Litvinenko's wife testified at a subsequent inquiry.[107] "[Litvinenko] and the others talked about corruption, criminalization of the FSB, and the fact that a system that was set up to protect the people was turning into a system from which people needed to be protected."[108] Instead of seeing the press conference as a first step toward reforming the FSB, the FSB viewed it as a threat to its authority.[109] In December 1998, Litvinenko and the other officers involved in the press conference were dismissed from the FSB; in March 1999, Litvinenko was arrested for staging the press conference and for "exceeding his authority."[110] He was eventually aquitted.[111]

Fearing for his safety and that of his family, Litvinenko fled Russia in November 2000.[112] Landing at England's Heathrow Airport, he approached the first police officer he saw and said, "I am KGB officer and I'm asking for political asylum."[113] In May 2001, Litvinenko and his family were given political asylum in the UK; in October 2006, they became naturalized British citizens.[114]

In 2002, Litvinenko was convicted in Russia in absentia on corruption charges.[115] Working in the UK as a consultant, Litvinenko assisted MI6, the British spy agency, and Spanish authorities on Kremlin links to organized crime in their respective countries.[116] In addition, he continued his vocal criticisms of Putin, now the president of Russia, for being responsible for the murders of Russian journalist Anna Politkovskaya and Armenian prime minister Vasgen Sargsyan, the seizure of the Moscow theater in 2002, and the Beslan school siege in 2004.[117]

On November 1, 2006, less than three weeks after becoming a British citizen, Litvinenko let his guard down and had tea with a former Russian FSB operative and a former Russian soldier at a bar in London's Millennium Hotel. Three weeks later, he was dead.

Conclusions

In 1898, Marie Curie discovered polonium-210, a rare and extremely deadly radioactive element that is up to a trillion times more toxic than hydrogen cyanide; Curie named it after her native country, Poland.[118] Having a very short half-life of only 138 days, the time for the radioactivity to decay by 50 percent, the radioisotope does not accumulate in nature to any significant degree, but it can be artificially made by bombarding atoms of bismuth with neutrons—subatomic particles without an electric charge, similar to protons.[119] Since polonium's alpha particles can travel only for short distances, they are easily absorbed by other materials, such as sheets of paper, thereby making polonium-210 difficult to detect with radiation detectors, including Geiger counters.[120] This explains why, on November 15, 2006, Virchis, Litvinenko's treating physician at Barnet Hospital failed to detect radioactivity being emitted from Litvinenko.

As long as polonium-210 remains outside of the body, it cannot damage internal organs since its alpha particles cannot pass through the skin.[121] However, if ingested, it can damage DNA, reduce white blood cell count, and damage hair follicles and internal organs, such as the liver, kidneys, spleen, gastrointestinal tract, and bone marrow—symptoms experienced by Litvinenko.[122]

Polonium had been produced in the United States until 1971, but since then, only one place in the world has had a nuclear facility capable of recovering polonium-210 from irradiated bismuth—the closed town of Sarov, in Nizhny Novgorod Oblast, five hundred miles south-east of Moscow, the center of Russia's nuclear research industry.[123] When it was determined Litvinenko had been poisoned with radioactive polonium-210, all indications immediately pointed to Russia as the obvious source of the radioisotope.[124]

After thorough tests by forensic scientists and law enforcement agencies in the UK, it was conclusively established that Litvinenko was poisoned by Lugovoy and Kovtun on November 1, 2006, when he ingested green tea contaminated with polonium-210 at the Pine Bar of the Millennium Hotel.[125] Alpha radiation was detected on the table at the Pine Bar where Lugovoy, Kovtun, and Litvinenko dined, as well as on one of the chairs at the adjacent table where they sat.[126] Most importantly, the hotel's white teapot, which was used to pour tea for Litvinenko, was identified, and the inside of its spout was highly contaminated with polonium-210.[127] It was concluded that "at some stage polonium … [had] been poured out of the spout."[128] Extensive radioactive contamination was also detected in Lugovoy's and Kovtun's hotel rooms, as well as in the bathroom of Kovtun's hotel room and in the U-bend sediment trap below the plughole of his bathroom sink.[129] Other locations linked to the two Russian agents, including restaurants, automobiles, airplanes, hotel restrooms, and office boardrooms, were also contaminated with radioactivity.[130] "The evidence points resolutely to Lugovoy and Kovtun and no one else as having administered the poison which killed Litvinenko," a representative of London's Metropolitan Police Service said.[131]

"I have no doubt whatsoever that this was done by the Russian Secret Services," Litvinenko declared after he was poisoned.[132] "Having knowledge of the system, I know that the order about such a killing of a citizen of another country on its territory, especially if it [is] something to do with Great Britain could have been given by only one person," he added.[133] When Litvinenko was asked who that person was, he replied, "That person is the President of the Russian Federation, Vladimir Putin."[134]

Lugovoy and Kovtun had attempted to poison Litvinenko on a previous occasion—October 16, 2006—when they all sat together for a meeting at Erinys, a security firm in London.[135] It was a "normal, very peaceful evening," Litvinenko's wife said, recalling the evening of October 16, but later that night, Litvinenko suddenly began to feel ill and vomited, his symptoms lasting about two days.[136] Subsequent testing detected high levels of polonium-210 contamination in Erinys's boardroom, as well as in Lugovoy's room and bathroom at the Best Western Hotel and in the U-bend sediment trap below the plughole of the bathroom sink in his hotel room.[137] Most likely, the reason Litvinenko did not die after ingesting polonium-210 on October 16 was because his exposure to the radioisotope was too low—one hundred times less than on November 1.[138]

Ten days after the meeting at Erinys, Lugovoy accidentally spilled the polonium-210 radioactive solution in his hotel room at London's Sheraton Hotel.[139] He mopped up the spill with two towels, which were later found in the hotel's laundry; both towels were highly contaminated with radioactivity.[140] Radioactive contamination was also detected in the bathroom of Lugovoy's hotel room and in a garbage can in his bathroom.

Apparently Lugovoy and Kovtun knew they were using a deadly "very expensive poison" to kill Litvinenko, but they most likely were unaware of its name or nature of the poison's properties.[141] "I really can't imagine that he would put my children in danger," Marina Wall, Kovtun's first wife, said when she found out her apartment in Hamburg, Germany, had been contaminated by Kovtun when he spent the nights of October 28 and 31 there while visiting their children.[142] Alexei Kondaurov, a former KGB general, explained. "Let's for the sake of argument, assume that I had been in charge of such an operation ... and let's assume Luguvoy was involved. I would have told him as little as possible. Agents are used all the time

341

without knowing the full details of an operation," Kondaurov said.[143] Because of their ignorance about the properties of the poison in their possession, Lugovoy and Kovtun failed to take proper precautions, pouring the remainder of the radioisotope solution down the sink of their hotel bathrooms on October 16 and November 1, and in the process contaminating themselves and their families. "Those arseholes have probably poisoned us all," Kovtun told his former mother-in-law when he became ill with radiation poisoning.[144]

In September 2021, the European Court of Human Rights in Strasbourg, France, issued its ruling, agreeing with the UK inquiry's conclusion. "The planned and complex operation involving the procurement of a rare deadly poison, the travel arrangements for the pair [Lugovoy and Kovtun], and repeated and sustained attempts to administer the poison indicated that Litvinenko had been the target of the operation."[145] The court further noted, "… there was a strong prima facie case that in poisoning Mr. Litvinenko, Mr. Lugovoy and Mr. Kovtun had been acting as agents of the Russian State."[146]

The Russian government has had a long history of "killing … prominent critics of Putin and his administration," said Robert Service, professor of Russian History at Oxford University.[147] In 2002, Ibn al-Khattab, an Islamist guerrilla leader, was killed after he licked an envelope smeared with poison.[148] In the same year, Vladimir Golovlev, founder of the Liberal Russia party, was shot and killed while walking his dog in a Moscow park.[149] Chechen vice president Zelinkhan Yandarbiev, a strong critic of the Putin administration, was killed in an explosion as he left a mosque in February 2004.[150] And in September of the same year, Roman Tsepo, a Russian businessman, died after drinking a cup of tea that probably was laced with a radioactive substance.[151]

Of the many Russian state-sponsored poisonings, perhaps the best known recent cases are those of Georgi Markov, a Bulgarian defector who was stabbed in 1978 with a ricin-tipped umbrella on London's Waterloo Bridge as he waited to catch a bus to the BBC station where he worked as a broadcaster; the 2018 poisoning of former Russian spy Sergei Skripal and his daughter, Yulia, with Novichok nerve agent smeared on the front door handle of their home; and Alexei Navalny in 2020, a Russian opposition leader who was poisoned with the same Novichok nerve agent planted in his underpants. There was additionally the release of a gas containing carfentanil, an opioid drug ten thousand times more powerful than morphine, into a Moscow theater in 2002, knocking unconscious nearly all the Chechen terrorists and their hostages, and the killing of 120 hostages and most of the guerrillas in the military raid that followed.[152] In light of all of the killings and poisonings of Russian opposition leaders and so-called "enemies of Russia," it should be no surprise that Litvinenko's poisoning was state-sponsored by Russia.

CHAPTER 28

Evel Knievel

Died November 30, 2007

Stunt Performer

SOME MIGHT CALL Evel Knievel a stunt performer, while others might describe him as a daredevil. No matter what the label, for most, the idea of flying on a motorcycle over fourteen Greyhound buses with only a helmet and a leather jumpsuit for protection is beyond imagination.[1] And yet for Knievel, it was all in a day's work.

On May 6, 1975, three weeks before his scheduled jump over thirteen single-decker British buses, Knievel arrived at London's Wembley Stadium to inspect the venue.[2] "He was a little wacko" but "I kind of admired him," Frank Gifford, a former running back for the New York Giants and broadcaster for Wide World of Sports, said of Knievel.[3]

On the day of the jump, Knievel looked out at the AEC Merlin buses lined up side by side and told Gifford, "I can't do this."[4] Unlike American Greyhound buses, the British buses were six inches wider, adding up to an additional 6.5 feet, for a total jump of 120 feet.[5] Knievel feared there was not enough room on the takeoff ramp to get up to speed to clear the buses.[6] With ninety thousand spectators counting on him, somehow he would have to find the speed.[7]

After two practice runs, Knievel gave the thumbs up sign that he was ready.[8] Traveling on his Harley-Davidson XR-750 motorcycle at nearly ninety-five miles per hour, Knievel came down hard on the plywood extension covering the top of the thirteenth bus.[9] Bouncing high in the air, he tried to hold on to the handlebars but was unable to do so, the momentum forcing him to tumble forward over the front of the bike.[10] After rolling several yards, he finally came to rest, his motorcycle on top of him.[11]

"Oh, my God," Gifford cried out into his live microphone, "he's down and he is hurt."[12] A bone was sticking out of Knievel's hand, an obvious compound fracture, and blood was coming from his mouth.[13] Knievel was put on a stretcher, and while being carried toward an ambulance, he asked to be helped up. "I walked in and I want to walk out," he told Gifford.[14]

With an arm over the shoulder of his promoter, John Daly, Knievel approached the microphone.[15] "Ladies and gentlemen of this wonderful country," he said, "I have to tell you that you are the last people in the world who will see me jump, because I will never, ever, ever jump again. I'm through."[16]

At the Royal London Hospital in Whitechapel, a district in East London, Knievel was diagnosed with a broken right hand, a compound fracture of the fourth and fifth vertebrae, a fractured left pelvis, and a nearly eight-inch split in his right pelvis.[17] Nevertheless, despite the announcement of his impending retirement, Knievel was at Kings Island theme park in Mason, Ohio, only five months later, ready to jump over fourteen Greyhound buses, a distance of 133 feet.[18] This time he cleared the buses without suffering any injuries.[19] It was the last big jump of Knievel's career, setting a record he held for twenty-four years.[20]

In 1981, Knievel officially retired as a stunt performer, telling reporters he was "nothing but scar tissue and surgical steel."[21] A recipient of the Guinness World Record for the "most broken bones in a lifetime—four hundred and thirty-three," Knievel was the "bionic man," held together with aluminum plates in both arms, titanium in his hip, and numerous pins in his remaining bones and joints.[22] In the ensuing years, his health deteriorated significantly.

In 1999, Knievel underwent a liver transplant after nearly dying of hepatitis C, most likely contracted during one of his many blood transfusions.[23] In 2005, he was diagnosed with idiopathic pulmonary fibrosis (IPF), an incurable terminal disease causing lung scarring.[24] A year later, a morphine pump was surgically implanted to help relieve the excruciating pain in Knievel's lower back.[25] Compounding his health problems further were his diagnoses of diabetes and arthritis, as well as having two strokes in the following years.[26]

Days before he died, Knievel gave an interview in which he struggled to breathe through a nose tube connected to an oxygen tank.[27] "All my life people have been waiting around to watch me die," he told the interviewer.[28] "[Well,] I'm dying. This may be the last interview I ever do."[29]

On November 30, 2007, Knievel was at his condominium apartment in Clearwater, Florida, having difficulty breathing.[30] He died before an ambulance could transport him to a hospital.[31] He was sixty-nine years old.[32]

The Autopsy

No autopsy or toxicology testing was performed after Knievel died.

Cause and Manner of Death

After I reviewed the circumstances surrounding Knievel's death, as well as published lay articles and the scientific literature, I concluded that the immediate cause of death was IPF; diabetes was a contributing factor. The manner of death was natural.

Life and Career

Knievel was born in 1938 in the copper-mining town of Butte, Montana.[33] His parents divorced when he was two years old, and he was raised by his paternal grandparents.[34] When he was eight, he attended a Joie Chitwood auto daredevil show, which inspired him many years later to become a motorcycle daredevil.[35]

At thirteen years of age, Knievel was arrested for stealing a Harley-Davidson motorcycle.[36] Three years later, his grandmother bought him a Triumph motorcycle.[37] In 1956, he was charged with reckless driving after crashing his motorcycle while being chased by police.[38]

While at Butte High School, Knievel excelled in track and field and in ice hockey, even winning the Northern Rocky Mountain Ski Association Class A Men's Ski Jumping Championship.[39] Struggling academically, he dropped out of school.[40] "He was no dummy," said Sonny Holland, Knievel's high school classmate and former Montana State football star and coach.[41] "I'll never forget a poem that he made up … about his friends and the people he hung out with. It was incredible. Everybody was just astounded when he recited it in front of the whole school."[42]

After leaving high school, Knievel held a job in the copper mines as a diamond drill operator with the Anaconda Mining Company.[43] Later, while working with an earth mover, he was fired when he attempted to do "wheelies" and collided into Butte's main power line, causing a major blackout for several hours.[44]

In the late 1950s, Knievel joined the army, volunteering for paratrooper school and making thirty jumps.[45] After his discharge from military service, he played semiprofessional and professional hockey with the Charlotte Clippers of the Eastern Hockey League, formed the Butte Bombers semiprofessional hockey team, and took up motorcycle racing, stopping in 1962 after falling in a race and breaking several bones.[46]

Knievel's subsequent jobs were as an insurance salesman and in hunting.[47] In the mid-1960s, he moved to Moses Lake, Washington, where he opened the Moses Lake Honda motorcycle dealership.[48] Unable to sell an adequate number of Japanese motorcycles because of steep competition from American automakers, he closed the shop and went to work at Don Pomeroy's motorcycle shop in Sunnyside, Washington.[49] To attract customers, he promised to jump on a motorcycle fifty feet over a box of rattlesnakes and two caged mountain lions.[50] One thousand new customers saw Knievel land short, but he managed to land safely.[51] "Right then, I knew I could draw a big crowd by jumping over weird stuff," Knievel later said.[52] It was the beginning of a new career as a stunt performer.[53]

In January 1966, with backing from Bob Blair, the West Coast distributor for Norton Motorcycles, the Evel Knievel and His Motorcycle Daredevils show was born.[54] Knievel recruited motorcyclists to perform at county fairs by doing wheelies, riding through burning walls of plywood, standing on the seats of their bikes, and jumping over vehicles.[55] It was a popular and entertaining show, but after several crashes and more broken bones, he disbanded the group.[56]

Knievel next began a solo act, jumping over cars.[57] To encourage people to come to his shows, he added more cars with each jump.[58] On June 19, 1966, while attempting to jump over twelve cars and a cargo van, Knievel crashed his motorcycle, suffering a severely broken arm and several broken ribs.[59] On May 30 of the following year, he successfully rode his motorcycle over sixteen cars in California.[60] When he attempted the same jump on July 28, 1967 in Graham, Washington, he crashed, suffering a serious concussion.[61] Not to be outdone, he returned to Graham about a month later only to crash again, this time breaking his left wrist, right knee, and two ribs.[62] Nonetheless, the publicity kept bringing more people to Knievel's daredevil shows, everyone wondering whether Knievel would survive his next jump. "They always expected more," Knievel said several years later.[63]

On New Year's Eve 1967, Knievel attempted his longest jump, which spanned 141 feet over the fountains at Caesar's Palace in Las Vegas, Nevada.[64] While he cleared the fountains, he came up short, tumbling like a ragdoll over the handlebars of his motorcycle and across the pavement, suffering a concussion, a crushed pelvis and femur, and fractures to his hip, wrist, and both ankles.[65] "It was terrible," Knievel said afterward.[66] "I lost control of the bike. Everything seemed to come apart. I kept smashing over and over and ended up against a brick wall."[67] Nonetheless, Knievel became more famous than he had ever been, with ABC-TV buying the rights to air the film of his jump on *Wide World of Sports*.[68]

By the time of his Snake River Canyon jump in Twin Falls, Idaho, in 1972, Knievel had broken his right leg and foot while attempting to jump fifteen Ford Mustangs in Scottsdale, Arizona (May 1968); had broken his hip for a second time in Carson City, Nevada (October 1968); had set a new world record (February 28, 1971) by jumping over nineteen cars in Ontario, California; had broken his collarbone and had suffered compound fractures of his right arm and both legs while attempting to jump thirteen Pepsi delivery trucks in May 1971; and had suffered a broken back and a concussion in Dale City, California (March 1972).[69]

The much-hyped jump over the canyon in a jet-powered rocket that took off from an inclined metal runway was a complete failure.[70] The parachute malfunctioned and deployed prematurely, and the wind caused the rocket to drift back toward the canyon, landing on the rocks a few feet from the river's edge.[71] When asked what went wrong, Knievel replied, "I was on the cover of *Sports Illustrated*. What more do you want?"[72] After the Snake River Canyon fiasco, Knievel turned away from rocket jumps and back to motorcycle jumping. His next jump, at Wembley Stadium, was to be a major televised event on *Wide World of Sports*.[73] Unfortunately, it did not go as planned.

Conclusions

What makes a man like Knievel jump on a motorcycle over fountains, buses, and cars, breaking numerous bones in the process and then rising again and going back for more? "I wanted to fly through the air. I was a daredevil, a performer," Knievel told *Maxim* magazine in 2007.[74] "I loved the thrill, the money, the whole macho thing. All those things made me Evel Knievel."[75] Stuart Barker, the author, noted, "His fame had little to do with the stunts he successfully pulled off and everything to do with the epic failures and wipeouts."[76]

To get the adulation he so desperately needed, Knievel paid a heavy price in injuries and damage to his body.[77] "You know, I had a couple hundred jumps in my career," he said, "and I made most of them, but the ones they show over and over are the ones when I crashed."[78] In his last interview before he died, Knievel observed, "Those extreme-sports kids today are good but they have it easy. Try falling off of a motorcycle going seventy or eighty miles per hour on asphalt. Believe me, nothing equals it."[79] Said Pat Williams, who represented Montana in the US House of Representatives from 1979 to 1997, "He was an amazing athlete … He was sharp as a tack, one of the smartest people I've ever known and finally, as the world knows, no one had more guts than Bobby. He was simply unafraid of anything."[80]

In 1976, Knievel promised to jump over "the world's largest indoor saltwater pool, which will be filled with man-eating killer sharks."[81] In a practice run at the Chicago International Amphitheater, he crashed and broke his right forearm and left collarbone.[82] It was the final jump in his long professional career as a stunt performer.

By the time he died, Knievel had a new liver and was suffering from diabetes and arthritis, but it was IPF that finally caused his death.[83] Unlike COPD, which is fairly common and includes emphysema and chronic bronchitis, IPF is a rare chronic, progressive, and terminal "interstitial lung disease," affecting the alveoli and disrupting gas exchange, making it difficult to breathe, ultimately leading to respiratory failure and death.[84]

There are two main types of pulmonary fibrosis: IPF, the type Knievel had, whose cause is unknown and whose clinical course is unpredictable; and familial pulmonary fibrosis, a rare type of pulmonary fibrosis with a better prognosis than IPF, mainly because it can be diagnosed at a much earlier stage.[85]

The risk of IPF is higher in smokers, but Knievel claimed he never smoked.[86] The risk is also greater in men between the ages of fifty and seventy, those with a family history of IPF, people who have specific gene mutations or breathe certain toxic chemicals, and those with comorbidities, such as GERD and sleep apnea.[87] Since scar tissue in the lungs interferes with oxygen exchange, the brain receives much less oxygen than normal, raising the risk for stroke, of which Knievel had two.[88]

Knievel was not the only famous person to suffer from pulmonary fibrosis. Others include comedian Jerry Lewis, actors Marlon Brando and James Doohan—"Scotty" of *Star Trek*—and singers Robert Goulet and Odetta.[89]

Knievel redefined what it meant to be a celebrity. "It's easy to be famous today," he said, reminiscing about his best days as a daredevil.[90] "People pay a million dollars to be recognized, but nobody cares about them. They cared about me because I did things other men were afraid to do."[91]

Wide World of Sports made Knievel a hero to young boys across the globe.[92] The kids imitated his stunts on bicycles and with Evel Knievel toys.[93] A new term—"Evel Knievel Syndrome"—was coined to explain the "imitative and aggressive behavior exhibited by children as a result of televised violence, especially during sporting events and news reporting."[94]

In 1994, the Smithsonian Institution displayed Knievel's customized Harley-Davidson XR-750 motorcycle and his star-spangled leather jumpsuit, cape, and boots in a special exhibition titled *America's Legendary Daredevil.*[95]

In his heyday, Knievel "spent money faster than he could earn it," Barker observed.[96] Said Knievel in 1998, "I made 60 million dollars in my lifetime and spent 61 million. I created the character called Evel Knievel and he sort of got away from me."[97] In a 2006 interview with the Associated Press, Knievel reflected on his life, regretting he had not set aside more money to take care of his family. "No king or prince has lived a better life," Knievel said.[98] "You're looking at a guy who's really done it all. And there are things I wish I had done better, not only for me but for the ones I loved."[99]

Part of Knievel's legacy is that he was a strong supporter of mandatory helmet laws.[100] "Anytime you see anybody riding a motorcycle without a helmet on, you're looking at a goddamned fool," he told *Big Bikes* magazine.[101] Said Richard Floyd, a California State Assemblyman who served from

1980 until 1992, "Mr. Knievel has broken virtually every bone in his body, but his head has always been protected."[102]

Another one of Knievel's core values was his anti-drug message, something he spoke about before every one of his jumps.[103] In 1971, he fought members of Hell's Angels for "being drug dealers," sending three of them to the hospital with significant injuries.[104]

In time, Knievel became a folk hero.[105] "Evel Knievel ... may be the last great gladiator," wrote David Lyle in *Esquire* magazine in 1970.[106] Always the showman, Knievel agreed, describing himself as "the last gladiator in the new Rome."[107]

CHAPTER 29

Dawn Brancheau

Died February 24, 2010
SeaWorld Trainer

"SPEND AN UNFORGETTABLE day at SeaWorld Orlando," screams the SeaWorld website.[1] "SeaWorld Orlando offers exciting rides and roller coasters, up-close animal encounters, and more."[2] Visitors to the water park got much more than they had bargained for on Wednesday, February 24, 2010.

Believe, The Spectacular Shamu Show had just ended, and the *Dine with Shamu Show* was already ongoing in the faux rock–lined, 1.6 million gallon "G-pool."[3] Wrapped around the north side of the pool was an open-air restaurant, ensuring families could view the show while eating a buffet lunch.[4]

On the south side of the pool, Dawn Brancheau, a vivacious blonde trainer, was putting Tilikum, a male orca, through some of the many routines he had learned over his nearly twenty-seven years in captivity.[5] Weighing six tons and measuring twenty-two feet long, Tilikum was the largest killer whale at SeaWorld.[6]

Since Tilikum had previously been involved in two drownings, one in 1991 of an assistant trainer at Sealand of the Pacific in British Columbia, Canada, and another in 1999 of a twenty-seven-year-old man who climbed into the pool at SeaWorld Orlando, all the SeaWorld trainers were acutely mindful to never get in the water with Tilikum.[7]

"We did not treat [Tilikum] as though he was one of our animals that we could get in the water and swim with," said Cuck Tompkins, curator of zoological operations at SeaWorld.[8] "We were much more careful with him."[9]

At the end of the show, Brancheau fed Tilikum herring and doused him a few times with a bucket of water, something he especially liked.[10] She then moved to a shallow concrete slab built into the side of the pool and lay down on her stomach, allowing the orca to float over and to rest his nose inches from her shoulder.[11] Smiling, Brancheau talked to Tilikum, stroking his head and, at one point, even hugging and kissing his nose, in what is known as a "relationship session."[12] "This was an interaction she had done thousands of times with Tilikum," Tompkins explained.[13]

Jan Topoleski, a trainer and spotter, was sitting on rocks a short distance to the west of Brancheau, monitoring her interaction with the killer whale, while Lynne Schaber kept a close watch from the east.[14]

Meanwhile, in the underwater viewing area, about fifty people had gathered in front of a huge glass, waiting for Tilikum to dive down for a photo op.[15] At the designated hour, Schaber, who had come down to the viewing area, signaled Brancheau to instruct Tilikum to dive down to the window.[16]

It was then that Brancheau's ponytail brushed the orca's nose and her hair floated into his mouth.[17] Seeing Brancheau struggling to free her hair, Topoleski immediately pushed an alarm button behind him; however, when he turned around again, Brancheau was no longer in sight.[18] "Within the span of two seconds, she was pulled into the pool, unable to get her hair released from his mouth," Topoleski later told authorities.[19]

When Schaber saw Tilikum pull Brancheau into the water, she knew her friend and colleague was in trouble.[20] "This whale is very possessive. It never releases things," Schaber later declared.[21] "He got her down and that was it—she wasn't getting out," Jonathan Smith, a former trainer, said.[22]

Stacy Nichols, who was employed by SeaWorld to assist with the photo tours, and Susanne DeWit, a tourist from the Netherlands who had booked an animal photo tour with lunch, were in the underwater viewing area when they saw Tilikum do a deep dive with Brancheau in his mouth.[23]

"Tilikum was shaking the trainer violently and moving extremely fast," DeWit remembered.[24]

359

Shocked by what they saw, visitors were quickly ushered out of the underwater viewing area by SeaWorld personnel.[25] Topside, Topoleski saw Brancheau's sandals floating on top of the water.[26]

At some point, Brancheau, who was a strong swimmer, broke free from Tilikum's jaws. As she began to swim toward the surface, the orca "impacted her squarely in the chest," according to Jessica Wilder, who saw what was happening from the underwater viewing area.[27] "He looped around and came back with his mouth open" and retrieved the trainer, Wilder said.[28]

SeaWorld trainers tried to rescue Brancheau by slapping the water and "asking for control," but Tilikum did not respond to their slaps and would not release Brancheau.[29] "He started pushing her with his nose like she was a toy," said Paula Gillespie, one of the visitors.[30]   Utilizing nets, the trainers next redirected Tilikum to the "F-pool" and then to the larger "E-pool," but the orca still would not release Brancheau.[31] He was then redirected to the much smaller medical "D-pool," where, after raising the pool's false bottom, the whale was finally beached.[32]

It took nearly thirty harrowing and chaotic minutes before Brancheau's lifeless body was extracted from Tilikum's mouth.[33] She was pronounced dead at poolside. Brancheau was forty years old.[34]

The Autopsy

At 8:20 a.m. the day following the accident, Dr. Joshua D. Stephany, associate medical examiner, conducted the autopsy.[35] "Forty year old white female, animal trainer, attacked by a killer whale (*Orcinus orca*) at work," Stephany wrote in the autopsy report.[36]

Topoleski, described as "a friend and coworker," identified the body as belonging to Brancheau.[37] It weighed 123 pounds, was sixty-nine inches long, and was clothed in the same black-and-white wet suit Brancheau had worn when she last performed with Tilikum.[38] In the oral cavity were two clear, transparent orthodontic Invisalign mouth guards used to "transform a smile."[39] On the fifth digit of the left hand was a yellow metal ring.[40]

Received separately by the coroner's office were black footwear and a whistle attached to a white rope, both of which were retrieved from the E-pool.[41] Also received was a portion of the scalp with attached hair and a fragment of red-pink muscle.[42]

On external examination, the scalp was covered with up to forty-three centimeters of long, brown hair.[43] Both earlobes were pierced; there were no tattoos either on the torso or on the arms and legs.[44] The green/hazel eyes, nose, and teeth were all without trauma.[45]

That Brancheau was in excellent physical shape before she died was evident from the internal examination. The cardiovascular system was free of plaque, the heart valves were thin and pliable, the aorta was elastic with no evidence of atherosclerosis, and the coronary arteries had the normal distribution.[46] In addition, at 245 grams, the heart's weight was well within the normal range.[47] As for the liver, it was smooth, tan-brown, and within the normal weight range.[48]

The gallbladder contained approximately five milliliters of viscous dark green bile, about a teaspoonful, not an unusual finding.[49] The spleen was normal.[50]

The stomach contained approximately twenty milliliters (four teaspoonfuls) of tan fluid but otherwise was unremarkable.[51] The small and large intestines had no palpable masses; the kidneys were smooth, each weighing ninety grams; the urinary bladder was empty, and the endocrine system was normal.[52]

Examination of the head failed to find any skull fractures.[53] As for the brain, it was free of hemorrhage, with no evidence of cancer or necrosis.[54]

What was most distressing and disturbingly horrifying were the numerous blunt-force injuries Brancheau had sustained to her head, neck, torso, arms, and legs that undoubtedly contributed to or caused her death. The scalp was torn away from the head (avulsion) and the left upper arm was avulsed from the body.[55]

Several fractures were apparent, including fractures of the jaw; the seventh cervical vertebra; the ninth, tenth, and eleventh left ribs; the sternum; and the proximal left humerus, the bone forming the joint in the shoulder.[56] In addition, the left elbow and left knee were dislocated.[57]

Besides the liver, mouth, and right ear, all of the numerous abrasions, contusions, and lacerations were on the left side of the body.[58] The abdominal cavity was filled with about seventeen ounces of blood.[59]

One anatomical change that supported a finding of drowning was the heavier-than-normal lung weights, with each lung weighing 61 to 71 percent more than the average weight of a corresponding normal lung.[60] Another diagnostic indicator of drowning was the presence of approximately four milliliters of fluid in the sphenoid sinuses, two hollow spaces in bones behind the nose and between the eyes.[61]

It was clear Brancheau died by drowning and that she had suffered extremely violent injuries. Nevertheless, for completeness, it was important that I review the toxicology report.

Cause and Manner of Death

Drugs did not play a role in Brancheu's death, as none was detected in the blood by an immunoassay toxicology screen or by a gas chromatography and mass spectrometry confirmatory toxicology test.[62]

Some of Bancheau's injuries were probably sustained while she was alive. However, considering how long she remained underwater, many of her traumatic blunt-force injuries most likely were inflicted after she had already drowned.

After I reviewed the circumstances surrounding Brancheau's death, the autopsy and toxicology reports, published lay articles, and the scientific literature, I concluded that the immediate cause of death was drowning combined with traumatic blunt-force injuries. The manner of death was accident.

Life and Career

Brancheau was born in 1969 in Cedar Lake, Indiana, the youngest of her five siblings.[63] When she was nine years old, she went on a family vacation to Orlando.[64] It was then that she set her sights on becoming a "Shamu" trainer.[65] The original Shamu, a female orca, died in 1971, but the stage name Shamu has since been trademarked and used by SeaWorld to designate all of its star orcas.[66]

After graduating from the University of South Carolina with degrees in psychology and animal behavior, Brancheau spent two years working with dolphins at Six Flags Great Adventure in Jackson, New Jersey.[67] In 1994, she joined SeaWorld Orlando, where she first worked with otters and sea lions and then with killer whales.[68] In 2011, after working for fifteen years with orcas, Brancheau was promoted to senior animal trainer.[69]

A longtime avid animal lover, Brancheau had been a volunteer at an animal shelter and had raised birds, rabbits, chickens, and ducks.[70] During her appearance in 2000 on an NBC-affiliate television station in Florida, she spoke about the importance of staying physically fit while working with orcas.[71] To keep in shape, Brancheau ran marathons, lifted weights, and pursued cycling and running.[72]

A highlight of any Shamu show at SeaWorld was the interaction between trainers and orcas. On more than one occasion, Brancheau acknowledged it was dangerous working with killer whales in such proximity.[73] "You can't put yourself in the water unless you trust them and they trust you," she told a reporter.[74] Tragically, she was right.

Conclusions

It was Ted Griffin, the owner of the Seattle Marine Aquarium and the first man to swim in 1965 with a killer whale in a public exhibition, who introduced orcas to audiences around the globe.[75] In October of the same year, Griffin and his partner, Don Goldsberry, captured a two-thousand-pound, fourteen-foot female orca they named "Shamu" near Tacoma, Washington, and sold it to SeaWorld San Diego, a marine park in California.[76] With that sale, Griffin and Goldsberry began what ultimately became a billion-dollar franchise operation, capturing and shipping killer whales to marine parks all over the world.[77]

"It was good catching animals," recalled Goldsberry.[78] "It was exciting. I was the best in the world. There is no question about it."[79]

Goldsberry soon recognized that Iceland had many orcas, so by October 1976, he shipped the first Icelandic orca to SeaWorld.[80] Not to be outdone, Sealand of the Pacific purchased Tilikum, a male Icelandic killer whale, in late 1984.[81] "Tilikum was our favorite," said Eric Walters, a former trainer at Sealand.[82] Youthful, energetic, and eager to learn, "he was the one we all really liked to work with."[83]

In 1991, SeaWorld Orlando agreed to purchase Tilikum and two female orcas after Sealand of the Pacific closed its doors as a result of the bad publicity it received when an assistant trainer was killed by the three killer whales.[84] That Tilikum was a sexually mature male orca who had impregnated the two females "was not the only reason [SeaWorld] had interest, but [it was] definitely part of the decision," said Mark Simmons, a former trainer at SeaWorld.[85]

Once Tilikum arrived at SeaWorld, the company decided that since he had already been involved in one killing, it would be too great a risk to put trainers in the water along with the orca. SeaWorld focused instead on showcasing Tilikum's immense size and power.[86]

"One of the things we always talked about at Sea World was you never want to get totally comfortable with any animal," said Thad Lacinak, former vice president of animal training.[87] "The safety of our trainers and animals is paramount," said Flaherty Clark, SeaWorld's head trainer.[88] Nonetheless, in 1991, a twenty-seven-year-old man had hidden at SeaWorld and was found drowned the next day in Tilikum's pool.[89]

In 2006, Kenneth Peters, a trainer at SeaWorld San Diego, was attacked by a seventeen-foot orca called Kasatka and nearly drowned when he was repeatedly held below the surface of the water for as long as a minute at a time.[90] A year later, and after numerous incidents and several accidents, the Occupational Safety and Health Administration (OSHA) warned that "swimming with captive orcas is inherently dangerous and if someone hasn't been killed already, it is only a matter of time before it does happen."[91]

Brancheau had more experience than most of the other trainers, especially with Tilikum, with whom she had worked for sixteen years.[92] Said Clark, "There's not one of us who wouldn't say that she was one of the best."[93] Tompkins, the curator of zoological operations, agreed. "Dawn spent her entire career taking care of these animals," he said, adding "she loved doing it, she loved working with these killer whales … She was very comfortable in their presence."[94]

After Brancheau's death, many people thought SeaWorld should retire Tilikum, but Tompkins quickly disabused them of that notion.[95] Tilikum was "going to be a part of our family for a long time to come," Tompkins said.[96] John Jett, a visiting research professor at Stetson University in Deland, Florida, and a former trainer at SeaWorld Orlando, said the reason was simple—"money, money and money."[97] Jeffrey Ventre, a former SeaWorld trainer, agreed. "He [Tilikum] is huge, he's impressive, people just see him and they go 'Wow!' He's a money stream as well."[98] Jett declared, "SeaWorld is the new Ringling Brothers Circus, only now the draw is pretty girls in tight wetsuits interacting with large carnivores in environments that are in no way related to their natural history … except maybe the salt water."[99]

Putting Tilikum down was not the answer, Naomi Rose, a marine mammal scientist with the Humane Society, said.[100] "It's not his [Tilikum's] fault what happened, just as it wasn't Dawn Brancheau's. The fault lies with using these wild animals as entertainment. This was an accident waiting to happen."[101] Russ Rector, a former dolphin trainer in Fort Lauderdale, noted, "Tilikum is a casualty of captivity; it has destroyed his mind and turned him demented. If he was a horse, dog, bear, cat, or elephant he would already have been put down after the first kill, and this is his third."[102]

According to Jack Hanna, director emeritus of the Columbus Zoo and Aquarium in Ohio, Brancheau would have wanted her work to continue despite her fatal accident.[103] "She loved the whales like her children, she loved all of them," Diane Gross, Brancheau's sister, said, adding that she would not have wanted to see Tilikum destroyed.[104] Gross did not have to worry. After living in marine park pools for thirty-three years, and suffering from a persistent bacterial infection, Tilikum finally died on January 6, 2018.[105] He was thirty-six years old.[106]

CHAPTER 30

Andrew Breitbart

Died March 1, 2012

Conservative Journalist

THE BRENTWOOD RESTAURANT and Lounge in an affluent neighborhood of Los Angeles, California, had amazing food and a great wine cellar.[1] The ambience was just right, a little dark and moody, which gave the establishment a great vibe.[2] Andrew Breitbart, a conservative journalist and founder of *Breitbart News*, apparently thought so too, because sometime after ten o'clock on the last night in February 2012, he went to the lounge and sat next to Arthur Sando, a publicity and marketing executive he had never met.[3]

"He was on his BlackBerry a lot," Sando recalled.[4] "He wasn't drinking excessively."[5]

Over the next ninety minutes, Breitbart and Sando spent their time together in deep conversation intermingled with sips of pinot noir wine and occasional laughter.[6]

"We talked politics, television, college, and living in Los Angeles," Sando remembered.[7] "He said that conversations like ours were why he liked to go to bars and talk with people who had different political beliefs."[8] Other patrons soon joined in the conversation.[9]

Breitbart settled his bill at about 11:30 p.m. and headed home, but minutes after leaving the restaurant, he collapsed in front of a Starbucks.[10] A bystander saw him fall and called paramedics, who found Breitbart not breathing.[11] They attempted to restart Breitbart's heart with four doses of epinephrine and shocked him four times with electrodes.[12] After being rushed by ambulance to the emergency room at Ronald Reagan University of California Los Angeles Medical Center, Breitbart was pronounced dead at 12:19 a.m. by Dr. J. Feldman.[13] He was forty-three years old.

The Autopsy

Dr. Juan M. Carrillo, Deputy Medical Examiner of the County of Los Angeles, conducted the autopsy.[14] At seventy-five inches long and weighing 251 pounds, the body was moderately obese.[15] A healing ulceration was present on the right hand. A minor contusion on the forehead and an abrasion on the scalp and on the left shoulder had probably occurred when Breitbart collapsed on the sidewalk.[16] No tattoos were identified.[17]

The standard Y-incision was performed to view the internal organs, all of which were present and located in their normal positions.[18] There was no fluid in the abdominal cavity or evidence of peritonitis, an inflammation of the tissue that lines the abdomen.[19]

Approximately one year before he died, Breitbart was diagnosed with shortness of breath and congestive heart failure.[20] He did not smoke, was considered a "light drinker," and had been exercising and dieting, but nevertheless was under a lot of stress.[21]

Based on the circumstances surrounding Breitbart's death, which suggested he had probably died from a heart-related event, I was especially interested to review the autopsy findings related to the cardiovascular system.

Upon opening the body cavity, it was immediately apparent Breitbart had an enlarged heart.[22] At 720 grams, the heart was more than twice the average weight of a normal heart.[23] This was mainly due to "left ventricular hypertrophy," an enlargement of the heart's left ventricle.[24] Compared to the right ventricle, the left was more than seven times thicker than the right.[25] In addition, the septum of the heart, the dividing wall between the right and left sides of the heart, was also thickened.[26]

There was up to 60 percent narrowing of the anterior descending branch of the left coronary artery due to atherosclerosis; however, no evidence of heart muscle death was apparent.[27] The lack of evidence of heart muscle death suggested Breitbart may have died from an arrhythmia, an electrical abnormality in the heart which can cause death within minutes, rather than a heart attack due to blockage of coronary arteries.[28]

Although the lungs were congested, they were without thromboembolism or a blood clot.[29] When lung tissue was examined under a microscope, "heart failure cells" were detected, a diagnostic indicator of congestive heart failure.[30] These "hemosiderin laden macrophages" are present in the alveolar spaces of the lungs when high blood pressure in the lungs causes red blood cells to pass through the vascular wall.[31]

The stomach contained partially digested food but no pill fragments.[32] The esophagus was normal, the appendix was present, and the pancreas was unremarkable.[33] The descending colon showed evidence of diverticulosis (pockets).[34]

The liver was of normal size, but when it was examined under the microscope, some fatty changes were apparent.[35] Nevertheless, there was no evidence of cirrhosis, a chronic liver disease that is often seen in alcoholics.[36]

The gallbladder was present, the kidneys were congested, the urinary bladder contained 200 milliliters of urine that was free of glucose (sugar), the prostate was not enlarged or nodular, the spleen was of average size, and the endocrine system was unremarkable.[37]

Evidence of subcutaneous (below the skin) hemorrhage was noticeable on the scalp, undoubtedly due to Breitbart's fall the night he died.[38] However, the skull was not fractured, and the brain was normal, with no contusions, hemorrhage, or discoloration.[39]

Having reviewed the autopsy findings, it was clear Breitbart had suffered a heart-related event. However, since he had been drinking wine the night he died, it was important that I investigated whether alcohol contributed to his death. With that in mind, I next reviewed the toxicology report.

Cause and Manner of Death

According to Mario Sainz, an investigator at the Department of the Coroner in the County of Los Angeles, no foul play was suspected in Breitbart's death.[40]

Toxicology testing detected a blood alcohol level .04 gram percent.[41] That amount of alcohol was 50 percent lower than the legal limit for driving while intoxicated.

No drugs of abuse were identified in Breitbart's blood.

After I reviewed the circumstances surrounding Breitbart's death, the autopsy findings and results of toxicology testing, as well as published lay articles and the scientific literature, I agreed with the coroner's conclusion that the immediate cause of death was heart failure, possibly in combination with an arrhythmia. Contributing factors included cardiomegaly and atherosclerosis.[42] The manner of death was natural.[43]

Life and Career

Breitbart was born in 1969 to Irish American parents in Los Angeles, California, but when he was three weeks old, he was adopted by a Jewish couple.[44] As a young child, Breitbart attended Hebrew school; when he turned thirteen, he had a bar mitzvah, the Jewish coming-of-age ritual.[45]

After Breitbart died, Joel B. Pollak, editor-in-chief and general counsel for Breitbart's online media empire, said of Breitbart, "He was the best kind of Jew and human being you could ever meet. He carried his faith as he carried all his convictions: with a lighthearted touch but a deep commitment."[46] In true Jewish fashion, Breitbart called a follower "a putz" (a jerk) in his final message on Twitter.[47]

Breitbart attended the Brentwood School, one of the top private secular K–12 day schools in the country.[48] His first satirical article, published in the *Brentwood Eagle*, the school's newspaper, was about the difference between the school's senior and junior parking lots; the senior lot had Mercedes and BMWs in it.[49] It was then that Breitbart discovered he not only enjoyed writing but also that he could do it in a funny, politically incorrect way.[50]

In 1991, Breitbart graduated from Tulane University with a major in American studies.[51] Like many other college graduates, he had no idea what he wanted to do with his life. "I was so excruciatingly bored after college," he said.[52] His early jobs included waiting tables, coding for the online magazine *E! Entertainment Television*, and film production.[53]

Breitbart discovered the internet in the early nineties, marveling at weather sites and at monitoring earthquakes in real time.[54] The digital environment held a special attraction for Breitbart, and he decided to pursue a career in that field.

One of Breitbart's early internet-related jobs was in 1995 as Matt Drudge's first assistant on The Drudge Report.[55] Ten years later, Drudge introduced Breitbart to author and conservative syndicated columnist Arianna Huffington.[56] Upon meeting Huffington, Breitbart decided to join *The Huffington Post*, where he helped turn the blog into a news site advocating right-wing political views.[57] "I didn't want to exist in Drudge's shadow in perpetuity," Breitbart said.[58]

Huffington recalled that "[Breitbart] brought two things to the blog. He knew when a big story was about to happen. But more important, he could find stories buried in the thirteenth paragraph, link them with other things and put a spotlight on them."[59] In an interview with the *New Yorker*, Breitbart said Huffington was "the closest thing I ever had to a collaborator who was working on the same energy levels and with the same kind of skill set."[60]

Breitbart's time at *The Huffington Post* was short-lived, however.[61] After only one month, he left to launch his own website, Breitbart.com, providing a conservative perspective for people in the Los Angeles entertainment industry.[62] In its first month of operation, Breitbart.com reported 2,640,000 visitors.[63] "With the internet, I have communication with large amounts of people, in perpetuity," Breitbart declared.[64]

David Carr of the *New York Times* observed, "Mr. Breitbart, as much as anyone, turned the Web into an assault rifle. Less watchdog than pit bull, Mr. Breitbart altered the rules of civil discourse."[65]

In 2007, Breitbart launched a video blog called Breitbart.tv; after that, he launched BigHollywood.com, BigGovernment. com, and Big Journalism.com.[66]

A darling of the political right, Breitbart often appeared as a guest commentator or as a panelist on television shows, including Fox News late night programs.[67] He regularly attended Tea Party events, wrote columns for the *Washington Times*, penned a book titled *Righteous Indignation: Excuse Me While I Save the World*, and was featured in a 2012 documentary titled *Occupy Unmasked*.[68]

One of Breitbart's most significant pieces of reporting was in 2011. The Breitbart websites noted that then US Democratic congressman Anthony Weiner of New York was sending women revealing photographs of himself.[69] This reporting eventually led to Weiner's resignation.[70]

Matt Labash of the *Weekly Standard* described Breitbart as "half right wing Yippie, half Andy Kaufman [the comedian]."[71] Breitbart's own description of himself was as "a raucous, opinionated, red meat-eating libertarian who refuses to be relegated to a conservative ghetto."[72]   "I love fighting for what I believe in," Breitbart once said.[73] "At the end of the day, I can look at myself in the mirror, and I sleep very well at night."[74]

Conclusions

"Andrew Breitbart was a conservative political combatant who was unafraid of his critics," tweeted Donna Brazile, a Democratic Party strategist, when she heard of Breitbart's death.[75] "[He was a] powerful force, constantly out there driving and pushing," former Senator Rick Santorum said.[76]

Breitbart specialized in taking what seemed like a small, inconsequential report and expanding it until it grew to become a very significant and important headline-grabbing story. Taking advantage of the internet, he extended the news cycle, keeping a story alive by incrementally publishing the facts, one fact at a time, over days and weeks.[77]

In his book *Righteous Indignation*, Breitbart wrote, "If you do a good enough job, you can force them to make a mistake," referring to politicians on the left.[78] "When they do, you must be ready to exploit it."[79]

"Andrew Breitbart was the most creative conservative in the country, in his use of technology, in his understanding of how to wage cultural war using the new media," said Newt Gingrich, former Speaker of the House.[80]

Tucker Carlson of Fox News and founder of the *Daily Caller*, a conservative website, noted, "My strong sense was that he loved the performance aspect, the drama of it all, and lived for those moments of provocation."[81] Greg Gutfeld, host of *Red Eye* on Fox News, agreed. "He was the least serious, serious person I ever met."[82]

Shocked and devastated by Breitbart's death, Pollak, editor-in-chief for Breitbart's online media empire, assured everyone that the work Breitbart had started would go on.[83] "He continues to inspire us, and we'll be moving forward … as he would have wanted," Pollak said.[84]

In 2012, Breitbart shared an evening's conversation with Sando, the public relations executive. An hour later, he died from a heart-related event. In 2019, Sando also died from a heart-related event.[85] That both men died from heart disease may be a coincidence, but it will be the tie that forever binds the two of them together.

CHAPTER 31

Tamerlan Tsarnaev

Died April 19, 2013
One of the Boston Marathon Bombers

MONDAY, APRIL 15, 2013, was the deadline for Americans to file their federal income tax and to avoid incurring a substantial penalty. However, in Boston, Massachusetts, that was the last thing on many people's minds. On that beautiful spring day, nearly everyone's attention was focused on over twenty-three thousand runners participating in the 117th Boston Marathon, the world's oldest annual marathon.[1]

The race began at 9:32 a.m., when the elite women runners started the twenty-six-mile course.[2] They were followed at 10:00 a.m. by top male runners and the first wave of thousands of other runners.[3] Additional groups of runners took off at 10:20 a.m. and again at 10:40 a.m.[4] All along Boylston Street, more than five hundred thousand spectators waited anxiously behind guardrails for the runners to cross the finish line.[5]

At approximately 2:45 p.m., Tamerlan's nineteen-year-old brother, Dzhokhar, wearing a white baseball cap, walked over and set his backpack down in front of the Forum restaurant, in the seven hundred block of Boylston Street.[6] Pretending to be checking his emails, he raised his cell phone to his ear and began walking away, slowly at first and then more quickly.[7]

Four minutes later, an improvised explosive device (IED) planted by Tamerlan about a block away, exploded in front of Marathon Sports.[8] Within twelve seconds of the explosion, the IED inside Dzhokhar's backpack also detonated.[9] The chaos and horrifying moments that followed were forever ingrained in the consciousness of all Americans.

Tamerlan and Dzhokhar had been preparing for this day for some time.[10] In late 2012, after finding instructions on the internet, they made a bomb out of a pressure cooker filled with explosive powder and shrapnel.[11] A few months before the race, Dzhokhar obtained a nine-millimeter handgun and a Ruger semiautomatic pistol.[12] And on March 20, 2013, the brothers practiced shooting at a firing range in New Hampshire.[13] By April 15, they were ready to put their plan into action.

Fortunately, on the day of the bombing, a temporary medical tent staffed by physicians, paramedics, nurses, and physical therapists erected at the finish line of the Boston Marathon provided immediate medical care to the injured.[14] Those severely wounded were transported to area hospitals or to one of five adult level-one trauma centers; children were taken to one of four pediatric trauma centers.[15] Despite heroic efforts by the onsite medical team, three people died at the scene and more than 260 were injured.[16]

Speaking to reporters at the White House, President Barack Obama declared, "We will find out who did this. We'll find out why they did this. Any responsible individuals, any responsible groups, will feel the full weight of justice."[17] FBI special agent Richard DesLauriers vowed, "[We will] go to the ends of the Earth" to find those responsible.[18]

By Wednesday, April 17, based on eyewitness accounts and video surveillance footage, the FBI was focusing on Tamerlan and his brother.[19] Photos of the suspects were released to the media at approximately five o'clock the following evening.[20]

Sometime between ten thirty and eleven o'clock at night on Thursday, April 18, the Tsarnaev brothers killed a police officer on the campus of the Massachusetts Institute of Technology in Cambridge in an unsuccessful attempt to steal his service revolver.[21] At about midnight, Tamerlan hijacked a Mercedes-Benz SUV, taking the driver, Dun Meng, hostage.[22] After withdrawing cash from an ATM with Meng's debit card, Tamerlan stopped at a convenience store to buy snacks.[23] Seeing an opportunity to escape, Meng ran to a nearby Mobil gas station, where he called police.[24] By the time help arrived, the Tsarnaev brothers had already driven off. Nevertheless, police were able to track their movements using the GPS installed in the stolen automobile.[25]

At 12:42 a.m. on Friday, police located the stolen Mercedes in Watertown, Massachusetts.[26] After the police fired numerous shots at the two suspects, the brothers retaliated by hurling explosive devices at the police.[27] In the ensuing skirmish, Tamerlan was severely wounded and tackled to the ground as police attempted to handcuff him.[28] Dzhokhar tried to run over the officers, but they dived out of the way, and he ran over his brother instead, dragging Tamerlan's body approximately fifty feet.[29]

Dzhokhar sped away from the scene and abandoned the Mercedes about half a mile away. Running through a quiet neighborhood and seeing a dry-docked twenty-two-foot boat in the backyard of one of the houses, he climbed into the boat and hid.[30] Later that evening, David Henneberry, the owner of the boat, went to investigate why the tarp covering his boat was loose.[31] When he pulled back the tarp, he found Dzhokhar lying inside the boat. Covered with blood, he had gunshot wounds to the head, neck, legs, and hand.[32]

Police arrived, and after an intense firefight, hostage negotiators convinced Dzhokhar to surrender. He was arrested at 8:45 p.m.[33] A note written by Dzhokhar was found inside the boat claiming that the Boston Marathon bombing was in retaliation for US wars in Muslim countries.[34] "Stop killing our innocent people and we will stop," Dzhokhar wrote.[35]

Meanwhile, at Beth Israel Deaconess Medical Center, doctors were unable to save Tamerlan, and he died from his wounds.[36] He was twenty-six years old.

The Autopsy

Neither the autopsy nor the toxicology report was available for review. However, based on the death certificate and published reports, Tamerlan suffered gunshot wounds to the body and the extremities, as well as blunt trauma to the head and torso.[37]

Cause and Manner of Death

After I reviewed the circumstances surrounding Tamerlan's death, the death certificate, and published lay articles, I concluded that the immediate cause of death was either gunshot wounds after being shot by police or blunt trauma after being run over and dragged by a motor vehicle driven by Dzhokhar.[38]

At Dzhokhar's subsequent trial, prosecutor William Weinreb claimed that while "Tamerlan's bullet wounds also contributed to his death ... [Dzhokhar] killed [Tamerlan] by running him over with the Mercedes."[39]

The manner of Tamerlan's death was homicide, either by Dzhokhar or justifiable homicide by police.[40]

Life Experiences

Tamerlan was born on October 21, 1986, in the Republic of Kalmykia, located north of the Caucasus in Eastern Europe.[41] As a young child, his family moved to Krygyzstan, a former Soviet republic in Central Asia, and then to Chechnya, where they spent a few months in the late 1990s before fleeing the Russian military invasion in 1999 to Dagestan, on the Caspian Sea.[42]

In 2002, Tamerlan's father was granted political asylum in the United States. The following year, Tamerlan, who was sixteen years old at the time, immigrated to America.[43]

After settling in a run-down neighborhood of Cambridge, a city in Massachusetts known for welcoming immigrants and refugees, Tamerlan enrolled in the "English as a Second Language" program at the Cambridge Rindge and Latin School, a prestigious public high school from which he graduated in 2006.[44]

Having trained as a boxer in Dagestan, Tamerlan's goal was to represent the United States in the Olympics, and then to turn pro.[45] Tom Lee, president of the South Boston Boxing Club, thought otherwise.[46] "He was an underachiever because he did not dedicate himself to the proper training regimen," Lee said.[47] In 2009, notwithstanding Lee's views, Tamerlan won the New England Golden Gloves championship in the 201-pound division.[48]

In 2010, Tamerlan won the New England Golden Gloves championship for the second time.[49] Since he was not an

American citizen, he was blocked from advancing to the nationals.[50] Married to Katherine Russell, an American-born home health aide who had converted to Islam, and with an infant daughter, Tamerlan decided to drop out of boxing competitions altogether, as well as from Bunker Hill Community College, and instead he became more devoted to Islam.[51]

In 2011, the FSB, Russia's Federal Security Service, requested information about Tamerlan from the FBI because he was about to travel to Russia for what the FSB suspected were meetings with extremist groups.[52] "[Tamerlan] was a follower of radical Islam and a strong believer," the FSB claimed.[53] The FBI and Central Intelligence Agency (CIA) investigated the FSB claim but failed to turn up any ties between Tamerlan and militant extremists. In mid-January 2012, the FBI cleared Tamerlan to visit Russia, Chechnya, and Dagestan.[54]

Upon returning to the United States, Tamerlan sported a long, thick beard.[55] Two months later, he applied for citizenship. His application was held up by the Department of Homeland Security owing to federal investigations of his recent travels.[56] It was never approved.

On the morning of April 15, 2013, Tamerlan shaved his long, flowing beard and traveled to the Boston Marathon. He wore dark sunglasses, carried a backpack over his shoulder, and had a cell phone in his pocket. A week later, he was dead, but not before he inflicted the greatest carnage Boston had endured on Patriots' Day since the start of the American Revolution.

Dzhokhar was only eight years old when he arrived in the United States in 2002.[57] A likable young man, he easily made friends.[58] "He was soft-spoken," recalled Sierra Schwartz, a former classmate.[59] "Very funny, very sweet, very sociable."[60] Like his older brother, Dzhokhar also attended Cambridge Rindge and Latin School, where he played soccer and was captain of the wrestling team.[61]

Having earned a $2,500 scholarship from the city of Cambridge, Dzhokhar decided to attend the University of Massachusetts Dartmouth.[62] He dropped out of the university after he received several failing grades during the three semesters in which he was enrolled.[63]

On September 11, 2012, Dzhokhar became an American citizen, but over the following seven months, he dramatically changed, so much so that on April 15, 2013, he and his brother detonated two bombs at the Boston Marathon.[64]

"I used to warn Dzhokhar that Tamerlan was up to no good," Zur, Dzhokhar's cousin, later said.[65]

On April 22, 2013, Dzhokhar was charged with using a weapon of mass destruction.[66] His defense attorney, Judy Clarke, claimed, "It was Tamerlan who ... planned and orchestrated and enlisted his brother into these series of horrific acts."[67] Prosecutor Weinreb thought otherwise.[68] "[Dzhokhar] acted that way because he believed that what he had done was good, was something right," Weinreb said in his opening statement at Dzhokhar's trial.[69] "They agreed to do these crimes together, and they carried them out together."[70]

After eleven and a half hours of deliberation, a jury found Dzhokhar guilty of all thirty charges.[71] He was sentenced to death by lethal injection in June of 2015.[72]

In 2020, an appeals court ruled that Dzhokhar should be given a new penalty trial because the trial judge, George O'Toole, failed to exclude potentially biased jurors.[73] The court also set aside three of Dzhokhar's thirty convictions.[74] "Make no mistake," Judge Ojetta Rogeriee Thompson wrote in the ruling, "Dzhokhar will spend his remaining days locked up in prison, with the only matter remaining being whether he will die by execution."[75]

The Supreme Court agreed to review Dzhokhar's case in March 2021 after the Justice Department argued that the "victims, the potential jurors, the district court, the government, and the nation" should not have to bear the burdens associated with having to reinstate the capital sentence.[76]

Conclusions

"How is it [possible] that someone could grow up in a place like this [Cambridge] and end up in a place like that?" asked Jeffrey Young, the schools superintendent in Cambridge, a place he described as "beyond tolerant."[77] John Curran, Tamerlan's former boxing coach, said after learning that one of his former boxers was involved in the Boston Marathon bombing, "I am shocked beyond belief today."[78] Tamerlan's wife released a statement through her attorney saying, "The reports of involvement by her husband and brother-in-law came as an absolute shock to them all."[79] Unfortunately, it is not unusual to hear such sentiments expressed about murderers by unsuspecting friends and relatives.

Considering all the early warning signs, including that Tamerlan's name was added to the federal government Terrorist Identities Datamart Environment (TIDE), a database of known and suspected terrorists, eighteen months before the Boston Marathon bombing, as well as the alert the FBI received in 2011 from the FSB, it is surprising the bombing wasn't preventable.[80]

To understand what may have motivated Tamerlan, one need only review the timeline of his activities since he immigrated to the United States. In 2004, Tamerlan was very upbeat about his prospects, telling the *Lowell Sun* he "liked the USA ... America has lots of jobs ... You have a chance to make money here if you are willing to work."[81] Within four years, he dramatically changed, regularly attending the Islamic Society of Boston mosque, a place associated with terrorism suspects and becoming more obsessed with violent Islamic extremism.[82] Then, in 2009, he was arrested for aggravated domestic assault and battery against his then live-in girlfriend, Nadine Ascencao.[83] By 2011, subsisting on income from odd jobs supplemented with food stamps, and with his dream of becoming a famous boxer dashed because he wasn't an American citizen, Tamerlan visited Russia for what the FSB suspected to be meetings with extremist groups.[84] Finally, in January 2013, Tamerlan had a couple of heated outbursts at his local mosque.[85] Disillusioned with the American dream and with his application for American citizenship not approved, Tamerlan, now completely radicalized, detonated an IED at the Boston Marathon in April 2013.

As to what motivated Dzhokhar, a naturalized American citizen, to commit such an atrocity, Weinreb said, "He believed he was a soldier in a holy war against Americans."[86] According to Weinreb, Dzhokhar started reading terrorist writings and posting online messages about the persecution of Muslims in 2011. In 2012, he began to listen to terrorist lectures and songs. Then, in 2013, he created an online identity to spread radical Muslim ideas.[87] By April 19, 2013, the day he was apprehended for his crimes, Dzhokhar, now completely radicalized, wrote, "The U.S. government is killing our innocent civilians ... I can't stand to see such evil go unpunished."[88]

At his trial, Dzhokhar's defense attorney tried to portray her client as a typical teenager. "While Tamerlan Tsarnaev was looking and immersed in death and destruction and carnage in the Middle East," Clarke said, "[Dzhokhar] spent most of his time on the Internet doing things that teenagers do: Facebook, cars, girls."[89] A similar defense was presented at the Nuremberg trials of Nazi Party officials and high-ranking military officers. "It was him," Clarke conceded, pointing at Dzhokhar, who, along with his brother, committed the bombing at the Boston Marathon, but she then claimed

Dzhokhar wasn't to blame.[90] "Tamerlan had a special kind of influence [over Dzhokhar] dictated by his age, their culture, and [his] sheer force of personality," Clarke said.[91] With Dzhokhar's parents having recently moved back to Russia and his grades plummeting, "[he] became much more vulnerable," she said.[92] It was Tamerlan who was the driving force and mastermind behind the attack, not Dzhokhar.[93] Dzhokhar was simply drawn into his brother's passion and plan and followed his brother's wishes.[94] The jury didn't buy it.

The concept of suicide bombers and terrorists, the most extreme examples of asymmetrical warfare in modern times, can be traced back to the Japanese kamikaze pilots during World War II who rammed fully fueled fighter planes into more than three hundred ships.[95] According to Yuki Tanaka of the Hiroshima Peace Institute, kamikaze pilots rationalized their deaths as being in defense of their country.[96] What ensured that they completed their mission was their strong solidarity with their flight-mates, a contempt for cowardice, and having no hatred for their enemy.[97] This is in contrast to today's terrorists, who rationalize their deaths as being in defense of religion.[98] It is the terrorists' strong desire to enter paradise that ensures they complete their mission, not their camaraderie with other terrorists.[99]

Since the Koran, the Islamic sacred book, forbids the taking of one's own life and cautions against killing civilians, some Muslim leaders and extremist groups, such as Hamas, a Palestinian Sunni-Islamic fundamentalist, militant, and nationalist organization, declare jihad, or struggle, to justify the existence of suicide bombers and terrorists, referring to them as "martyrs," a term indicative of an honorable and heroic sacrifice for the faith that is rewarded rather than condemned.[100]

To attract recruits, Muslim clerics preach the "honor of martyrdom" as the noblest deed a Muslim can perform.[101] Martyrdom, they claim, brings not only victory but also the assurance of eternal life in paradise with all of its rewards, including "tents in heaven, each one made of pearl sixty miles high and sixty miles wide … rivers of water, milk, honey, and wine … immediate atonement of all sins … seventy-two hours (virgins) … and the potency of seventy men."[102] Other factors that may influence a terrorist's decision to become a martyr include revenge; a fatalistic-altruistic desire; a belief that it is his solemn duty; a yearning for adventure; economic, social, and personal rewards, especially for his family; and a way of gaining instant fame and respect.[103]

That Dzhokhar, and presumably Tamerlan, believed he was doing something honorable for his faith can be appreciated from his writings. As he declared, "The United States government is killing our innocent civilians … I can't stand to see such evil go unpunished. We Muslims are one body. You hurt one, you hurt us all."[104]

It is interesting to note that most of the rewards for becoming a martyr, such as aid and credit to a martyr's family and the earning of respect from one's peers, are not rewards enjoyed by the martyr in life; instead they are rewards left behind for others to enjoy once the martyr is dead. What captures a martyr's imagination are the rewards he will obtain in the afterlife, in particular the seventy-two virgins who will be waiting for him in paradise.[105] As the Bali bomber, Amrozi, said at his trial in 2003, smiling broadly and raising two thumbs up, "It's a martyr's death I am looking for."[106]

It is impossible to know whether Tamerlan expected to die in the course of his terroristic acts. However, in his writings, Dzhokhar, Tamerlan's brother, expressed an interest in becoming a martyr, which would happen only if he died in defense of Islam.[107] Presumably, Tamerlan had the same aspiration. As Weinreb, the prosecutor at Dzhokhar's trial, said, Dzhokhar bombed the Boston Marathon because he thought it would "help him [secure] a spot in heaven."[108] Clarke, Dzhokhar's defense attorney, agreed, saying, "He was jealous of his brother who had achieved martyrdom and his wish that he would as well."[109]

Academics often neglect the strong influence the promise that sexual rewards in paradise can have on young men, such as Tamerlan and Dzhokhar. It goes without saying that sex sells, both in advertising of consumer goods and in recruitment of terrorists.[110]

A report from the Library of Congress and an article by Amos Harel of *Haaretz* both note that suicide bombers range in age from seventeen to twenty-eight, the average age being twenty-one to twenty-four.[111] Tamerlan was twenty-six years old when he committed the Boston Marathon bombing; Dzhokhar was nineteen. At these ages, "The promise of seventy-two virgins waiting in heaven … offers the bomber considerable motivation," Harel wrote.[112] "Attackers anticipate personal rewards in the afterlife following 'martyrdom'," Gregor Bruce wrote in the *Journal of Military and Veterans' Health*.[113] "These can include … a welcome by virgins who are available for their pleasure."[114]

There is little doubt in my mind that for Tamerlan and Dzhokhar, the promise of sexual gratification in paradise with seventy-two virgins was a strong motivating factor for becoming martyrs. Apparently they never considered the possibility that by their heinous act, they would go to hell.

CHAPTER 32

Tom Petty

Died October 2, 2017

Member of Tom Petty and the Heartbreakers

TOM PETTY AND the Heartbreakers were on their fortieth anniversary tour on September 25, 2017, playing their third and final show at the Hollywood Bowl in Los Angeles, California.[1] With the last two concerts scheduled in New York City in November, it was almost time to go home for a much-needed break.[2] "We're all on the backside of our sixties," Petty said prior to the tour.[3] "I have a granddaughter now I'd like to see as much I can."[4]

The band had already played sixteen songs in a two-hour set as well as its first encore.[5] And yet, not surprisingly, the audience was clapping enthusiastically for more.[6] "We're almost out of time," Petty told the sold-out crowd after he introduced his bandmates and thanked his fans.[7] "We've got time for this one [though]," he added, strumming the familiar first guitar chords of "American Girl." Everyone went wild, the cheers and applause deafening.

A week later, on Sunday, October 1, Petty was informed by his physician that a hip fracture with which he had been performing for months "had graduated to a full-on break."[8] In a statement later released, the Petty family announced, "Despite this painful injury, [Petty] insisted on keeping his commitment to his fans and he toured for fifty-three dates with a fractured hip and, as he did, it worsened to a more serious injury."[9]

That evening, in their Malibu, California, home, Petty fell asleep on the living room couch next to his wife, Dana.[10] At about 10:45 p.m., Petty's wife got up and went into the kitchen. When she returned, she found Petty not breathing and unresponsive.[11] She immediately called 911, and the dispatcher tried to get her to administer cardiopulmonary resuscitation (CPR) to Petty until Emergency Medical Services arrived.[12]

Petty was transported to the UCLA Santa Monica Hospital, but on the way there, he went into cardiac arrest.[13] He was put on life support as soon as he arrived at the hospital.[14]

At 10:30 a.m. the following morning, a chaplain was called to administer the last rites to Petty.[15] Petty died that night, at about 8:40 p.m., surrounded by his family, his bandmates, and his friends.[16] He was sixty-six years old.[17]

The Autopsy

While the autopsy was conducted on October 3, 2017, the autopsy report was not available for review.[18]

According to a statement issued by the Los Angeles County Medical Examiner-Coroner, Petty suffered from a narrowing of the coronary arteries due to atherosclerosis, as well as from emphysema.[19] Other ailments included knee problems and a fractured hip, neither of which contributed to his death.[20]

Cause and Manner of Death

Brian Elias, the chief of coroner investigations at the Los Angeles Medical Examiner-Coroner, confirmed Petty had a mixture of the opioids fentanyl, oxycodone, acetyl fentanyl, and despropionyl fentanyl, as well as the benzodiazepine tranquilizers temazepam and alprazolam, and citalopram, in his system.[21]

Without additional information, it is impossible to determine whether any of the drugs found in Petty's system were in the overdose range. However, since Petty had been suffering from depression throughout his life, it seems likely he was being treated with citalopram, an antidepressant medication, before he died.[22] It is also likely he was prescribed alprazolam to treat the anxiety that often accompanies depression and temazepam for his insomnia.[23]

Petty's wife and daughter both confirmed Petty was prescribed a fentanyl transdermal patch for his hip pain, so the presence of fentanyl, a synthetic opioid drug that is fifty to one hundred times more potent than morphine, in Petty's system was not unexpected.[24] What was surprising, however, was the presence in Petty's blood of oxycodone, an opioid analgesic medication, and two illicit opioid drugs—acetyl fentanyl and desproprionyl fentanyl.[25]

Acetyl fentanyl is an illegal designer drug that is five to fifteen times more potent than morphine. Often mixed with oxycodone, the drug is sold as "oxycodone" on the internet.[26] Desproprionyl fentanyl is another illicit opioid drug used as a precursor to manufacture acetyl fentanyl. It is eighty times more potent than morphine and is sometimes found as an impurity in acetyl fentanyl preparations.[27] That all three opioid drugs—oxycodone, acetyl fentanyl, and desproprionyl fentanyl—were found in Petty's system suggests that Petty probably consumed oxycodone adulterated with acetyl fentanyl and desproprionyl fentanyl.[28] If so, the circumstances surrounding Petty's death are very similar to how Prince died.[29] Like Petty, Prince died after he ingested a counterfeit medication, Vicodin, that was adulterated with fentanyl.[30]

According to the CDC, there has been a rise in fatalities associated with acetyl fentanyl since 2012.[31] As with other opioids, death from an acetyl fentanyl overdose results from respiratory depression.[32] When several central-nervous-system-depressant drugs, such as fentanyl, acetyl fentanyl, despropionyl fentanyl, oxycodone, temazepam, and alprazolam, are ingested at the same time, their combined toxicological effects can easily reach the toxic range, with death from respiratory depression following soon thereafter.

After I reviewed the circumstances surrounding Petty's death, the autopsy findings and results of toxicology testing, published lay articles, and the scientific literature, I concluded that the immediate cause of death was respiratory depression due to polypharmacy—the combined ingestion of benzodiazepine and several central-nervous-system-depressant opioid drugs, all with similar toxicological properties. Atherosclerosis was a contributing factor.[33] The manner of death was accident.[34]

Life and Career

Petty was born on October 20, 1950, in Gainesville, Florida.[35] When he was ten years old, his uncle took him to the set of the film *Follow That Dream*.[36] It was there that Petty met Elvis Presley, and he quickly became a huge fan.[37] Another turning point in Petty's life was when he saw the Beatles on *The Ed Sullivan Show*.[38] "It looked like so much fun," Petty said.[39] "It was something I identified with."[40]

In high school, Petty played bass with a local band called the Epics.[41] When he was seventeen years old, he became the face of the newly formed band Mudcrutch.[42]

Petty's musical career began to take off when Mudcrutch disbanded and he formed a new band, Tom Petty and the Heartbreakers.[43] After signing a contract with Shelter Records, the band's debut album in November 1976 did poorly at first, but it eventually landed on the British charts when the band toured England with Nils Lofgren.[44]

By the time Petty died in 2017, he had recorded two albums with Mudcrutch, thirteen with Tom Petty and Heartbreakers, two with the Traveling Wilburys—a group that included Petty, Bob Dylan, George Harrison, Roy Orbison, and Jeff Lynne—and three solo albums, and he sold millions of records worldwide.[45] In addition to the recordings, Petty produced music videos, collaborated with Stevie Nicks on her album *Bella Donna*, and appeared in several films.[46]

In 2002, Tom Petty and the Heartbreakers were inducted into the Rock and Roll Hall of Fame as the "quintessential American individualists."[47]

Conclusions

While rehearsing for his fortieth anniversary tour, Petty slipped and cracked his hip just as the tour was about to get started, but he decided to do the tour anyway.[48] "It is our feeling that the [hip] pain was simply unbearable and was the cause of [Petty's] over use of medication," Petty's wife and daughter said after Petty died.[49] They were probably right. "His feeling was, 'I can't do that to my crew," Petty's wife said.[50] "I can't do that to the fans. I can't do that to my band.""[51]

A hip fracture is a serious injury that can be very painful.[52] Left untreated, it can lead to various complications, including death.[53] Petty was already being treated for his hip pain with a fentanyl transdermal patch when he went on tour, but apparently it wasn't enough, especially after he broke his hip.[54] Fentanyl transdermal patches are used to treat moderate to severe chronic pain around the clock when other pain treatments, such as non-opioid pain medications or immediate-release opioid medicines do not treat the pain well enough or the pain can no longer be tolerated.[55] With oxycodone, acetyl fentanyl, and desproprionyl fentanyl being added to Petty's already potent pharmaceutical cocktail of fentanyl, temazepam, and alprazolam, the combined toxicological effects of the six potent central-nervous-system-depressant drugs invariably pushed Petty over the pharmacological limit to a point where he suffered respiratory depression and death, a toxic effect the coroner labeled "cardiopulmonary arrest."[56]

"If he hadn't gone on tour and [instead] had the hip replacement surgery," Petty's wife said, "he would still be with us."[57] I agree, mainly because if Petty had undergone the hip replacement surgery, he may not have ingested what appears to have been adulterated oxycodone.

In the 1960s and 1970s, Petty experimented with alcohol and marijuana; in the 1980s, he experimented with cocaine; and in the mid-1990s, he was addicted to heroin.[58] "Using heroin went against my grain," Petty said in 2001, after he underwent a detoxification program and was treated for heroin addiction.[59]

That Petty was "sober" when he died is supported by the absence of alcohol, cocaine, and heroin from his system.[60] "Many people who overdose begin with a legitimate injury or simply do not understand the potency and deadly nature of these medications," Petty's wife said.[61] Petty may have been one of those people.

In death, Petty joined several other entertainers who succumbed to the toxic effects of polypharmacy, including Elvis Presley, Anna Nicole Smith, Heath Ledger, and Philip Seymour Hoffman.[62]

As a rock 'n' roll musician, Petty was the real deal. "Music is probably the only real magic I have encountered in my life," he once said.[63] "There's not some trick involved with it. It's pure and it's real. It moves, it heals, it communicates and does all these incredible things."[64]   I must admit, it was only after I heard Petty sing "I Won't Back Down" that I became a fan. The haunting sound of his voice and the "direct, and to the point" lyrics were everything I had heard about Petty. "He was very stubborn," his wife said.[65] In my mind, "I Won't Back Down" is the rock 'n' roll equivalent of Frank Sinatra's "My Way." Just as Scott McKenzie's "San Francisco" is recognized today as a song representing the 1960s, I am confident "I Won't Back Down" will become a song identified with millennials.

CHAPTER 33

Anthony Bourdain

Died June 8, 2018
Celebrity Chef

PARTS UNKNOWN WAS a travel and food television show hosted by Anthony Bourdain, an American celebrity chef. Traveling the world, often to lesser-known places, Bourdain introduced viewers to cultures and cuisines and, in the course of doing so, made the world a smaller place through a common interest—food. "More than anything, Anthony Bourdain wanted us to not feel isolated — to not feel alone in the world," David Fienberg, a television critic, said.[1]

On June 8, 2018, Bourdain was filming an episode of the twelfth season of *Parts Unknown* in Kayserberg-Vignoble, a historical town in the northeastern Alsace region of France, near Strasbourg.[2] After the shoot, he skipped dinner and went straight to his room at the luxury hotel Le Chambard.[3]

The next morning, Bourdain did not come down for his scheduled breakfast with his best friend, chef Eric Ripert, so Ripert went up to Bourdain's room to investigate.[4] According to Christian de Rocquigny du Fayel, the French public prosecutor, Bourdain was found hanging in the bathroom with a bathrobe belt and was declared dead by suicide.[5] He was sixty-one years old.[6]

The Autopsy

The medical examiner concluded there were no signs of violence on Bourdain's body.[7] The autopsy report was not available for review.

Cause and Manner of Death

Bourdain did not leave a suicide note when he died.[8] Nonetheless, de Rocquigny declared, "There is no element that makes us suspect that someone came into the room at any moment."[9] Also, according to de Rocquigny, the death appeared unplanned and was an "impulsive act."[10] No foul play was suspected.[11]

The toxicology report was not available for review. However, de Rocquigny announced that no opioids were detected in Bourdain's system, only "a nonnarcotic medicine in a therapeutic dose."[12]

After I reviewed the circumstances surrounding Bourdain's death, the autopsy findings and results of toxicology testing, and published lay articles, I concluded that the immediate cause of death was asphyxiation due to hanging. The manner of death was suicide.

Life and Career

Bourdain was born in 1956 in New York City, but he was raised in Leonia, New Jersey, an affluent suburb of New York.[13] "As a child growing up in New Jersey … your purpose in life was looking across the bay to New York City and figuring out a way to end up there," Bourdain said.[14]

The son of French parents, Bourdain's mother was a copy editor for the *New York Times*.[15] She was an "enthusiastic amateur chef," which may explain where Bourdain got his love of food.[16] Bourdain "always had this interest in good taste, good smells. From a very young age, he loved to try new things," even eating snails, his mother remembered.[17]

Bourdain's father, an executive for a record company, thought food was either "marvelous" or not worth mentioning.[18] Chris, Bourdain's brother, explained: "A thing that was particularly nice that influenced Tony was our parents influencing us to try new things."[19]

Bourdain graduated from the Dwight Englewood School for Boys in Englewood, New Jersey, in 1973, after which he attended Vassar College, working at seafood restaurants in Cape Cod during the summers.[20] But after two years, Bourdain decided to drop out of Vassar and pursue a career in cooking, transferring to the Culinary Institute of America, from which he graduated in 1978.[21]

When he was twenty-four years old, Bourdain purchased his first bag of heroin on the Lower East Side of New York.[22] "I just like heroin, it feels really good," Bourdain said.[23] In time, Bourdain became addicted to the drug, and then to crack cocaine.[24] "I should have died in my twenties," Bourdain said in a 2016 interview.[25]

According to the Substance Abuse and Mental Health Services Administration, the food services industry has the highest rate of illicit drug use of any occupation.[26] "It's part of the culture," chef John Puckett said.[27] "It's a combination of the hours and the accessibility."[28]

In his 2000 *New York Times* best-selling book, *Kitchen Confidential: Adventures in the Culinary Underbelly*, based, in part, on his 1997 article *Don't Eat before Reading This* for the *New Yorker* magazine, Bourdain described what it was like working in the kitchens of restaurants in the 1980s.[29] "[They were] drenched in drugs and alcohol and accompanied by constantly loud Rock and Roll music. We were high all the time, sneaking off to the walk-in refrigerator at every opportunity to 'conceptualize.' Hardly a decision was made without drugs," Bourdain said.[30]

It was only after Bourdain had been addicted to heroin for seven years that he realized, "Only one in four has a chance of making it and right there, I knew that if one of us was getting off dope, and staying off dope, it was going to be me. I was going to live. I was the guy."[31] However, while he detoxified from heroin and "finally ended a lifelong love affair with cocaine," Bourdain continued to drink alcohol.[32] "You see me drink myself stupid on my show all the time. And I have a lot of fun doing that ... When I indulge, I indulge," Bourdain said, "but I don't let it bleed over into the rest of my life."[33]

After working as a dishwasher, a line cook, a sous chef, and a chef for several years, Bourdain became executive chef in 1998 at Brasserie Les Halles, a French-brasserie-style restaurant in Manhattan.[34] "I was a happy dishwasher," Bourdain reminisced in a 2016 interview on NPR.[35]

In 2001, Bourdain combined his interests in food and travel and published *A Cook's Tour: Global Adventures in Extreme Cuisines*, even hosting a television show, *A Cook's Tour*, on the Food Network.[36] In *A Cook's Tour*, Bourdain traveled to exotic locations worldwide, sampling different types of local foods and cuisines.[37]

In 2005, Bourdain took his food and travel show to the Travel Channel, where he hosted *Anthony Bourdin: No Reservations*, a show similar to *A Cook's Tour*; it ran for nine seasons.[38] "At the end of the day, the TV show is the best job in the world," Bourdain said.[39] "I get to go anywhere I want, eat and drink whatever I want. As long as I just babble at the camera, other people will pay for it. It's a gift."[40]

Between 2006 and 2010, Bourdain published three more books—*The Nasty Bits: Collected Varietal Cuts, Usable Trim, Scraps, and Bones, No Reservations: Around the World on an Empty Stomach*, and *Medium Raw: A Blood Valentine to the World of Food and the People Who Cook*.[41] In the years prior to his death, he hosted *The Layover* for the Travel Channel and *Anthony Bourdain: Parts Unknown* for CNN, was a guest judge on several seasons of *Top Chef* and a main judge on *Top Chef All Stars*, and wrote essays and articles for the *New York Times, Gourmet, Maxim, and Town & Country*, among others.[42]

Bourdain's career as an author and television host garnered him many honors, including Food Writer of the Year (2001), eight Emmy Awards and a Peabody Award.[43] "He's irreverent, honest, curious, never condescending, never obsequious," the judges said when they presented Bourdain with the Peabody Award.[44] "People open up to him and, in doing so, often reveal more about their hometowns or homelands than a traditional reporter could hope to document."[45] Chef Gordon Ramsay said Bourdain "brought the world into our homes and inspired so many people to explore cultures and cities through their food."[46]

In 2017, Bourdain received an honorary doctorate of humane letters from the Culinary Institute of America.[47] The Smithsonian Institution called Bourdain "the original rock star" of the culinary world, "the Elvis of bad boy chefs."[48] In true Bourdain fashion, he responded, "I'm not a chef, I'm not bad, and I'm not a boy."[49]

Conclusions

Bourdain has been described as "blunt" with a "liberal use of swear words and sexual innuendo when describing food."[50] He was "notorious for his negative comments on vegetarianism and veganism" and "unabashedly candid about his past addiction to cocaine, heroin and cannabis."[51] Well-known for insulting other chefs, Bourdain once said, "Bad food is made without pride, by cooks who have no pride, and no love. Bad food is made by chefs who are indifferent, or who are trying to be everything to everybody, who are trying to please everyone."[52]

The one word that most people use to describe Bourdain is "storyteller."[53] Bourdain was "One of the great storytellers of our time who connected with so many," his friend, Ripert, said after Bourdain died.[54] And yet, when John Lurie, the artist, heard that Bourdain's death was a suicide, he wondered, "How does a storyteller check out without leaving a note?"[55]

Many people have speculated Bourdain's suicide was due to depression; however, I was unable to locate any evidence he had ever been professionally diagnosed with or treated for the disorder. A hint of Bourdain's despondency was revealed in a 2016 episode of *Parts Unknown* in which he admitted to psychotherapists in Buenos Aires, Argentina, "I'd like to be happy. I'd like to be happier. I should be happy, I have incredible luck. I'd like to be able to look out the window and say, 'Yay, life is good.'" But he couldn't.[56] As an example, Bourdain revealed to the therapists, "I ate [a hamburger] at *Johnny Rockets* in an airport once and it opened up an abyss of depression and self-loathing, a spiral of self-hatred, rage, and despair that lasted weeks."[57]

To film his show, Bourdain traveled more than 250 days a year.[58] "I stay in a lot of beautiful places and look out the window at a lot of beautiful views, but I am usually alone," he said.[59] "His travel schedule was grueling and he often seemed quite beat-up from it," one of his assistants told *People* magazine.[60] "He'd put everything into the shoots and then go back to his room to isolate."[61]

There were nearly two and a half times as many suicides in the United States in 2019 as there were homicides.[62] Mental disorder, such as depression, is the number-one cause of suicide; alcoholism or drug addiction is number two.[63] People with active substance abuse, depression, and suicidal thoughts are six times more likely to kill themselves than the general population.[64]

In a study of over thirty-seven thousand adults, 7 percent of former illicit opioid drug users still experienced suicidal thoughts one year after they stopped using opioids, as compared to 3 percent of those who had never used illicit opioids at all.[65]

Of all suicides in the United States in 2019, suffocation due to hanging was the second method of choice, lagging only behind firearms.[66] Poisoning was a distant third, constituting approximately 13 percent of all suicides.[67] While death from judicial hanging is usually instantaneous because of fracture and/or dislocation of the cervical vertebrae and vasovagal shock, death from suicidal hanging is often a slow process, taking about eight to ten minutes.[68] This is because in suicidal hanging, death is secondary to hypoxia, a lack of oxygen, and cerebral ischemia, a lack of blood flow to the brain, due to compression of the airways and major blood vessels in the neck and not from fracture of the vertebrae.[69]

"People may think that death by hanging is immediate and painless, but people struggle … I am sure it is not painless by any means," said Susan Baker, founding director of the Johns Hopkins Center for Injury Research.[70] When people who attempt suicide by hanging are rescued, they often develop respiratory and neurological complications immediately after the incident.[71]

In his final year, Bourdain became an advocate for the #MeToo movement, especially after his girlfriend, Italian actress Asia Argento, accused former Hollywood producer Harvey Weinstein of rape.[72]

Five days before Bourdain died, photos emerged in the tabloids suggesting Argento had been cheating on Bourdain.[73] "I understand that the world needs to find a reason" for Bourdain's death, Argento said in a tearful interview with the *Daily Mail* when she was accused of being the cause of Bourdain's suicide.[74] Two years later, still mourning her loss, she posted a photo on Instagram of her puffy face with the caption, "You want pain? Here's the pain. No filter needed. Two years without my love."[75]

Bourdain's career was all about communication, but speaking of his personal life, Bourdain said, "I'm terrible with communicating with people I care about." [76] Nonetheless, there is no denying that the two things Bourdain cared most about were food and people. And so, despite any of his shortcomings, Bourdain will always be remembered for the way he changed public perception about food and its relationship to humanity. "Meals make the society, hold the fabric together in lots of ways that were charming and interesting and intoxicating to me," Bourdain said.[77] "The perfect meal, or the best meals, occur in a context that frequently has very little to do with the food itself."[78]

CHAPTER 34

Aretha Franklin

Died August 16, 2018
Singer-Songwriter

THREE WEEKS PRIOR to the presidential inauguration in January 2009, Barack Obama, the first African American to be elected president of the United States, invited Aretha Franklin, the "Queen of Soul," to sing at his outdoor swearing-in ceremony.[1] "Oh my God! It was like … Oh, my God," Franklin recalled, "I couldn't hardly sleep at night. I was, like, jumping, just excited, and I couldn't hardly settle down after the first night or two."[2]

Before she left her home, Franklin checked the temperature.[3] "I rarely sing outside," she said.[4] It was twenty-eight degrees and "very, very cold, extremely cold," seven degrees colder than four years earlier, when George Bush became the forty-third US president.[5] In an interview with Larry King, Franklin later explained, "Some singers it doesn't bother and others it does. I don't care for it. It affected my voice."[6]

Bundled up against the bitter cold in a gray coat and matching gloves, Franklin's rendition of "My Country 'Tis of Thee" was compelling and memorable.[7] But the next day, what everybody was talking about was Franklin's gray felt pillbox hat with its huge Swarovski rhinestone–bordered bow, created by Luke Song of Mr. Song Millinery in Detroit, Michigan.[8] Ten years after his inauguration, Obama formally requested that the hat be donated to the Barack Obama Presidential Library.[9] "I think that is exactly where it should be," Song said.[10] "[Franklin] loved Obama, I know, and I personally couldn't think of any better place for it."[11]

Franklin's health began to deteriorate in 2010. She canceled two free concerts in New York in March and April of that year due to "fractured ribs and pain in the abdomen;" in December, she was rumored to have undergone surgery for pancreatic cancer.[12] But in 2014, having lost almost one hundred pounds, Franklin returned to performing with an appearance at New York's Radio City Music Hall.[13]

At the Kennedy Center Honors in 2015, Franklin paid tribute to Carol King, one of the honorees, by singing "(You Make Me Feel Like) A Natural Woman," a song written by King and Jerry Wexler but identified with Franklin.[14] Dressed in a full-length fur coat and carrying a diamond-studded purse and the largest sparkling jewelry imaginable on her fingers and earlobes, Franklin's exuberant performance brought the audience to its feet.[15] Many, including Obama, shed a tear or two.[16] It was "one of the three or four greatest nights of my life," Franklin told the *New Yorker* magazine.[17]

In February 2017, looking very frail, Franklin announced she would stop touring.[18] At her final performance in November, Franklin, appearing very thin, nevertheless was in fine voice, delivering a nine-song set at the Elton John AIDS Foundation gala in New York.[19]

On Monday August 13, 2018, Franklin was reported to be under hospice care, "comfortable at home," but "gravely ill" and "not doing well."[20] She passed away from advanced pancreatic cancer five days later.[21] Franklin was seventy-six years old.[22]

The Autopsy

No autopsy or toxicology testing was performed after Franklin died.

Cause and Manner of Death

After I reviewed the circumstances surrounding Franklin's death, as well as published lay articles and the scientific literature, I concluded that the immediate cause of death was advanced pancreatic cancer of the neuroendocrine type.[23] The manner of death was natural.

Life and Career

Franklin was born in 1942 in Memphis, Tennessee, to a Baptist preacher father and a gospel singer mother.[24] When she was five years old, her family relocated to Detroit, where her father founded the New Bethel Baptist Church.[25] When she was six, her parents separated; four years later, her mother died from a heart attack.[26]

Franklin taught herself to play the piano "by ear" when she was eight years old.[27] Regarded as a gifted pianist with a powerful voice, she began singing in front of her father's congregation at the age of ten.[28] "Someone found a footstool in the office and put it here on the stage, and they put it there for me to be seen because I was so small," she told an interviewer on the television show *Morning Edition* in 2004.[29]

Recognizing his daughter's musical talents, Franklin's father began to manage her musical career.[30] In a 1988 interview on *American Masters*, Franklin recalled her father's coaching technique.[31] "He would give me different records to listen to, to see if I could emulate them on the piano, different vocalists to listen to."[32]

In 1956, when she was fourteen years old, Franklin recorded songs at her father's church, releasing them as an album entitled *Songs of Faith*.[33] Four years later, she released a single, "Today I Sung the Blues."[34]

Franklin's debut pop album, *Aretha: With The Ray Bryant Combo*, was released in 1961. It included the hit single "Rock-a-bye Your Baby with a Dixie Melody," which reached number 37 on the pop charts.[35] But it wasn't until 1967 and 1968 that Franklin topped the R&B charts with the album *I Never Loved a Man the Way I Love You* and the Billboard Hot 100 with the hit single "Respect," for which she was awarded her first two Grammy Awards.[36] Jerry Wexler, Franklin's producer, said of "Respect," "There are songs that are a call to action. There are love songs. There are sex songs. But it's hard to think of another song where all those elements are combined."[37]

Other Top 10 hits soon followed, including "Baby I Love You," "Think," "Chain of Fools," "I Say a Little Prayer," and "(You Make Me Feel Like) A Natural Woman."[38] Franklin incorporated the piano into much of her work, including in arranging and songwriting.[39] "If I'm writing and I'm producing and singing, too, you get more of me that way, rather than having four or five different people working on one song," she said in 2003.[40]

In 1968, Franklin, now dubbed the "Queen of Soul," performed at the funeral of Dr. Martin Luther King Jr., a longtime friend; in the same year, she sang the national anthem at the Democratic National Convention in Chicago.[41] In later years, Franklin sang at the funeral for civil rights pioneer Rosa Parks.[42]

In 1972, Franklin released the album *Amazing Grace*.[43] It was recorded live at New Temple Missionary Baptist Church in South Central Los Angeles, California, sold more than two million copies, and became the best-selling gospel album at the time.[44]

417

Over her musical career, Franklin recorded 112 charted singles on Billboard, including seventy-three Hot 100 entries, seventeen top-ten pop singles, 100 R&B entries, and twenty number-one R&B singles.[45] She won eighteen Grammy Awards and is one of the best-selling music artists of all time, having sold more than 75 million records worldwide.[46] In 1987, Franklin became the first female performer to be inducted into the Rock and Roll Hall of Fame.[47]

Franklin sang for three American presidents—at the 1977 presidential inauguration of Jimmy Carter, at the 1993 inauguration ceremony of Bill Clinton, and at the 2009 presidential inauguration of Barack Obama.[48] She received many accolades, including a Grammy Lifetime Achievement Award, a Presidential Medal of Freedom, an honorary doctorate from the University of Detroit, and an honorary doctor of fine arts from New York University; she was also a Kennedy Center honoree.[49]

In a February 2017 interview on Detroit radio station WDIV Local 4, Franklin announced her retirement.[50] "I feel very, very enriched and satisfied with respect to where my career came from and where it is now," she said.[51] "I'll be pretty much satisfied, but I'm not going to go anywhere and just sit down and do nothing. That wouldn't be good either."[52] Eighteen months later, gravely ill and surrounded by her family, Franklin passed away.[53]

Conclusions

The pancreas is about six inches long and lies in the abdomen, behind the lower part of the stomach and near the intestines.[54] Unlike other glands, it has two functions: hormonal secretion, by endocrine cells (also called islet cells) that produce insulin and glucagon, both of which are secreted into the blood, where they regulate glucose levels; and digestion, by exocrine cells that produce enzymes, including lipase, protease, and amylase, that are secreted into the small intestine.[55]

Pancreatic cancer is most curable when it is detected early; however, it often does not cause symptoms until it has already metastasized to nearby organs.[56] The most common type of pancreatic cancer, pancreatic ductal adenocarcinoma, occurs in the exocrine pancreas.[57]

Neuroendocrine cancers (NET cancers) begin in specialized cells that have traits similar to nerve cells and hormone-producing cells.[58] NET cancers can be found in various parts of the body, such as the lungs, appendix, small intestine, rectum, and pancreas.[59] When NET cancer is formed from neuroendocrine or islet cells in the pancreas, as was the case with Franklin, it is called pancreatic NET cancer.[60]

Pancreatic NET cancer is rare, making up less than 2 percent of all pancreatic cancers.[61] One major risk factor for pancreatic NET cancer is a genetic disorder known as "multiple endocrine neoplasia type 1 syndrome."[62] Other risk factors include inherited syndromes, such as von Hippel Lindau syndrome and neurofibromatosis type 1.[63] The biological behavior of pancreatic NET cancer is unpredictable.[64] A higher tumor grade, lymph node and liver involvement, and a larger primary tumor generally portend a less favorable prognosis.[65] Extensive liver metastasis is the most common cause of death for people with pancreatic NET cancer.[66]

Pancreatic NET cancer has a five-year relative survival rate of 93 percent if it is localized and 25 percent if it has metastasized to distant sites.[67] Since pancreatic NET cancer is slow growing, it has a potential to be cured surgically if the tumor is removed before it metastasizes to the liver.[68] "Survival for many years or even decades with endocrine cancer is not surprising," said Leonard Saltz, of Memorial Sloan-Kettering Cancer Center.[69] Like Franklin, Steve Jobs, one of two founders of Apple computers, also was diagnosed with pancreatic NET cancer.[70] And just like Franklin, Jobs died eight years after his diagnosis.[71]

Pancreatic cancer of the exocrine pancreas, including pancreatic ductal adenocarcinoma, has a worse prognosis than pancreatic NET cancer, with a five-year relative survival rate of 39 percent if the cancer is localized and 3 percent if it has metastasized.[72] Some famous people who were diagnosed with pancreatic ductal adenocarcinoma include Alex Trebek, host of *Jeopardy!*, actor Patrick Swayze, opera singer Luciano Pavarotti, astronaut Sally Ride, football great Gene Upshaw, and Supreme Court justice Ruth Bader Ginsburg.[73] With the exception of Ginsburg, who survived ten years, all the other celebrities died within two years of their diagnoses.[74]

Ginsburg "beat the odds, and it was a remarkable fight," said Dr. Timothy Donahue of UCLA's Jonsson Comprehensive Cancer Center in Los Angeles, California.[75]

Pancreatic cancer "has remained one of the most, if not the most difficult cancer for us to treat," said Dr. Brian Wolpin, director of the Gastrointestinal Cancer Center and Hale Family Center for Pancreatic Cancer Research at Dana-Farber Cancer Institute in Boston, Massachusetts.[76] According to the American Cancer Society, of the fifty-seven thousand people who will be diagnosed with pancreatic cancer this year, about 82 percent will die of their disease.[77] "You can have a tiny little cancer, and you can operate on it, but it still has a high risk of coming back," said Dr. Mary Mulcahy of Lurie Cancer Center at Northwestern Memorial Hospital in Chicago, Illinois.[78]

Upon hearing of Franklin's death, record producer Clive Davis said she "was truly one of a kind. She was more than the Queen of Soul. She was a national treasure to be cherished by every generation throughout the world."[79] Former first lady Hillary Clinton and former president Bill Clinton agreed, saying Franklin "stirred our souls. She was elegant, graceful, and utterly uncompromising in her artistry."[80] Former first lady Michelle Obama and former president Barack Obama remembered Franklin this way: "Every time she sang, we were all graced with a glimpse of the divine."[81]

In a 2008 interview, Franklin described herself as follows: "Music is my thing, it's who I am. I'm in it for the long run.

I'll be around singing, 'What you want, baby I got it.' Having fun all the way."[82] Said Michelle and Barack Obama, "Aretha may have passed on to a better place, but the gift of her music remains to inspire us all."[83]

CHAPTER 35

Jeffrey Epstein

Died August 10, 2019

Financier and Convicted Sex Offender

"TERRIFIC GUY," DONALD Trump, the future president of the United States, told *New York* magazine in 2002 when describing Jeffrey Epstein, a financier.[1] "He's lots of fun to be with. It is even said that he likes beautiful women as much as I do, and many of them are on the younger side."[2]

By 2019, Trump's opinion of Epstein had changed, especially after they had a falling out when they both bid on the same oceanfront property in Palm Beach, Florida.[3] "I was not a fan of his, that I can tell you," Trump said of the now convicted sex offender.[4]

Epstein's downfall began in 2005, when a woman claimed he molested her fourteen-year-old stepdaughter at a large mansion in Palm Beach.[5] Over the next year, police investigated the allegation, and when they were done, Barry Krischer, the Palm Beach state attorney, referred the case to a grand jury.[6]

The FBI opened its own investigation of Epstein in July 2006, interviewing potential victims and witnesses.[7] At the same time, Epstein's legal team was in delicate negotiations with the Palm Beach State Attorney's Office for a favorable plea deal.[8]

In 2008, Epstein pled guilty in state court to two counts of solicitation of prostitution, one of which involved a minor.[9] Sentenced to eighteen months in prison and required to register as a sex offender, Epstein served only thirteen months in a private wing of the Palm Beach County Stockade, nearly ten months of which were in a work-release program in his office at twelve hours a day, six days per week, followed by a year's probation.[10] US attorney Alexander Acosta, who was later appointed Secretary of Labor, negotiated the plea agreement the *Miami Herald* called "the deal of a lifetime." In 2019, Acosta was forced to resign from the president's cabinet.[11]

Epstein's legal troubles did not end with his state conviction. On Saturday, July 6, 2019, he was arrested at New Jersey's Teterboro Airport after flying in from France.[12] In the indictment, the Manhattan US Attorney's Office claimed Epstein "enticed and recruited ... minor girls [to] engage in sex acts with him, after which he would give the victims hundreds of dollars in cash."[13] Two days later, Epstein was charged by federal prosecutors of the Southern District of New York with one count of sex trafficking of a minor and one count of conspiracy to commit sex trafficking.[14] Pleading not guilty in federal court to allegations he "sexually exploited and abused dozens of minor girls" between 2002 and 2005, Epstein offered to put up more than $100 million in bail.[15] In denying Epstein bail, Manhattan federal judge Richard Berman said, "The government has established danger to others and to the community by clear and convincing evidence. I doubt that any bail package can overcome a danger to the community."[16]

Epstein spent his first night in jail among the general prison population, but the following morning, he was transferred to a special housing unit.[17] Forced by inmates to overpay for snacks, sodas, and special meals, and fearing for his safety, Epstein contemplated hiring an intimidating inmate for protection.[18]

In the early hours of July 23, 2019, Epstein was found unconscious on the floor of his cell with marks on his neck and a strip of bedsheet wrapped around his neck in an apparent failed suicide attempt.[19] He was placed on a suicide watch for six days, and guards were assigned to check on him every thirty minutes to ensure his safety.[20]

On August 9, Epstein's cellmate was transferred out of his cell; contrary to prison protocol, he was not replaced.[21] That night, two cameras positioned in front of Epstein's cell malfunctioned, and the two guards who were supposed to monitor Epstein every thirty minutes fell asleep.[22]

At six thirty the following morning, Epstein's body was discovered, a bedsheet tied around the neck in an apparent suicidal hanging.[23] According to published reports, it appeared Epstein had tied bedsheets to a bunk bed and had hurled himself off the top bunk.[24] Video surveillance footage from the single functioning camera showed that no one other than Epstein had entered his cell after 10:30 p.m. the night he died.[25]

Epstein was rushed in cardiac arrest to a local hospital, where he was pronounced dead.[26] He was sixty-five years old.

On August 29, 2019, nearly three weeks after he died, a judge dismissed all criminal charges against Epstein, a standard procedure since Epstein no longer was able to mount a defense against the criminal charges.[27]

The Autopsy

The autopsy was conducted on August 11, 2019, by Dr. Kristin Roman, a New York City medical examiner.[28]

The external examination revealed a ligature furrow of the neck, contusions on both wrists, an abrasion on the left forearm, and deep muscle hemorrhaging in the left shoulder muscle.[29] In addition, there was an injury to the back of the neck, a cut on the lip, and an injection mark on the arm.[30] Presumably, some of the injuries occurred during resuscitation attempts by EMS personnel.[31]

Petechial hemorrhages, or small burst capillaries, were present on the face, mouth, and eyes.[32]

Of special significance to the identification of cause of death were fractures of the left and right thyroid cartilage and left hyoid bone.[33]

Cause and Manner of Death

In her several interviews with the media, Dr. Barbara Sampson, the New York City chief medical examiner, noted, "In forensics, it's a general principle that all information from all aspects of an investigation must be considered together. Everything must be consistent and nothing can be inconsistent, and no one finding can be taken in isolation. You can't draw a conclusion from one finding. Everything about the case has to be considered."[34]

Sampson carefully reviewed all of the available investigative information, including the autopsy findings, video surveillance from security cameras, and Epstein's prior attempt at suicidal hanging, and concluded that the cause of death was asphyxiation due to hanging. She labeled the manner of death a suicide.[35]

Dr. Michael Baden, an independent pathologist, was retained by Epstein's brother to observe the autopsy and to review its findings.[36] He concluded that Epstein's injuries "are extremely unusual in a suicidal hanging and could occur much more commonly in homicidal strangulation … the evidence points to homicide rather than suicide."[37]

Baden claimed that petechial hemorrhages like those found on Epstein's face, mouth, and eyes are often an indication of a homicidal hanging and strangulation.[38] However, this opinion is contrary to a 2020 study of thirty-six cases of hanging deaths in which no difference was found in the incidence (over 50 percent) of petechial hemorrhage in suicidal, homicidal, and accidental hangings.[39]

Baden further noted that autopsy photos showed fractures of the left and right thyroid cartilage and of the left hyoid bone, a small horseshoe-shaped bone located between the root of the tongue and thyroid cartilage. He claimed these were unusual findings in suicidal hanging and more common in homicidal hanging.[40] "I have never seen three fractures like this in a suicidal hanging," Baden said, "going over a thousand jail hanging suicides in the New York City state prisons over the past forty to fifty years, no one had three fractures."[41] Sampson disagreed. "In general, fractures of the hyoid bone and the cartilage can be seen in suicides and homicides," she said.[42]

Fractures of the hyoid bone are most common in men over forty; Epstein was sixty-five years old when he died, so it is not unusual that he had this bone fracture.[43] Also, in the 2020 study of thirty-six cases of deaths due to hanging, fractures of the thyroid cartilage and hyoid bone were present both in suicidal hanging as well as in homicidal hanging.[44] In a separate, prospective study of forty cases of suicidal hanging between 1996 and 1999, fractures of the thyroid cartilage combined with fractures of the hyoid bone were found in

15 percent of the deaths.[45] Taken together, these two studies do not support Baden's claim that Epstein's fractures of the thyroid cartilage and hyoid bone were unusual findings in suicidal hangings.

Baden suggested that, based on his review, the evidence indicated Epstein's death was a homicidal hanging, a conclusion with which I disagree.[46] Epstein was alone in a locked cell the night he died, and no one other than Epstein had entered his cell after 10:30 p.m. that night. In addition, petechial hemorrhaging and fracturing of the hyoid bone and thyroid cartilages are present both in suicidal hanging as well as in homicidal hanging. Moreover, Epstein was sixty-five years old when he died, an age when fractures of the hyoid bone are most likely to occur. Lastly, Epstein had attempted suicide by hanging about two weeks prior to his death, an important fact that is always considered in a psychological autopsy.

Several forensic pathologists claimed that knowing the position in which Epstein was found in his cell would clarify certain aspects of the autopsy, such as the location of the ligature around his neck and the way blood settled and pooled after he died.[47] They note that without such evidence or photographs, it is difficult to determine the cause of Epstein's death with certainty.[48] Such photographs, however, were not publically available.

After I reviewed the circumstances surrounding Epstein's death, the autopsy findings and results of toxicology testing, his prior attempt at suicidal hanging, published lay articles, and the scientific literature, I concluded that the immediate cause of death was asphyxiation due to hanging. The manner of death was suicide.

Life and Career

Epstein was born in 1953 in Brooklyn, New York.[49] His mother was a homemaker and a school aide while his father was a groundskeeper and gardener for the New York City Department of Parks and Recreation.[50]

A product of local public schools, Epstein began learning to play the piano when he was five years old, even attending the National Music Camp at the Interlochen Center for the Arts in Michigan during the summers.[51] Upon graduating from high school in 1969, he enrolled at Cooper Union, but two years later he transferred to the Courant Institute of Mathematical Sciences at New York University; he left college in 1974 without earning a degree.[52]

After leaving New York University, Epstein became a physics and mathematics teacher at the Dalton School, an exclusive private school on the Upper East Side of Manhattan.[53] While there, he met Alan Greenberg, the CEO of Bear Stearns, whose children were students at the school.[54] Impressed with Epstein's intelligence and financial acumen, Greenberg offered him a job in 1976 as a junior assistant to a floor trader, which Epstein gladly accepted after he was dismissed from the Dalton School for poor performance.[55]

At Bear Stearns, Epstein quickly rose through the ranks, becoming an option trader, working in the special products division, and advising the bank's wealthiest clients, including Edgar Bronfman, president of Seagram.[56] In 1980, he became a limited partner at Bear Stearns. A year later, he was asked to leave for "Regulation D violations."[57]

In 1982, Epstein founded Intercontinental Assets Group Inc., a company specializing in recovering embezzled money.[58] Some of the company's clients included the very wealthy, such as Spanish actress and heiress Ana Obregón and Saudi Arabian businessman Adam Khashoggi.[59] In the course of his efforts at finding wealthy clients, Epstein travelled extensively throughout Europe and Southwest Asia.[60] On one such occasion, he met Steven Hoffenberg, chairman of Tower Financial Corporation, a debt collection agency.[61] In 1987, Hoffenberg recruited Epstein as a consultant for his company, and together they unsuccessfully attempted to take over Pan American World Airways and Emery Air Freight Corporation.[62] Within six years of hiring Epstein, Tower Financial lost its investors $450 million in what is considered one of the biggest Ponzi schemes in American history.[63]

In 1988, Epstein founded J. Epstein & Company, a financial management firm for clients with net worths of more than a billion dollars.[64] One of the company's most important clients was Leslie Wexner, chairman and CEO of the Limited, Inc. and Victoria's Secret.[65] Epstein not only made millions of dollars in fees managing Wexner's finances but also often attended Victoria's Secret fashion shows, hosted its models at his New York City home, and helped aspiring models get employment at Victoria's Secret.[66]

In 1996, Epstein relocated J. Epstein & Company to St. Thomas, an island in the US Virgin Islands, thereby reducing his taxes by 90 percent.[67] In 2003, Epstein attempted to acquire *New York* magazine; in 2004, he invested millions of dollars in various hedge funds, much of which he lost in the "Great Recession" of 2007–2009.[68]

While under investigation for sexual offenses with minors in 2006, Epstein invested $57 million in a Bear Stearns hedge fund; in May 2007, the fund began to fail.[69] By then Epstein and his attorneys were in the middle of delicate negotiations with the Palm Beach State Attorney's Office for a favorable plea deal.[70]

Conclusions

Epstein lived in that rarified atmosphere where high-powered millionaires and billionaires reside. His hospitality was bestowed upon, and his lavish parties were attended by, princes, presidents, prime ministers, hotel chain owners, and well-known scientists and celebrities. Beautiful young women, some underage, from Europe, Russia, and Brazil and other South American countries were often flown in for Epstein's parties. In an attempt to ingratiate himself with powerful men, Epstein allegedly provided the women to his male guests for sexual activity.[71] "In those days, if you didn't know … Epstein, you were a nobody," Dershowitz, a former professor at Harvard Law School, told the *New York Times*.[72]

Certainly many of Epstein's famous acquaintances had motive to wish him ill. Had he gone to trial, their association with Epstein would have been splashed all over the front pages of newspapers and magazines, and their good names would have been forever tarnished. Who knows how such revelations would have affected their personal lives and careers? With Epstein dead, all their worries and concerns had undoubtedly diminished if not faded away.

In the United States, hanging is the second leading cause of suicide, following firearms.[73] Aside from "judicial hanging" due to state or federal executions, hanging can be divided into three categories—suicide, homicide, and accidental.[74] Of the three, suicidal hanging is the most common, with accidental hanging the most rare.[75] Unable to obtain a firearm while in prison, Epstein, once a close friend of royalty, billionaires, and politicians, chose to undertake the next most popular form of suicide in America—hanging.

On February 19, 2022, Jean-Luc Brunel, a former French modeling agent who had been charged with raping minors and trafficking young girls for Epstein, was found hanging in his cell at La Santé, a prison in southern Paris, France, in an apparent suicide.[76] Was Brunel's death an eerie coincidence or was it a homicide arranged by "powerful men?" Paris police opened an investigation, but the answer may never be known.

CHAPTER 36

Naya Rivera

Died July 8, 2020

Actor in *Glee*

"THERE ARE NO limits to fun at Lake Piru!" boasts the website for Lake Piru.[1] The reservoir, created by the Santa Felicia Dam, is located in Los Padres National Forest, approximately fifty miles northwest of downtown Los Angeles, across the Ventura County line.[2] The "picturesque Lake Piru offers an escape from city life, with a tree-shaded campground, fishing, boating, and water sports," notes the website.[3]

Trees, brush, and other debris below the surface, as well as strong currents, poor visibility, high winds, and changing water depths, make swimming in Lake Piru very dangerous.[4]

Although Bill Auyb, the Ventura County sheriff, said at a news conference that swimming is allowed in the lake, more than two dozen people have drowned, including five children, three teenagers, and seventeen adults, many of whom were considered "good swimmers"; some had even worn life vests.[5]

On Wednesday, July 8, 2020, Naya Rivera, an actor and cast member of the television show *Glee*, took her four-year-old son, Josey, to Lake Piru for some recreational activities.[6] Arriving at the boating dock at about 1:00 p.m., she rented a pontoon boat and took her son out to the northern end of the lake.[7] Approximately two hours later, after counting "one, two, three," Rivera and her son jumped off the boat and began to swim.[8]

The pontoon boat Rivera had rented was not equipped with an anchor, so with the wind at about twenty-one miles per hour, it drifted away.[9] Rivera managed to help her son back into the boat, but she was unable to get into the pontoon herself.[10] Raising her arms, she cried out for help as she tried to avoid drowning, but tragically, she soon disappeared below the surface of the water.[11]

Sometime after 4:38 p.m., a boater found Rivera's son asleep in the boat.[12] He was wrapped in a towel and wearing a life vest.[13] Rivera's body, which was without a life vest, was discovered at 9:10 a.m. on July 13, floating in the northern portion of the lake known as the "Narrows," an area with heavy brush, fifteen to twenty feet tall, that had grown when the lake was dryer.[14]

When asked why it took five days to discover Rivera's body, Ayub explained, "We believe she was concealed within some of the shrubbery on the floor bed of the lake,"[15] adding, "There's decomposition [and] the body fills with gas, becomes more buoyant, and then surfaces on its own."[16] Rivera was thirty-three years old.

The Autopsy

The autopsy was performed the day after Rivera's body was discovered; however, neither the autopsy nor the toxicology report was available for review.[17] Dental records were used to identify the body as belonging to Rivera.[18]

"There was no indication of foul play and no indication this was a suicide," Ayub said.[19]

The body was x-rayed, but no signs of traumatic injury were identified.[20] And while Rivera had suffered from vertigo and a recent sinus infection, neither of these ailments contributed to the drowning.[21]

"The autopsy findings are consistent with a drowning and the condition of the body is consistent with the time that she was submerged," the medical examiner said.[22]

Cause and Manner of Death

Toxicology tests detected a therapeutic amount of phentermine, an appetite suppressant, in Rivera's blood, as well as caffeine and low therapeutic levels of amphetamine and diazepam, an antianxiety medication.[23] None of these drugs was in the overdose range nor sufficiently elevated in Rivera's blood to have contributed to her death.[24]

Rivera had a BAC of 0.016 percent, a relatively insignificant amount and 80 percent lower than the legal limit for drivers in the United States.[25] "Some or all of the ethanol detected may have been due to postmortem production," the medical examiner said.[26]

After I reviewed the circumstances surrounding Rivera's death, the autopsy findings and results of toxicology testing, published lay articles, and the scientific literature, I concluded that the immediate cause of death was drowning. The manner of death was accident.

Life and Career

Rivera was born on January 12, 1987, in Valencia, California, to a half-black, half–Puerto Rican mother and a father of Puerto Rican and German descent.[27] In December of that year, the town merged with three other unincorporated towns to form the city of Santa Clarita, becoming the second largest and the sixth most populated city in Los Angeles County.[28]

When she was eight months old, Rivera began appearing in commercials for Kmart; at four, she performed as Hillary Winston in the television sitcom *The Royal Family*, for which she was nominated for a Young Artist Award.[29] Small parts in *Baywatch*, *The Fresh Prince of Bel-Air*, *Smart Guy*, *Family Matters*, and *Even Stevens* soon followed.[30]

In 2005, Rivera graduated from Valencia High School; she described her high school experience as "terrible."[31] "Every time I'm on a show that has a school atmosphere, I'm, like, these schools are so great," Rivera said.[32] "I would've loved high school if I could go to these schools."[33]

As an older teenager, Rivera couldn't find suitable acting roles, so instead she sold memberships at Lake Elizabeth Golf & Ranch Club, worked as a nanny, was a greeter at Abercrombie & Fitch, and even took up songwriting, cutting single records, appearing in a music video, and auditioning for *American Idol*.[34]

It wasn't until 2009, when she was twenty-two years old, that Rivera got the big break she had been hoping for when she was cast as Santana Lopez, a lesbian high school cheerleader in the musical comedy *Glee*. The role gave Rivera an opportunity to sing, dance, and act, as well as to perform as a cheerleader, something she couldn't do when she was in high school because her parents could not afford the additional expense.[35]

Santana is "really your typical high school cheerleader, for the most part," Rivera said after she was cast for the part.[36] "She's really mean and loves boys. She's really witty so I love playing her."[37] She added, "It's kind of cool," being a lesbian sex symbol.[38] "I get more girls than my boyfriend. They always tweet me about my booty."[39]

In 2010, Rivera and actor Ryan Dorsey briefly dated.[40] In her autobiography, *Sorry Not Sorry: Dreams, Mistakes, and Growing Up*, Rivera revealed she had had an abortion after splitting with Dorsey.[41] "No matter what [anyone] says to you, every girl wants to get married. I want to get married," she said at the time.[42] Rivera's thoughts about an ideal guy were, "He's nice. I don't know. I like people that are kind. And people who like me."[43]

Despite their differences, Rivera and Dorsey reconnected, and in 2014, they married in Cabo San Lucas, Mexico.[44] In September 2015, their son, Josey, was born; by November 2016, they filed for divorce.[45]

After *Glee*, Rivera appeared in a recurring role in the Lifetime drama series *Devious Maids*.[46] Most recently, she starred on the YouTube Red series *Step Up: High Water*.[47]

Rivera was "considered to be a good swimmer," had "strong swimming skills," and was in "exceptional fitness" for her age.[48] Nevertheless, on July 8, 2010, the current at Lake Piru was just too strong for her to handle, and tragically, she drowned after "she mustered enough energy to get her son back into the boat, but not enough to save herself," Ayub said.[49]

"No matter the year, circumstance, or strife, everyday you're alive is a blessing," Rivera said in one of her last Instagram posts.[50] "Make the most of today and every day you are given. Tomorrow is not promised."[51] It was very prophetic.

Conclusions

Rivera isn't the only actor to have drowned. In 1981, Natalie Wood drowned in the Pacific Ocean while on a Thanksgiving weekend sailing trip with her husband, actor Robert Wagner, and her costar Christopher Walken.[52] And in 2012, Whitney Houston, the Grammy Award–winning singer and actress, drowned in the bathtub of her Beverly Hilton Hotel room the night before she was to attend the 54th Annual Grammy Awards.[53]

Rivera's life was more than her character on *Glee*. She was a philanthropist, working with many charitable organizations including the nongovernmental media monitoring organization; GLAAD; the Trevor Project, a nonprofit organization that focuses on suicide prevention among the LGBTQ community; Stand Up to Cancer; the Elephant Project, an organization that addresses the threats posed to the survival of elephants; and the Sunshine Foundation, an organization that helps answer the dreams of chronically ill, seriously ill, physically challenged, and abused children.[54]

While Rivera played a lesbian character on *Glee*, she, in fact, was bisexual.[55] "Getting hit on by both genders is such a champagne problem," she once said.[56] When asked for her reaction to how Santana, her character on *Glee*, is a favorite among gays, Rivera replied, "I love my gay bars ... I don't get recognized anywhere except in gay bars."[57]

Rivera was "an amazing talent, but was an even greater person, mother, daughter, and sister," her family said.[58] "We are forever grateful for the indelible contribution she made to *Glee*," said Ryan Murphy, Brad Falchuk, and Ian Brennan, the creators of the show.[59] They and the rest of the *Glee* team remembered Rivera as warm and caring, fiercely protective of the rest of the cast, tough and demanding, fun, kind, and generous.[60] "She could turn a bad day into a great day with a single remark," said Chris Colfer, one of Rivera's costars on *Glee*.[61]

Regrettably, Rivera was the third among a group of *Glee* cast members who died in their thirties.[62] Exactly seven years earlier, Cory Monteith died at the age of thirty-one from a mixture of alcohol and heroin.[63] Both drugs are central nervous system depressants and in combination can cause sedation and death from respiratory depression.[64] In 2018, after pleading guilty to child pornography charges, Mark Sailing, whom Rivera had briefly dated, committed suicide; he was thirty-five years old.[65]

At her death, Rivera joined the "Thirties *Glee* Club," a group of cast members of *Glee* who died in their thirties, similar to the "The 27 Club," a group of music legends who died at the age of twenty-seven, including Amy Winehouse, Kurt Cobain, Janis Joplin, and Jimi Hendrix.[66]

CHAPTER 37

Conclusions

FOURTEEN OF THE thirty-six famous and infamous people I investigated for this book (39 percent) died of natural causes; seven (19 percent) of the deaths were accidental, and six (17 percent) were suicides. Three cases each of homicide and justifiable homicide by police, one of court-mandated execution, and three in which the manner of death was undetermined constituted the remaining deaths. In total, seventeen of the thirty-six deaths (47 percent) were of people in the entertainment industry.

Seven of the fourteen people who died from natural causes had a history of drug abuse, smoking cigarettes, or exposure to toxic or carcinogenic chemicals. These risky behaviors and chemical exposures slowly, and over many years, inevitably contributed to the so-called "natural" deaths.

The first president of the United States, George Washington, died of epiglottitis, an infection of the throat. Though it could not be cured in the eighteenth century, the disease is easily treatable today with antibiotics.

Various respiratory ailments took the lives of two famous people: Carson, who died from emphysema and COPD, a disease strongly linked to chronic smoking; and Knievel, who died from idiopathic pulmonary fibrosis, a rare progressive lung disease whose cause is unknown. Others who suffered from emphysema but died from other causes include Liston, Gibb, and Petty.

Gibb's death from ischemic congenital malrotation of the small intestine with volvulus, a life-threatening intestinal condition, occurred with little advance warning. Unrelated to his death was the presence of 60 percent narrowing of one of his coronary arteries. Had Gibb not died from his congenital intestinal condition, he may have eventually suffered from heart disease or a heart attack.

Cancer took the lives of four famous people I reviewed for this book. Bonaparte died from stomach cancer caused by arsenic, Mantle's death was from liver cancer due to alcoholism and hepatitis C, Harrison succumbed to lung cancer due to his long-term smoking, and Franklin passed away from pancreatic cancer, the cause of which is unknown. While the number of cancer deaths in this group of famous people is small, the fact that three of the four cancers were caused by exposure to chemicals the US National Toxicology Program (NTP) labeled "known human carcinogens" should give everyone pause.[1] In total, the NTP has listed 256 substances that are "known or reasonably anticipated to cause cancer in humans."[2] The International Agency for Research on Cancer (IARC) of the World Health Organization (WHO) has similarly identified more than 500 substances that are "carcinogenic and probably or possibly carcinogenic to humans."[3] Thus, exposure to toxic chemicals and carcinogens—especially in the workplace, where airborne concentrations potentially are much higher than in the general environment, should be limited or avoided entirely by maintaining adequate indoor ventilation and wearing gloves and respirators, when needed.

Seven deaths were due to heart-related events—heart attack, heart failure, or aortic dissection. Candy had always been concerned he would die young from a heart attack. His grandfather had heart disease, his brother suffered a heart attack, and his father died at an early age from a heart attack. Besides his genetic predisposition to cardiovascular disease, increasing Candy's risk further was his weight of 350 pounds, his heavy smoking, and his history of drug use. As for Garcia, Hatfield, and Lay, all three had significant atherosclerosis with 75 to 90 percent narrowing of one, two, or three coronary arteries. In addition, Garcia had an enlarged heart, and Lay had an enlarged heart and two stents in his coronary arteries. With such drastically occluded atherosclerotic coronary arteries (Garcia, Hatfield, and Lay), enlarged hearts (Garcia and Lay), and a genetic predisposition to heart disease, obesity, and chronic smoking (Candy), it was just a matter of time before they were all due to suffer a heart attack. Sadly, when they did, it was fatal.

Of the two people who died from heart failure, Liston had been diagnosed with hardening of the heart muscle prior to his death, making it much more difficult for his heart to pump blood. As for Breitbart, he had already been diagnosed with heart failure, had an enlarged heart and 60 percent narrowing of one of his coronary arteries, and the wall between the right and left sides of his heart was thickened—anatomical changes that affected the functioning of his heart. Eventually, the added strain on Liston's and Breitbart's weakened hearts made their deaths from heart failure almost inevitable.

With the exception of Lay and Breitbart, the four remaining famous people who died of heart disease—Candy, Garcia, Hatfield, and Liston—had all been chronic abusers of illicit drugs, especially cocaine, a drug that is toxic to the heart. Although none died from a cocaine overdose, their long-term abuse of cocaine contributed to the severity of their atherosclerosis and the formation of cardiomyopathy, a disease of the heart muscle that makes it harder for the heart to pump blood to the rest of the body, as well as to the malfunctioning of their hearts and ultimately to their deaths.

As for Ritter, by the time he began to complain of chest pain and had surgery to repair his aortic dissection, it was already too late. Aortic dissection is rarely diagnosed early, since it often occurs without any symptoms. Regrettably,

Ritter died at the young age of fifty-four and at the height of his career.

Unlike cocaine, which is cardiotoxic and can cause death from an arrhythmia, death from an overdose of heroin and other opioids, fentanyl, benzodiazepine tranquilizers, and polypharmacy is due to respiratory depression. Farley, who was already at a significant risk for a heart attack because of his enlarged heart and severe narrowing of three coronary arteries, died from respiratory depression and cardiotoxicity after ingesting an overdose of a speedball, a combination of heroin and cocaine. Ramone died from respiratory depression due to an overdose of heroin. As for Petty, who suffered from severe atherosclerosis, he died from respiratory depression due to polypharmacy—ingestion of several opioids and other central nervous system depressants.

Homicide was the manner of death of Rasputin and Anastasia, both of whom died from gunshot wounds. State-sponsored poisoning with radioactive polonium-210 led to the death of Litvinenko, a former Russian FSB Officer.

Seven deaths were due to suicide. Barbiturate intoxication in combination with suffocation with a plastic bag was the cause of death of Applewhite, the cult leader of Heaven's Gate. Foster's and Cobain's deaths were from gunshot wounds, as were the deaths of Harris and Klebold, two students responsible for the Columbine High School massacre. Suicidal hanging was the method of choice of Bourdain and Epstein.

Gunshot wounds were the cause of death of six of seven mass murderers reviewed for this book. These include Jim

Jones, cult leader of the Peoples Temple responsible for the mass suicide in Jonestown, Guyana; Koresh, cult leader of the Branch Davidians, responsible for the death of his followers in Waco, Texas; Harris and Klebold, who commited the massacre at Columbine High School; Whitman, the University of Texas tower shooter; and Tsarnaev, one of the Boston Marathon bombers. McVeigh, the seventh mass murderer, responsible for the Oklahoma City bombing, was executed using a three-drug lethal injection protocol.

That Jim Jones and Koresh were able to blindly lead their cult members to their deaths is seemingly beyond comprehension. According to some experts, that is because cult members are very committed to their groups. "The cult leader has a certain degree of interpersonal intelligence which pulls people into his orbit," said Dr. Alexandra Stein, a former cult member who specializes in social psychology of ideological extremism.[4] "While he is not able to reflect on his own psychological state, he understands the state of his victims, listens to them and uses it to control them," Stein said.[5] Once the victims are isolated, the effort to charm them is replaced by a form of coercive control in which charisma and authoritarianism are enough and violence is rarely needed.[6] Soon the only perceived safe place for cult members is in the group.[7] Cult members become highly dependent on the group, allowing the cult leader to easily exploit them for his own purposes, including leading them to their deaths.[8]

This group of famous and infamous people included seven accidental deaths, three of which came about through drowning—Brian Jones in his swimming pool, Brancheau at SeaWorld Orlando, and Rivera while swimming at Lake Piru in California. Of these, only Brancheau's and Rivera's deaths were truly accidental. Brian Jones's drowning may have been preceded by an arrhythmia due to ingestion of amphetamine. As for Farley's, Ramone's, Hatfield's, and Petty's "accidental" deaths, they were caused by overdoses of illicit drugs, or polypharmacy.[9] In my opinion, deaths caused by self-administered illicit drugs should have their own separate category and should not be grouped along with other accidental deaths, such as drownings or car accidents.[10]

There is no question that real or perceived ambiguity in classifying manner of death only adds to the public discourse and stokes the flames of doubt and suspicion. Listing deaths as accidental when they are due to drug overdoses or polypharmacy is a misnomer in my view. Similarly, there is nothing natural about deaths caused or contributed to by long-term abuse of illicit drugs or alcohol, or by chronic exposure to toxic chemicals, carcinogens, or cigarette smoke. With time, such exposures exert their deleterious effects on the heart, lungs, and other organs, as well as on the induction of cancer, eventually leading to so called "natural" deaths.

Perhaps the most controversial autopsy finding was Whitman's aggressive brain tumor. Both the neuropathologist who conducted the autopsy and teams of seven pathologists and six psychiatrists concluded that scientific knowledge at the time about brain function was not sufficient to determine whether Whitman's glioblastoma multiforme contributed to his bizarre behavior when he began shooting from the tower at the University of Texas on August 1, 1966. Nevertheless, the massacre possibly could have been prevented since, weeks prior to the shooting, Whitman had confided in his psychiatrist that he was "thinking about going up on The Tower with a deer rifle and start shooting people."

Several anatomical changes unrelated to the immediate cause of death include Bonaparte's enlarged liver and chronic hepatitis, possibly due to excessive drinking of alcohol; Brian Jones's fatty liver, which was twice its normal size, most likely due to his chronic abuse of drugs; Mantle's hepatitis C and cirrhosis of the liver caused by his long-term promiscuity and alcoholism; Knievel's liver transplant; and Ramone's lack of an appendix.

Three people whose manners of death are listed as undetermined include Lee, who died from cerebral edema whose cause is unknown, and two mass murderers, Jim Jones and Koresh, who died from gunshot wounds that were either self-inflicted or caused by somebody else.

A cursory survey of over 230 mass murders in the past twenty years identified many in which the perpetrators committed suicide by self-inflicted gunshot wounds or were shot by police once their heinous deed was done.[11] In others, such as the 2018 shootings at the Marjory Stoneman Douglas High School in Parkland, Florida; at Santa Fe High School in Texas; and at the Tree of Life Synagogue in Pittsburgh, Pennsylvania, the shooters were apprehended.[12] After my review, I was left wondering why so many mass murderers chose to commit suicide rather than to surrender to authorities.

Jillian Peterson, a forensic psychologist and professor of criminology and criminal justice at Hamline University in St. Paul, Minnesota, studied mass shootings and observed that 98 percent of the perpetrators were male.[13] "Men just are generally more violent," she said.[14] A report by NPR noted, "Researchers say that men, more than women, tend to externalize their problems and look for others to blame, which can translate into anger and violence. When women do choose violence, guns are not typically their weapon of choice."[15]

According to Peterson and James Densley of the Violence Project, there are four common characteristics among mass shooters.[16] The vast majority experienced early childhood trauma and exposure to violence at a young age.[17] In addition, practically every mass shooter had reached an identifiable crisis point in the weeks or months leading up to the shooting, becoming angry and despondent because of a specific grievance.[18] Furthermore, most mass shooters had studied the actions of other shooters, modelling their actions after previous shootings and seeking validation for their motives.[19] Lastly, all had the means to carry out their plans, deciding that life was no longer worth living and that murdering others was a proper revenge.[20]

Adam Lankford, an associate professor of criminal justice at the University of Alabama who studied 185 cases of mass shootings between 1966 and 2010, both in the workplace and in schools, noted that hopelessness is one of the most common reasons why people seek death.[21] "Unlike most murderers and terrorists, mass shooters almost never escape the scene of their crimes," Lankford declared.[22] "They die 48 percent of the time, 38 percent by self-inflicted gunshot wounds with the remainder [10 percent] by 'suicide by cop.'"[23] According to Lankford, the likelihood a perpetrator of a mass killing will die is 1.2 times higher for each additional person who is killed and 1.76 times higher for each additional weapon the perpetrator brings to the scene of the crime.[24] "It's about self-loathing and perceived injustice. Those who have the most rage toward others, end up killing the most victims," Lankford explained.[25] Seeing so many dead victims, the perpetrators feel the most guilty and ashamed, and they are more likely to engage in "self-punishment" through suicide or suicide by cop.[26]

Dr. Antonio Preti, a psychiatrist in Italy, agreed.[27] "Suicide with hostile intent encompasses a wide range of behaviors, from self-killing by methods that can harm others ... to the suicide that generally follows a spree-killing raid," Preti said.[28] "The major determinant of these forms of lethal behavior ... is the will to express rage toward those who are seen as the source of one's misfortune."[29] Revenge is often a motivating factor. Preti concluded that since many mass murders often end up with the perpetrators killing themselves, it "implies some suicidal intention on the part of the perpetrators, who awaited or planned the action with the purpose of committing suicide after the execution of ... many victims."[30]

If there is one lesson to be learned from this book, it is that unlike manner of death, which is subject to interpretation, forensic analysis of cause of death is almost never disputed, as it is based on scientifically proven facts. For example, there is wide acceptance that Bruce Lee died from cerebral edema. However, even four very learned and experienced medical and scientific experts could not agree what caused the cerebral edema and how to label Lee's manner of death. Lycette, the medical pathologist who conducted the autopsy, thought it was accidental, caused either by cannabis or Equagesic; Langford and Wu, who treated Lee's first and second bouts of cerebral edema, respectively, were uncertain what caused the cerebral edema; and Teare, the expert retained by the judge at Lee's inquest, concluded it was accidental, caused by an allergic reaction to aspirin or meprobmate, two ingredients in Equagesic. Sometime after the inquest, Filking, a Chicago deputy medical examiner, suggested Lee's cerebral edema was due to SUDEP, while author Matthew Polly proposed it was due to anhidrosis. Had either Filking's or Polly's explanations for the cerebral edema been accepted by the jury at Lee's inquest, the manner of death would have then been labeled natural and not accidental.

Having reviewed the science behind the deaths of fifty-nine famous and infamous people in my two books on this subject, I am confident forensic analysis will continue to be an important and integral part of the determination of cause of death, with new methodologies potentially added in the area of neurotoxicology. I hope that with time, designation of manner of death will also evolve, possibly by adding new categories to account for drug-related deaths that are neither truly accidental nor natural.

FORMULARY

Acetaminophen (Tylenol)

Acetaminophen is an over-the-counter medication that relieves pain and lowers fever. The drug was discovered by accident in the late nineteenth century. The FDA first issued a patent for acetaminophen in 1951. Unlike aspirin, acetaminophen does not cause stomach ulcers or gastrointestinal upset. However, when taken long-term or in higher-than-recommended doses, it can damage the liver and may even cause death.

Acetyl fentanyl

Acetyl fentanyl is an analog of fentanyl, an opioid analgesic drug. It is weaker than fentanyl but fifteen times more potent than morphine and several times stronger than heroin. Acetyl fentanyl is manufactured, distributed, and sold illicitly. It may be mixed with heroin or other agents and marketed as heroin, oxycodone, or fentanyl to unsuspecting buyers.

Alcohol

Alcohol, also known as ethanol, depresses the central nervous system and can impair judgment, reduce inhibition and reaction time, diminish fine motor control, and cause sedation. Tolerance, physical dependence, and withdrawal symptoms may develop after long-term use. The BAC legal limit for drivers in the United States is eighty milligrams per deciliter.

Alprazolam (Xanax)

Alprazolam is an antianxiety medication of the benzodiazepine class of pharmaceuticals. The drug was first introduced to the US market in 1981. Alprazolam facilitates the action of gamma aminobutyric acid, an inhibitory biochemical neurotransmitter in the brain. The FDA specifically warns against the simultaneous use of benzodiazepine and opioid drugs, the combination of which can cause profound sedation, respiratory depression, coma, and death.

Amphetamine

Amphetamine is one of the most potent drugs that stimulate the central nervous system. It causes wakefulness, alertness, a decreased sense of fatigue, mood elevation, an ability to concentrate, elation, and euphoria. When taken in large doses over an extended duration, the stimulating effect of amphetamine is almost always followed by depression and fatigue.

Arsenic

Arsenic is a poison, but in the past it was widely used in medicine for the treatment of diseases such as diabetes, psoriasis, syphilis, skin ulcers, and joint diseases. Despite its proven therapeutic benefits, concerns due to its toxicity and carcinogenicity caused a decline in arsenic's medicinal use. While the exact biochemical mechanism of action of arsenic is not known, the chemical can interfere with biochemical reactions by replacing phosphate or reacting with critical thiol groups in proteins and thereby inhibiting their activity.

Aspirin

Aspirin is an over-the-counter medication that relieves pain and lowers fever. When taken long-term, it may cause gastrointestinal upset and ringing in the ears. The drug's popularity declined in 1956 after the development of acetaminophen and further declined in 1962 after the introduction of ibuprofen.

Barbiturate

Barbiturate is a class of pharmaceuticals that depress the central nervous system. Drugs in this class produce a wide range of effects, including sedation. Most barbiturate overdoses involve a combination of barbiturates with other central-nervous-system-depressant drugs, such as alcohol and opiates.

Benzodiazepine

Benzodiazepine is a class of psychoactive pharmaceutical drugs used to treat anxiety or as sedatives. The FDA specifically warns against the simultaneous use of benzodiazepine and opioid drugs, the combination of which can cause profound sedation, respiratory depression, coma, and death.

Benzoylecgonine

Benzoylecgonine is the major metabolite of cocaine. It is formed in the liver, is pharmacologically inactive, and is excreted in the urine. Drug testing for cocaine relies on the identification of benzoylecgonine in the urine.

Blisters of cantharides

Blisters of cantharides, a topical treatment of the Spanish fly, a "blister beetle," forms blisters within twenty-four to forty-eight hours. The degree of blistering is controlled by instructing the patient to wash the treated site with soap and water, usually every two to six hours. Healing is complete four to seven days after application.

Butalbital

Butalbital is a barbiturate medication with an intermediate duration of action. It is often combined with other medicines, such as acetaminophen and caffeine, to relieve symptoms of tension headaches. Most barbiturate overdoses involve a combination of barbiturates with other central-nervous-system-depressant drugs.

Caffeine

Caffeine is a drug with mild central-nervous-system-stimulant properties. It is present in over-the-counter cold preparations and some foods and drinks, and it is often added to pain relievers and products that keep a person alert. When taken in high doses, caffeine can cause restlessness, insomnia, a rapid heart rhythm, and anxiety.

Calomel

Calomel, also called "mercurous chloride," has been used in medicine since the sixteenth century. It was once the most popular of cathartics, but recognition of its potential toxicity, along with the development of superior and safer cathartics, has led to a decline in its use in internal medicine.

Cannabis

Cannabis, also known as marijuana, is a psychoactive drug. It contains the chemical delta-9-tetrahydrocannabinol, or THC, which is responsible for the psychoactive mind-altering state produced by cannabis. THC alters normal brain communication, especially in areas of the brain that influence pleasure, memory, thinking, concentration, movement, coordination, and sensory and time perception. The effects of cannabis begin almost immediately, but they last only one to three hours. However, THC can be detected in the body for days or even weeks after first use. When taken in large doses, cannabis can cause acute psychosis, including hallucinations, delusions, and a loss of a sense of personal identity.

Carfentanil (Wildnil)

Carfentanil is a synthetic opioid drug approximately ten thousand times more potent than morphine and one hundred times more potent than fentanyl. It is used as a tranquilizing agent for elephants and other large mammals. The drug has not been approved by the FDA for human use.

Chloral hydrate

Chloral hydrate is a central-nervous-system-depressant drug that is rapidly metabolized to trichloroethanol, which is largely responsible for the sedative and hypnotic properties of chloral hydrate. When taken in an overdose, chloral hydrate can cause respiratory depression, coma, arrhythmia, and death. In 2012, chloral hydrate was taken off the market due to oversedation in children and possible liver damage upon long-term use.

Chloroquine

Chloroquine is a medication used to prevent or treat malaria. It was discovered in 1934 and was introduced into medicine in the 1940s. Chloroquine is a relatively well-tolerated drug. The most common adverse reactions include stomach pain, nausea, vomiting, and headache. Other effects include an increased risk of arrhythmias, QT elongation, ventricular fibrillation, and ventricular tachycardia.

Ciprofloxacin (Cipro)

Ciprofloxacin is an antibiotic medication used to treat skin, bone, joint, respiratory, sinus, and urinary tract infections, as well as certain cases of diarrhea. The drug was first introduced to the United States in 1987. It is on the World Health Organization's List of Essential Medicines, which enumerates the safest and most effective medicines needed in a health system. Some of the more serious side effects of ciprofloxacin include tendon problems, nerve damage, and mood or behavioral changes.

Cisatracurium

Cisatracurium is an intermediate neuromuscular-blocking medication used to facilitate endotracheal intubation and to provide skeletal muscle relaxation during surgery or mechanical ventilation. As a paralytic drug, cisatracurium is one of three drugs used in lethal injections in some parts of the United States.

Citalopram (Celexa)

Citalopram is an antidepressant medication that affects biochemical neurotransmitters in the brain in people with depression. The drug selectively inhibits the reuptake of serotonin with little to no effect on the reuptake of two other chemicals, norepinephrine and dopamine.

Cocaine

Cocaine is a powerfully addictive drug that stimulates the central nervous system and increases the levels of dopamine, a biochemical neurotransmitter in the brain. Cocaine causes mental alertness; hypersensitivity to sight, sound, and touch; irritability; and paranoia. The effects of cocaine appear almost immediately and disappear within a few minutes to an hour, depending on whether it is injected, smoked, or snorted. Some of the most severe side effects of a cocaine overdose include arrhythmia, a heart attack, stroke, difficulty breathing, high blood pressure, hallucinations, and extreme agitation or anxiety. There is no specific antidote to revese a cocaine overdose.

Codeine

Codeine is an opioid drug that is seven to fourteen times less potent than morphine. It is used to treat coughs and to relieve mild to moderately severe pain. Some side effects of codeine include sedation, mental cloudiness, euphoria, agitation, abdominal bloating, nausea, vomiting, and constipation. When taken in higher than therapeutic doses, codeine is less likely to cause respiratory depression than morphine. However, when combined with other central-nervous-system-depressant drugs, especially at higher doses, codeine can cause respiratory distress and death.

Despropionyl fentanyl

Despropionyl fentanyl is an illicit opioid analogue of fentanyl, an analgesic drug. It is much more potent than fentanyl and is manufactured, distributed, and sold illegally in the United States.

Diazepam (Valium)

Diazepam is a drug in the benzodiazepine class of pharmaceuticals. It is used to treat various anxiety disorders and to alleviate the symptoms of alcohol withdrawal. Diazepam facilitates the action of gamma aminobutyric acid, an inhibitory biochemical neurotransmitter in the brain. The FDA specifically warns against the simultaneous use of benzodiazepine and opioid drugs, the combination of which can cause profound sedation, respiratory depression, coma, and death.

Diphenhydramine (Benadryl)

Diphenhydramine is an antihistamine medication that relieves the symptoms of the common cold or hay fever, including sneezing, itching, watery eyes, and runny nose, caused by histamine, a natural biochemical in the body. Because of its mild sedative properties, caution is advised when taking diphenhydramine with other central-nervous-system-depressant drugs.

Emetic tartar

Also known as tartar emetic, this compound of antimony potassium tartrate has irritant properties. Emetic tartar has long been known as a powerful emetic that induces vomiting. Emetic tartar may cause lethal cardiac toxicity, among its other adverse effects.

Epinephrine

Epinephrine is a vasoconstrictor medication that is used to treat severe asthma attacks and life-threatening allergic reactions, including anaphylaxis, caused by insect bites and stings. The drug acts quickly to improve breathing, stimulate the heart, raise a dropping blood pressure, reverse hives, and reduce swelling of the face, lips, and throat.

Equagesic

Equagesic is a pharmaceutical combination of meprobamate, a tranquilizer, and aspirin, a nonnarcotic analgesic. The drug is used in the short-term treatment of pain accompanied by tension or anxiety in patients with musculoskeletal disease.

Fentanyl

Fentanyl is a powerful opioid drug that is fifty to one hundred times more potent than morphine. The drug is typically used to treat severe pain and to manage pain after surgery. Fentanyl is sometimes used to treat patients with chronic pain who exhibit tolerance to other opioids. As with all opioids, when taken in an overdose, fentanyl slows or stops the breathing process, thereby decreasing the amount of oxygen reaching the brain. Coma, permanent brain damage, and death may follow.

Flunitrazepam (Rohypnol)

Flunitrazepam is a drug in the benzodiazepine class of pharmaceuticals. It is used to treat severe insomnia and to assist with anesthesia. The FDA specifically warns against the simultaneous use of benzodiazepine and opioid drugs, the combination of which can cause profound sedation, respiratory depression, coma, and death.

Fluoxetine (Prozac)

Fluoxetine is an antidepressant medication that affects biochemical neurotransmitters in the brain in people with depression, panic, anxiety, or obsessive-compulsive symptoms. The drug selectively inhibits the reuptake of serotonin with little to no effect on the reuptake of two other chemicals, norepinephrine and dopamine.

Fluvoxamine

Fluvoxamine is an antidepressant medication that affects biochemical neurotransmitters in the brain. The drug selectively inhibits the reuptake of serotonin with little to no effect on the reuptake of two other chemicals, norepinephrine and dopamine. Fluvoxamine is approved by the FDA for the treatment of obsessive-compulsive disorder and depression.

Glucose

Glucose is a simple sugar present in blood. Insulin, a hormone produced by the pancreas, assists in transporting glucose from the blood into cells for energy and storage. People suffering from diabetes have a higher-than-normal level of glucose in their blood.

Hashish

Hashish, often called hash, is a potent form of cannabis produced by collecting and compressing trichomes, the most potent material from cannabis plants. Hashish contains essentially the same active ingredients present in marijuana, but the THC level is much more concentrated. THC is responsible for the psychoactive mind-altering state produced by hashish. It alters normal brain communication, especially in areas of the brain that influence pleasure, memory, thinking, concentration, movement, coordination, and sensory and time perception. The effects of hashish begin almost immediately, but they last only one to three hours. However, THC can be detected in the body for days or even weeks after first use. When taken in large doses, hashish can cause acute psychosis, including hallucinations, delusions, and a loss of a sense of personal identity.

Heroin

Heroin is a highly addictive opioid drug that depresses the central nervous system. It is two to five times more potent than morphine. Heroin is rapidly metabolized to morphine, which binds to areas of the brain responsible for controlling pain, pleasure, heart rate, sleep, and respiration. When taken in an overdose, heroin slows or stops the breathing process, thereby decreasing the amount of oxygen reaching the brain. Coma, permanent brain damage, and death may follow. Naloxone is a specific antidote to reverse a heroin overdose.

Hydrocodone

Hydrocodone is an opioid drug that is equal in analgesic potency to morphine. As with all opioids, when taken in an overdose, hydrocodone can cause a severe drop in blood pressure. Death from respiratory depression may follow. Naloxone is a specific antidote for a hydrocodone overdose.

Mannitol

Mannitol is a diuretic drug that occurs naturally as a sugar in fruits and vegetables. It elevates blood plasma osmolality, a measure of the concentration of chemical particles in the fluid part of the blood, resulting in enhanced flow of water from tissues, including the brain and cerebrospinal fluid, into interstitial fluid and plasma.

Marijuana

Marijuana is a greenish-gray mixture of the dried flowers of the *Cannabis sativa* plant. It contains the chemical

466

delta-9-tetrahydrocannabinol, or THC, which is responsible for the psychoactive mind-altering state produced by marijuana. THC alters normal brain communication, especially in areas of the brain that influence pleasure, memory, thinking, concentration, movement, coordination, and sensory and time perception. The effects of marijuana begin almost immediately, but they last only one to three hours. However, THC can be detected in the body for days or even weeks after first use. When taken in large doses, marijuana can cause acute psychosis, including hallucinations, delusions, and a loss of a sense of personal identity.

Meprobamate

Meprobamate is a tranquilizer medication used to treat symptoms of anxiety. The drug works by slowing activity in the brain, allowing for relaxation. Although meprobamate is not commonly used anymore, it is still available commercially.

Mercury

Mercury was in use in the early sixteenth century and remained the primary treatment for syphilis, a sexually transmitted disease caused by the bacterium *Treponema pallidum*, until the early twentieth century. Mercury is no longer used for this purpose, owing to its toxicity.

Midazolam (Versed)

Midazolam is a drug in the benzodiazepine class of pharmaceuticals. It is used to sedate patients prior to minor surgery, dental work, or other medical procedures. Midazolam facilitates the action of gamma aminobutyric acid, an inhibitory biochemical neurotransmitter in the brain. The FDA specifically warns against the simultaneous use of benzodiazepine and opioid drugs, the combination of which can cause profound sedation, respiratory depression, coma, and death.

Morphine

Morphine is an opioid drug that depresses the central nervous system. It is also the active metabolite of heroin. Morphine relieves moderate to severe pain by binding to areas of the brain responsible for controlling pain, pleasure, heart rate, sleep, and respiration. When taken in an overdose, morphine can cause a severe drop in blood pressure. Death from respiratory depression may follow. Naloxone is a specific antidote for a morphine overdose.

Naloxone (Narcan)

Naloxone is a drug used to rapidly reverse an opioid overdose. It acts by competitively binding to opioid receptors.

Norcocaine

Norcocaine is a minor, pharmacologically active metabolite of cocaine. There is very little evidence to show that norcocaine plays an important role in cocaine toxicity in humans.

Oxycodone

Oxycodone is an opioid drug that is about 50 percent more potent than morphine. The drug is used to treat moderate to severe pain. When taken in an overdose, oxycodone can cause a severe drop

468

in blood pressure. Death from respiratory depression may follow. Naloxone is a specific antidote for an oxycodone overdose.

Pancuronium (Pavulon)

Pancuronium is a medication with muscle relaxant properties. It is used in some states as the second of three drugs administered during lethal injections. Pancuronium paralyzes skeletal muscles, but it does not affect the brain or nerves.

Penicillin

Penicillin is an antibiotic medication discovered in 1928 by Scottish scientist Alexander Fleming. It is one of the most widely used antibiotic drugs in fighting bacterial infection. Penicillin inhibits bacterial enzymes responsible for the synthesis of the bacterial cell wall, rendering the wall "leaky" so that material inside the cell is depleted, thereby killing the bacterium. Since human cells lack a cell wall, they are resistant to the action of penicillin. Penicillin is used in the treatment of throat infections, meningitis, syphilis, and various other infections caused by bacteria. The chief side effects of penicillin are hypersensitivity reactions including skin rash, hives, swelling, anaphylaxis, and allergic shock.

Pentobarbital (Nembutal)

Pentobarbital is a barbiturate drug that depresses the central nervous system. It has a rapid onset of effect, and its sedative action lasts three to four hours when given in therapeutic doses. When taken in an overdose, symptoms may include extreme drowsiness, slowed or shallow breathing, weak pulse, rapid heart rate, little or no urination, pinpoint or dilated pupils, and a feeling of coldness. Death from respiratory arrest may follow. Pentobarbital is utilized to initiate and maintain medically induced coma, especially in cases of brain injury, and as a means of lethal injection in humans. Most barbiturate overdoses involve a combination of barbiturate with other central-nervous-system-depressant drugs.

Phenobarbital

Phenobarbital is a barbiturate medication used to treat or prevent seizures. The drug is also used as a sedative. Most barbiturate overdoses involve a combination of barbiturates with other central-nervous-system-depressant drugs.

Phentermine

Phentermine is a drug that stimulates the central nervous system, increases the heart rate and blood pressure, and helps weight loss by decreasing hunger. Together with diet and exercise, phentermine is used to treat obesity, especially in people with risk factors, such as high blood pressure, high cholesterol, and diabetes.

Phenytoin (Dilantin)

Phenytoin is an antiepileptic or anticonvulsant medication that works by slowing down impulses in the brain that cause seizures. The drug is prescribed to treat and prevent seizures that may begin during or after surgery on the brain or nervous system.

Potassium chloride

Potassium is a mineral the body needs for proper functioning of the heart, muscles, kidneys, nerves, and digestive system. At therapeutic doses, potassium chloride is used to prevent or treat low potassium levels in the body, which may result from disease, from certain medications, or following a prolonged illness with diarrhea or vomiting. When administered at high doses, potassium chloride is one of three drugs in a lethal injection, producing death by stopping the heart from beating.

Promethazine (Phenergan)

Promethazine is a drug in the phenothiazine class of pharmaceuticals. It works by changing the actions of certain chemicals in the brain or by acting as an antihistamine, blocking the effects of histamine, a naturally occurring chemical in the body. Promethazine is used to combat motion sickness and to treat the symptoms of allergies, such as itching, runny nose, sneezing, itchy or watery eyes, hives, and itchy skin rashes. Phenergan can also be used as a sedative before or after surgery.

Quinine

Quinine is a natural cinchona alkaloid that has been used for centuries to treat malaria, but it should not be used to prevent the disease. The drug is also used for idiopathic muscle cramps. Quinine therapy has been associated with rare instances of hypersensitivity reactions, which can be accompanied by hepatitis and mild jaundice.

Sodium thiopental

Sodium thiopental is an ultra-short-acting barbiturate drug with a rapid onset. As one of three drugs used in lethal injections in the United States, sodium thiopental is used at a high dose that renders a person unconscious in fewer than thirty seconds.

Speedball

A speedball is a mixture of a stimulant, such as cocaine, and a depressant, such as heroin, an opioid drug. It is typically snorted, although it may also be injected. The combination of a stimulant and a depressant can create an intense euphoric rush. However, cocaine's stimulating effects cause the body to use more oxygen, while the depressant effects of heroin slow breathing rates. As cocaine's stimulating effects dissipate long before heroin's depressant effects, death from respiratory depression often follows.

Tartar emetic

Also known as emetic tartar, this compound of antimony potassium tartrate has irritant properties. Tartar emetic has long been known as a powerful emetic that induces vomiting. Tartar emetic may cause lethal cardiac toxicity, among its other adverse effects.

Temazepam (Restoril)

Temazepam is a drug in the benzodiazepine class of pharmaceuticals. It affects chemicals in the brain in people suffering from insomnia. The FDA specifically warns against the simultaneous use of benzodiazepine and opioid drugs, the combination of which can cause profound sedation, respiratory depression, coma, and death.

Trazodone

Trazodone is an antidepressant medication that belongs to a group of drugs called serotonin receptor antagonists and reuptake inhibitors. It works by balancing chemicals in the brain.

Verapamil

Verapamil is a drug belonging to a class of pharmaceuticals known as calcium channel blockers. The drug is used to treat high blood pressure, heart pain (angina), and certain heart rhythm disorders. Verapamil works by relaxing the muscles of the heart and blood vessels.

Vicodin

Vicodin is a combination medication consisting of hydrocodone, an opioid analgesic drug, and acetaminophen, a nonnarcotic pain reliever. It is used to treat moderate to moderately severe pain and is similar in potency to morphine. When taken in an overdose, Vicodin can cause a severe drop in blood pressure. Death from respiratory depression may follow. Naloxone is a specific antidote for a Vicodin overdose.

Wheat-bran poultice

A poultice is a moist, usually heated concoction that is spread on an injury, ache, or wound and held in place with a cloth. When the poultice is smeared on a bandage before application, it is often called a "plaster." A popular homemade poultice combines two parts wheat bran, one part Epsom salts, and enough water to moisten the mixture.

GLOSSARY

Abrasion

An abrasion, or excoriation, is a wearing away of the upper layer of skin as a result of an applied friction force.

Accidental hanging

Accidental hanging is rare, leading to difficulty in distinguishing its diagnosis from a diagnosis of suicidal hanging or even homicidal hanging. A common characteristic in almost all cases of accidental hanging is an immobile, fixed, and exposed suspension apparatus that causes death to unsuspecting victims.

Acute myocardial infarction

Acute myocardial infarction, also known as a heart attack, is a life-threatening medical emergency. It usually occurs when a clot blocks the flow of blood to the heart. Without an adequate blood flow, heart muscle does not receive sufficient oxygen and dies. Symptoms of acute myocardial infarction include tightness or pain in the chest, neck, back, or arms, as well as fatigue, lightheadedness, abnormal heartbeat, and anxiety. Women are more likely to have atypical symptoms of acute myocardial infarction than men. Treatment ranges from lifestyle changes and cardiac rehabilitation to medications, stents, and bypass surgery.

Acute respiratory failure

Acute respiratory failure occurs when fluid builds up in the alveoli, tiny air sacs in the lungs, so that the lungs cannot release oxygen into the blood. This, in turn, leads to an inadequate delivery of oxygen-rich blood to critical organs, and they cannot function properly. Conditions that affect breathing can cause respiratory failure. These conditions include lung disease, such as COPD; diseases and syndromes that affect nerves and muscles that control breathing, including amyotrophic lateral sclerosis (ALS), muscular dystrophy, spinal cord injuries, and stroke; spine problems, such as scoliosis, a curvature in the spine; smoke inhalation from fires or harmful fumes; and injury to the chest. Symptoms of acute respiratory failure include shortness of breath, sleepiness, and loss of consciousness.

Adenosine triphosphate

Adenosine triphosphate (ATP) is the primary organic compound that provides energy to drive many processes in living cells, such as muscle contraction, nerve impulse propagation, condensate dissolution, and chemical synthesis. When energy is needed by a cell, it is converted from storage molecules into ATP. ATP in turn delivers the energy to places within the cell where energy-consuming activities take place.

Alpha-1-antitrypsin deficiency

Alpha-1 antitrypsin deficiency is an inherited disorder that may cause lung disease and liver disease. People with alpha-1 antitrypsin deficiency usually develop the first signs and symptoms of lung disease between ages twenty-five and fifty. The earliest symptoms are shortness of breath following mild activity, reduced ability to exercise, and wheezing. Other signs and symptoms can include unintentional weight loss, recurring respiratory infections, and fatigue. Affected individuals often develop emphysema.

Alpha particles

Alpha particles are positively charged atomic particles consisting of two protons and two neutrons tightly bound together. Although alpha particles are very energetic, they are heavy and lose their energy over short distances so that they are unable to penetrate the skin. However, if they are inhaled, ingested, or enter the body through a cut, alpha particles can then be very harmful, causing substantial damage to sensitive tissues and organs.

Altruistic suicide

Altruistic suicide is always intentional and occurs when individuals are so well integrated into a group that they are willing to sacrifice their own lives in order to fulfill some obligation for the group.

Alveoli

Alveoli are tiny air sacs in the lungs at the end of bronchioles. It is in alveoli that oxygen breathed in from the air passes into the blood before it then travels to the tissues throughout the body while carbon dioxide, which is carried in the blood from the tissues, passes through the alveoli and is exhaled.

Amygdala

The amygdala is an almond-shaped mass inside the brain and is part of the limbic system of the brain. Along with the hippocampus, the amygdala plays a central role in behavior and emotional response, including feelings such as pleasure, fear, anxiety, and anger. By attaching emotional content to memories, the amygdala plays an important role in determining how memories are stored in the brain.

Anaerobic respiration

Anaerobic respiration is a type of respiration by which cells can break down sugars to generate energy in the absence of oxygen.

Angina

Angina feels like pressure, squeezing, heaviness, tightness, or pain in the chest. It is a symptom of heart disease.

Anhidrosis

Anhidrosis is the inability to sweat normally. When a person does not perspire, the body cannot cool itself, leading to overheating and potentially to heatstroke.

Antecubital fossa

The cubital fossa is an area between the arm and the forearm, located in a depression on the anterior surface of the elbow joint.

Aorta

The aorta is the large artery that carries oxygen-rich blood from the left ventricle, one of the lower chambers of the heart, to other parts of the body.

Aortic dissection

An aortic dissection is a serious condition in which a tear occurs in the inner layer of the aorta. Blood rushes through the tear, causing the inner and middle layers of the aorta to separate. Aortic dissection is lethal if the blood exits the aorta through the outside aortic wall. It is most common in men between the ages of sixty and seventy.

Arrhythmia

An arrhythmia is an abnormal and irregular heartbeat due to a fault in the electrical system of the heart. The most common life-threatening arrhythmia is ventricular fibrillation, an erratic, disorganized firing of impulses from the heart ventricles, the lower chambers of the heart. Irregular heart rhythm, which can also occur in normal, healthy hearts, can be caused by certain substances or medications, such as caffeine, nicotine, alcohol, cocaine, inhaled aerosols, diet pills, and cough and cold remedies, as well as by emotional states, such as shock, fright, or stress.

Arsenic poisoning

Arsenic is a poison. While the exact biochemical mechanism of action of arsenic is not known, the chemical can interfere with biochemical reactions by replacing phosphate or reacting with critical thiol groups in proteins and thereby inhibiting their activity. Symptoms of arsenic poisoning can include vomiting, abdominal pain, encephalopathy, and watery and bloody diarrhea. The US National Toxicology Program has designated arsenic a known human carcinogen that causes cancer of the gastrointestinal tract, including stomach cancer.

Arteriosclerosis

Arteriosclerosis is the buildup of fat and cholesterol, called plaque, in arterial walls, causing the arteries to narrow and harden, leading to poor circulation of blood throughout the body. Arteriosclerosis often has no symptoms until plaque buildup is severe enough to block blood flow.

Astrocytoma

Astrocytoma is a type of cancer that can occur in the brain or spinal cord. Some astrocytomas grow slowly, while others can be aggressive and grow quickly. Survival is dependent on tumor grade.

480

Atherosclerosis

Atherosclerosis is a disease characterized by a deposition of plaque—fats, cholesterol, and other substances—on the inner walls of coronary arteries. Plaque causes narrowing of the lumen of the arteries and blocks the flow of oxygen-rich blood to heart muscle, potentially leading to an infarct, or heart attack, and death of heart muscle.

Avulsion of the scalp

Avulsion of the scalp is a forcible detachment of the scalp from the head. While rare, avulsion of the scalp is a severe, life-threatening injury that most commonly occurs as an industrial accident by entrapment of long hair in high-speed rotary parts of industrial machinery. Rapid cessation of bleeding, wound compression and aggressive fluid resuscitation are imperative.

Benign reactive lymphoid hyperplasia

Benign reactive lymphoid hyperplasia is a rare and benign lesion found in organs of the gastrointestinal tract, as well as in the skin, lung, orbit, and liver.

Blood alcohol concentration

Blood alcohol concentration (BAC) is the percentage of alcohol in the bloodstream. In the United States, a driver of an automobile is legally intoxicated if his or her BAC is 0.08 percent or higher.

Blood–brain barrier

The blood–brain barrier is a highly selective semipermeable border of endothelial cells that prevents toxic substances in the blood from crossing into the extracellular fluid of the central nervous system, where neurons or nerve cells reside. Besides shielding the brain, the blood–brain barrier supplies brain tissue with nutrients and filters harmful compounds from the brain back into the bloodstream.

Bloodletting

Bloodletting is the withdrawal of blood from a patient to prevent or cure illness and disease. The practice of bloodletting began around three thousand years ago with the Egyptians, continuing with the Greeks, Romans, Arabs, and Asians, and spreading throughout Europe during the Middle Ages and the Renaissance. Bloodletting was based on an ancient system of disease represented by four basic elements—earth, air, fire, and water—which in humans were related to the four basic humors—blood, phlegm, black bile, and yellow bile. Being sick meant having an imbalance of the four humors. Treatment consisted of removing an amount of the excessive humor by various means, such as bloodletting, purging, catharsis, and diuresis. When Galen of Pergamum (AD 129–200) declared blood as the most dominant humor in humans, the practice of bloodletting gained even greater importance.

Capillaries

Capillaries, the smallest blood vessels in the body, help connect arteries and veins. It is where oxygen, nutrients, and cellular waste are exchanged between the blood and tissues.

Carbon dioxide

Carbon dioxide is one of the waste products of metabolism. Carbon dioxide is carried by blood to the lungs, where it is exhaled and exchanged for oxygen. Too much or too little carbon dioxide in the blood can indicate a health problem.

Cardiomegaly

Cardiomegaly is an enlarged heart and may be the result of short-term stress on the body, such as pregnancy, or a medical condition, such as weakening of the heart muscle, coronary artery disease, heart valve problems, or abnormal heart rhythm. Cardiomegaly is a frequent cause of sudden death and is highly associated with obesity.

Cardiomyopathy

Cardiomyopathy is a disease of the heart muscle, a major cause of which is a viral infection. Cardiomyopathy makes it harder for the heart to pump blood to the rest of the body and can lead to heart failure. Some people who have cardiomyopathy never have symptoms, while others may show signs as the disease progresses. Symptoms of cardiomyopathy include shortness of breath, fatigue, swelling in the ankles and legs, an irregular heartbeat, palpitations, and fainting.

Cardiopulmonary resuscitation

Cardiopulmonary resuscitation (CPR) is an emergency procedure performed when a person is in cardiac arrest. Cardiopulmonary resuscitation consists of chest compressions, often combined with artificial ventilation.

Cause of death

Cause of death is a scientific and biological explanation for why a person died. The primary underlying cause of death is the condition or injury leading directly to the death.

Cecum

The cecum is a pouch connected to the junction of the small and large intestines. The main function of the cecum is to absorb any remaining fluids and salts after intestinal digestion.

Central nervous system

The central nervous system consists of the brain and spinal cord. The brain plays a central role in the control of most bodily functions, including awareness, thoughts, memory, movements, sensations, and speech. Some reflex movements can occur by way of spinal cord pathways without participation of the brain.

Cerebral edema

Cerebral edema, or brain swelling, is a life-threatening condition that causes fluid to build up in the brain. Brain swelling can be the result of an injury, an illness, or an infection. A buildup of fluid in the brain increases pressure inside the skull, commonly referred to as intracranial pressure. Brain swelling is a serious problem that can cause death and is difficult to treat.

Cerebral hemispheres

The cerebral hemispheres are the two halves of the cerebrum, the parts of the brain that control muscle function, speech, thought, emotion, reading, writing, and learning. In general, the left hemisphere controls speech, comprehension, arithmetic, and writing, while the right hemisphere controls creativity, spatial ability, and artistic and musical skills.

Cerebral ischemia

Cerebral ischemia is a condition that occurs when there is not enough blood flow to the brain to meet metabolic demand. A medical emergency if left untreated, cerebral ischemia is a common mechanism of acute brain injury that can lead to limited oxygen supply, or cerebral hypoxia, and death of brain tissue, cerebral infarction, or ischemic stroke.

Chronic obstructive pulmonary disease

Chronic obstructive pulmonary disease (COPD) is a group of lung diseases that block airflow and make it difficult to breathe, the most common of which are emphysema and chronic bronchitis. Damage to the lungs caused by COPD cannot be reversed. Symptoms of COPD include shortness of breath, wheezing, or a chronic cough. To minimize damage to the lungs, treatment of COPD includes rescue inhalers and inhaled or oral steroids.

Cirrhosis of the liver

Cirrhosis is a chronic liver disease that occurs when scar tissue replaces healthy liver tissue. Cirrhosis is usually due to excessive alcohol consumption. While cirrhosis does not usually cause symptoms, when symptoms do occur, they often include fatigue, weight loss, and abdominal pain.

Colorectal cancer

Colorectal cancer starts in the colon or the rectum. Early cases of colorectal cancer can begin as noncancerous polyps. Colorectal cancers often have no symptoms, but they can be detected by screening. Some symptoms of colorectal cancer include changes in bowel habits, changes in stool consistency, blood in the stool, and abdominal discomfort. Treatment of colorectal cancer includes surgery to remove the cancer, as well as chemotherapy and radiation therapy.

Confirmatory toxicology tests

Confirmatory toxicology tests are highly specific tests that confirm the presence of a drug in biological fluids, such as blood and urine. Unlike an immunological toxicology screen, confirmatory tests also quantify the amount of a drug present in a biological sample.

Congestive heart failure

Congestive heart failure, also known as heart failure, occurs when the heart muscle pumps blood less efficiently than normal. Blood can then back up and become congested, and fluid can be retained in the lungs, causing shortness of breath.

Contusion

A contusion, or bruise, is a region of injured tissue or skin in which capillaries have been ruptured. It is one of the most common types of injuries occurring in active children.

Cranium

The cranium is the skull, especially the part enclosing the brain. It is made up of cranial bones that surround and protect the brain and facial bones—bones that form the eye sockets, nose, cheeks, jaw, and other parts of the face. An opening at the base of the cranium is where the spinal cord connects to the brain.

Cyanide

Cyanide is a chemical compound that contains a cyano group consisting of a carbon atom triple-bonded to a nitrogen atom. Soluble salts of cyanide, such as sodium cyanide and potassium cyanide, are highly toxic. Cyanide is a rapidly acting, potentially deadly chemical. It is sometimes described as having a bitter almond smell, but it does not always give off an odor, and not everyone can detect the odor.

Cyanocarbonate

Cyanocarbonate is a chemical formed as a result of the combination of cyanide with carbon dioxide.

Cynanche trachealis

Cynanche trachealis is a disease of the throat or windpipe that includes inflammation, swelling, and difficulty breathing and swallowing.

Cytochrome c oxidase

Cytochrome c oxidase is the terminal enzyme of the mitochondrial respiratory chain involved in the electron transport system. The enzyme plays a vital role in producing energy in the form of ATP.

Depression

Depression is a mental health disorder characterized by persistently depressed mood or loss of interest in activities, causing significant impairment in daily life. Possible causes of depression include a combination of biological, psychological, and social sources of distress. These factors may cause changes in brain function, including altered activity of certain neural circuits in the brain. The persistent feeling of sadness or loss of interest that characterizes major depression can lead to a range of behavioral and physical symptoms, including changes in sleep, appetite, energy level, concentration, daily behavior, or self-esteem. Depression can also be associated with thoughts of suicide.

Diabetic ketoacidosis

Diabetic ketoacidosis is a serious, life-threatening complication of diabetes. It is most common among people with type 1 diabetes. Diabetic ketoacidosis develops when the body does not have enough insulin to allow sugar in the blood to enter the cells for use as energy. A diagnosis of diabetic ketoacidosis requires a plasma glucose concentration above 250 milligrams per deciliter, although it usually is much higher, as well as a pH level less than 7.30 and a bicarbonate level equal to or less than 18 milliequivalents per liter.

Diverticulosis

Diverticulosis is a condition in which small bulging pouches or pockets are formed in the wall or lining of any portion of the digestive tract. They occur when the inner layer of the digestive tract pushes through weak spots in the outer layer. Diverticulosis is common in people over the age of forty. Symptoms do not appear unless the diverticula become inflamed or infected, which can result in fever and abdominal pain.

Duodenum

The duodenum is the first part of the small intestine, immediately beyond the stomach, leading to the jejunum.

Dysentery

Dysentery is an infection of the intestines resulting in severe diarrhea and the presence of blood and mucus in the feces. Dysentery can be caused by a bacterial infection, such as *Shigella, Campylobacter, Salmonella,* or *E. coli.* Shigellosis is the most common type of dysentery, with about five hundred thousand cases diagnosed in the United States each year.

Dysphagia

Dysphagia is a symptom of disease that includes difficulty or discomfort when swallowing.

Edema

Edema is swelling caused by excess fluid trapped in tissues. It can affect any part of the body.

Embalming

During the embalming process, blood is removed from the body through the veins and is replaced through the arteries with an embalming solution containing formaldehyde, glutaraldehyde, methanol, ethanol, phenol, and water. Embalming sanitizes and preserves the body, retards the decomposition process, and enhances the appearance of a body disfigured by traumatic death or illness.

Emphysema

Emphysema is one of the lung diseases comprised by COPD. It involves the gradual damage of the alveoli in the lungs, causing shortness of breath. Over time, the inner walls of the alveoli weaken and rupture, creating larger air spaces instead of many small ones. This reduces the surface area of the lungs and, in turn, reduces the amount of oxygen entering the bloodstream.

Endocarditis

Endocarditis is a life-threatening inflammation of the inner lining of the heart's chambers and valves. It usually occurs when bacteria attach to damaged areas of the heart, causing an infection. People with damaged or artificial heart valves or other heart conditions are most at risk of endocarditis. Symptoms of endocarditis include fevers, chills, and fatigue. The main treatment is antibiotics, although surgery may sometimes be needed.

Endocrine system

The endocrine system is a network of hormone-producing glands, including the hypothalamus, pituitary, pineal, thyroid, parathyroid, thymus, adrenals, pancreas, and ovaries or testes. Glands of the endocrine system release hormones into the bloodstream to control mood, growth and development, metabolism, organs, and reproduction.

Epiglottitis

Epiglottitis is a potentially life-threatening condition that occurs when the epiglottis, a small cartilage flap that covers the windpipe, swells, blocking the flow of air into the lungs. Factors that can cause the epiglottis to swell include burns from hot liquids, direct injury to the throat, and various infections. Symptoms of epiglottitis in adults include severe sore throat; fever; a muffled or hoarse voice; an abnormal, high-pitched sound when breathing; difficulty breathing and swallowing; and drooling.

Familial pulmonary fibrosis

Familial pulmonary fibrosis is defined as histologically confirmed idiopathic pulmonary fibrosis (IPF) occurring in two or more members of the same family. IPF is a progressive interstitial lung disease of unknown etiology.

Fatalistic suicide

Fatalistic suicide results from excessive regulations. Fatalistic suicide occurs when individuals are placed under extreme rules or high expectations, which removes their sense of self or individuality.

Fatty liver

Fatty liver is an increased buildup of fat in the liver, usually due to obesity or type 2 diabetes. While fatty liver does not usually cause symptoms, when symptoms do occur, they often include fatigue, weight loss, and abdominal pain.

Fibrosis

Fibrosis is the thickening and scarring of connective tissue, usually as a result of injury.

Foramen magnum

Foramen magnum is the large hole at the base of the skull that allows passage of the spinal cord. It functions as a passage of the central nervous system through the skull, connecting the brain with the spinal cord.

Formaldehyde

Formaldehyde is a strong-smelling, colorless gas used in making many household products and building materials, such as particleboard, plywood, fiberboard, glues and adhesives, permanent-press fabrics, paper product coatings, and certain insulation materials. The chemical has been shown to cause cancer in laboratory animals.

Fundus of the stomach

The fundus is the upper part of the stomach, which forms a bulge higher than the opening of the esophagus. The fundus is farthest from the pylorus, the opening from the stomach into the duodenum, the upper part of the small intestine. The function of the fundus is to store gas produced during digestion.

Gastric cancer

Gastric cancer, or gastric carcinoma, is a disease in which malignant cells form in the lining of the stomach. Symptoms of gastric cancer include indigestion and stomach discomfort or pain. While stomach cancer can occur in any part of the stomach, it is more likely to affect the gastroesophageal junction, the area where the esophagus meets the stomach.

Gastritis

Gastritis is an inflammation of the lining of the stomach. It can be caused by irritation due to excessive alcohol use, chronic vomiting, stress, or the use of certain medications, such as aspirin or other anti-inflammatory drugs. Gastritis can also be caused by a bacterial or viral infection or bile reflux. If left untreated, gastritis can lead to a severe loss of blood and may increase the risk of developing stomach cancer.

Gastroenteritis

Gastroenteritis is a short-term illness caused by a bacterial or viral infection and inflammation of the digestive system. Symptoms of gastroenteritis include abdominal cramps, diarrhea, and vomiting.

Gastroesophageal reflux disease

Gastroesophageal reflux disease (GERD) is a chronic disease that occurs when stomach acid or bile flows into and irritates the lining of the esophagus. Symptoms of GERD include burning pain in the chest, usually occurring after meals and worsening when lying down.

Gastrostomy

A gastrostomy is a surgical opening into the stomach from the abdominal wall. A tube inserted through the wall of the abdomen directly into the stomach allows air and fluid to leave the stomach. It can also be used to administer drugs and liquids, including liquid food.

Glabella

The glabella is the smooth part of the forehead above and between the eyebrows.

Glioblastoma multiforme

Glioblastoma multiforme is the most aggressive type of cancer that begins within the brain. It invades nearby brain tissue but generally does not spread to distant organs. In adults, glioblastoma multiforme occurs most often in the cerebral hemispheres, especially in the frontal and temporal lobes of the brain. It is a devastating brain cancer that can result in death in six months or less if left untreated. Signs and symptoms of glioblastoma multiforme are nonspecific and can include headaches, personality changes, nausea, and symptoms similar to stroke. Treatment includes surgery, chemotherapy and radiation.

Glioma

Glioma is one of the most common types of brain tumors. Glioma can affect brain function, and depending on its location and rate of growth, it can be life-threatening.

Glottis

The glottis is the part of the larynx, or voice box, consisting of the vocal cords and the opening between them. The glottis affects voice modulation by expanding and contracting.

Half-life

The half-life of a drug is the time it takes for the concentration of a drug in the blood to be reduced by half. When the term "half-life" is applied to radioisotopes, it refers to the time it takes for a radioisotope to decay by 50 percent.

Head and neck cancer

Head and neck cancers include cancers of the larynx, throat, lips, mouth, nose, and salivary glands. Tobacco use, heavy alcohol use, and infection with human papillomavirus (HPV) increase the risk of head and neck cancers.

Heart attack

A heart attack, also called acute myocardial infarction, occurs when an artery supplying the heart with blood and oxygen becomes blocked by fatty deposits and cholesterol (plaque). If a plaque ruptures, a clot can form, blocking the coronary arteries and causing a heart attack. The interrupted blood flow can damage or destroy heart muscle, potentially causing death.

Heart disease

Heart disease is the leading cause of death in the United States. The term "heart disease" refers to several types of heart conditions, the most common of which is coronary artery disease.

Heart failure

Heart failure, also known as congestive heart failure, is a condition that develops when the heart muscle does not pump enough blood. This can occur if the heart does not fill up with enough blood or is too weak to pump blood properly. When this happens, blood often backs up, and fluid can build up in the lungs, causing shortness of breath.

Heart failure cells

Heart failure cells are "siderophages" generated in the alveoli of the lungs in people with left heart failure or chronic pulmonary edema. Siderophages are nonspecific diagnostic indicators of heart failure.

Heart ventricles

Heart ventricles are involved in the pumping of blood. The right ventricle of the heart pumps oxygen-poor blood into the lungs to be oxygenated, whereas the left ventricle pumps oxygen-rich blood to the rest of the body.

Heatstroke

Heatstroke is the most serious heat-related illness. It occurs when the body is unable to control its temperature owing to a failure in the sweating mechanism, causing the body temperature to rapidly rise.

Hemophilia

Hemophilia is a rare inherited bleeding disorder in which the blood does not clot properly because it does not have enough blood-clotting proteins. This can lead to spontaneous bleeding as well as to bleeding following injuries or surgery.

Hemorrhagic shock

Hemorrhagic shock is a condition of reduced tissue perfusion, resulting in the inadequate delivery of oxygen and nutrients necessary for cellular function. The imbalance between oxygen demand of tissues and the body's inability to supply oxygen leads to shock. Classically, there are four categories of shock—hypovolemic, cardiogenic, obstructive, and distributive shock. Hypovolemic shock due to severe dehydration or from loss of blood can lead to cardiovascular compromise.

Hemosiderin laden macrophages

When blood leaves a ruptured blood vessel, the red blood cell dies and the hemoglobin of the red blood cell is released into the extracellular space. Phagocytic cells called macrophages engulf the hemoglobin and degrade it, producing hemosiderin and biliverdin. Pulmonary congestion with dilated capillaries and leakage of blood into alveolar spaces leads to an increase in hemosiderin-laden macrophages.

Hepatitis

Hepatitis is inflammation of the liver. When the liver is inflamed or damaged, its function can be affected. Hepatitis can be caused by chronic alcohol abuse, chemical toxins, some medications, and certain medical conditions. Hepatitis A is a highly contagious liver infection caused by the Hepatitis A virus.

Hodgkin's lymphoma

Hodgkin's lymphoma, formerly known as Hodgkin's disease, is a cancer of the lymphatic system, part of the immune system. Hodgkin's lymphoma is most common in people between the ages of twenty and forty years old and those over fifty-five. Of the two common types of cancers of the lymphatic system, non-Hodgkin's lymphoma is far more common than Hodgkin's lymphoma.

Homicidal hanging

Homicidal hanging is an extremely rare occurrence. Very few cases have been reported in which a person is rendered senseless and then hanged to simulate suicidal death, although there are a lot of cases in which a victim of a homicide has later been hanged.

Hospice care

Hospice care is a type of health care that prioritizes comfort and quality of life by reducing pain and suffering. Hospice care focuses on reducing or eliminating the pain associated with a terminal illness and attending to a patient's emotional and spiritual needs at the end of life.

Human papillomavirus

Human papillomavirus (HPV) is a viral infection that is passed between people through skin-to-skin contact during vaginal, anal, or oral sex. It is the most common sexually transmitted infection in the United States. There are over one hundred varieties of HPV, more than forty of which are passed through sexual contact. HPV can affect the genitals, mouth, or throat. Symptoms of HPV include warts on the genitals or surrounding skin, which may go away on their own. A vaccine that prevents the HPV strains most likely to cause genital warts and cervical cancer is recommended for boys and girls.

Humerus

The humerus is the bone of the upper arm or forelimb, forming joints at the shoulder and the elbow.

Hydrogen cyanide

Hydrogen cyanide is a colorless or pale blue liquid or gas with a bitter, almondlike odor. The chemical interferes with the body's use of oxygen and can be toxic to the brain, heart, blood vessels, and lungs. Exposure to hydrogen cyanide can be fatal.

Hyoid bone

The hyoid bone is a small U-shaped bone located in the midline of the neck at the base of the mandible (lower jaw), behind the fourth cervical vertebra, and near the thyroid cartilage. It is part of a functional system that provides attachments for the muscles of the tongue, the larynx, the mandible, and other structures in the mouth and throat.

Hyperthermia

Hyperthermia is an abnormally high body temperature caused by a failure of the heat-regulating mechanisms of the body to deal with heat generated by the environment. Heat fatigue, heat syncope (sudden dizziness), heat cramps, heat exhaustion, heat stroke, confusion, nausea and vomiting, and rapid breathing are common symptoms of hyperthermia.

Hypertrophy

Hypertrophy is an enlargement of any organ or part of the body due to the increased size of the constituent cells.

Hypotension

Hypotension, or low blood pressure, occurs when blood pressure drops below the normal range. Doctors generally define low blood pressure as 90/60 millimeters of mercury or below. Physicians usually do not treat hypotension unless it is severe enough to cause symptoms. Low blood pressure can be a sign of an underlying health problem, especially in the elderly, where it may cause inadequate blood flow to the heart, brain, and other vital organs.

Hypoxia

Hypoxia is a state in which oxygen is not available in sufficient amounts at the tissue level to maintain adequate homeostasis. Hypoxemia, on the other hand, is when the oxygen level in the blood is low. High altitude, asthma, or heart disease can result in hypoxemia, particularly under more extreme conditions, such as exercise or illness. Some symptoms of hypoxemia include shortness of breath, headache, confusion, and restlessness.

Idiopathic pulmonary fibrosis

Idiopathic pulmonary fibrosis (IPF) is a serious lung disease in which scar tissue grows inside the lungs, making it harder to breathe. IPF slows oxygen flow from the lungs to the blood, thereby substantially reducing the amount of oxygen reaching vital organs and affecting organ function. There is no cure for

IPF. Symptoms of IPF include shortness of breath, a dry, hacking cough that doesn't go away, chest pain or tightness, leg swelling, and a loss of appetite, among others.

Ileum

The ileum is the third portion of the small intestine, between the jejunum and the cecum. The ileum helps to further digest food and to absorb nutrients and water.

Immunological toxicology screen

An immunologic toxicology screen is a test to detect the presence of a drug in a biological fluid, such as blood or urine. The test does not quantify and is subject to false-positive and false-negative results.

Infarct

An infarct is a small localized area of dead heart muscle resulting from a failure of adequate blood supply due to a heart attack.

Innominate bone

The innominate bone, also known as the hip bone, is the fused bone of the pelvis on either side of the sacrum, the triangular bone just below the lumbar vertebrae.

Insanity defense

The insanity defense is based on the premise that a defendant is not responsible for his or her actions owing to an episodic or persistent psychiatric disease at the time of the criminal act.

Intestinal ischemic enteropathy

Intestinal ischemic enteropathy is the result of insufficient delivery of oxygen-rich blood to the small intestine due to a blocked blood vessel, usually an artery. Intestinal ischemic enteropathy is a serious condition that can cause pain, affect the function of the intestines, and, in severe cases, lead to death.

Intestinal malrotation

Intestinal malrotation is an abnormality in which the intestine has not formed properly in the fetus between the eighth and twelfth weeks of the pregnancy. The condition is congenital and present at birth. While it can lead to complications, intestinal malrotation is treatable in children when caught early. Cases of intestinal malrotation in adults, however, are rare, and they can have devastating consequences if not recognized early, including the onset of gangrene and death.

Ischemic enteropathy

Insufficient oxygen delivery through the mesenteric capillary circulation is the common precipitating factor in acute ischemic enteropathy. The syndrome may result from systemic circulatory failure or sudden vascular occlusion.

Jaundice

Jaundice is a condition in which the skin, whites of the eyes, and mucous membranes turn yellow because of a high level of bilirubin, a yellow-orange bile pigment in red blood cells. While jaundice is rare in adults, it has many causes, including hepatitis, gallstones, alcohol-related liver disease, blocked bile ducts, pancreatic cancer, and certain medications.

Jejunum

The jejunum is the middle part of the small intestine, between the duodenum and the ileum. The jejunum helps to further digest food and to absorb nutrients and water.

Judicial hanging

The cause of death in judicial hanging is controversial and is often attributed to "hangman's fracture" of the second cervical vertebra. Research has shown that such fractures are the exception in judicial hangings, and the cause of death can be attributed to a range of head and neck injuries, particularly compression or rupture of the vertebral and carotid arteries, leading to cerebral ischemia. The rapidity of loss of consciousness and death is highly dependent upon knot positioning and the length of drop.

Ketones

Ketones are byproducts of the breakdown of fatty acids. Ketone levels in the blood are elevated in a person with diabetes.

Laceration

A laceration tends to be caused by a sharp object, such as a knife or a shard of glass. "Cut" and "laceration" are terms for the same condition. Unlike an abrasion, none of the skin is missing in a laceration.

Laparotomy

Laparotomy is a surgical incision into the abdominal cavity allowing for examination of the abdominal organs. Possible complications of laparotomy include infection and the formation of scar tissue within the abdominal cavity.

Laryngeal diphtheria

Laryngeal diphtheria usually results from the spread of the infection downward from the nasopharynx to the larynx. In such a condition, the airway may become blocked, and it must be restored by inserting a tube or cutting an opening in the trachea.

Laryngitis

Laryngitis is an inflammation of the larynx from overuse, irritation, or infection.

Larynx

The larynx is the passageway for air between the pharynx or throat, above, and the trachea, below. The larynx is involved in breathing, producing sound, and protecting the trachea against aspiration of food.

Latency period

Latency period is the amount of time elapsed between an initial exposure to a carcinogen and a diagnosis of cancer.

Leukemia

Leukemia is a group of cancers of the blood-forming tissues, including the bone marrow. Many patients with slow-growing types of leukemia do not have symptoms. Rapidly growing types of leukemia may cause symptoms that include fatigue, weight loss, frequent infections, and easy bleeding or bruising. Treatment of slow-growing leukemia includes monitoring. Treatment of aggressive leukemia includes chemotherapy, which is sometimes followed by radiation and stem-cell transplant.

Liver cancer

Primary liver cancer, also known as hepatocellular carcinoma, tends to occur in livers damaged by birth defects, alcohol abuse, or chronic infection with diseases such as hepatitis B and C, hemochromatosis, a hereditary disease associated with too much iron in the liver, and cirrhosis, a scarring condition of the liver commonly caused by alcohol abuse. More than half of all people diagnosed with primary liver cancer have cirrhosis. Liver cancer is also linked to obesity and fatty liver disease.

Manner of death

Manner of death is a medicolegal interpretation of the events leading up to a death. There are five categories for manner of death, including natural, accident, suicide, homicide, and undetermined.

Medulla oblongata

The medulla oblongata, located at the base of the brain, where the brain stem connects the brain to the spinal cord, plays a critical role in transmitting signals between the spinal cord and the brain and in controlling autonomic activities, such as heartbeat and respiration.

Mesentery

The mesentery is a fold in the peritoneum, the tissue that lines the abdominal wall and covers most of the organs in the abdomen.

Metabolic acidosis

Metabolic acidosis is a clinical disturbance characterized by an increase in plasma acidity. It may be a sign of an underlying disease process or poorly functioning kidneys.

Multifocal myocardial fibrosis

Multiple myocardial fibrosis is an increased quantity of collagenous scar tissue in the heart. It can arise as a result of heart disease and can lead to heart failure and death.

Multiple endocrine neoplasia type 1 syndrome

Multiple endocrine neoplasia type 1 is a hereditary condition associated with tumors of the endocrine-hormone-producing glands. The most common tumors seen in multiple endocrine neoplasia type 1 syndrome involve the parathyroid gland, islet cells of the pancreas, and pituitary gland. Other endocrine tumors include adrenal cortical tumors, neuroendocrine tumors, and rarely pheochromocytoma, as well as tumors in other parts of the digestive tract.

Myocardial infarction

A myocardial infarction or a heart attack occurs when one or more areas of the heart muscle do not get enough oxygen owing to a blockage in blood flow to the heart muscle.

Myocardium

The myocardium is the muscular layer of the heart.

Nasal pharynx

The nasal pharynx is one of three parts of the pharynx, a cone-shaped passageway leading from the oral and nasal cavities in the head to the esophagus and larynx. The pharynx serves both respiratory and digestive functions, enabling breathing through the nose and mouth.

Neurofibromatosis type 1

Neurofibromatosis type 1 is a genetic condition that causes tumors to grow along nerves. Neurofibromas are often seen as raised bumps or multiple café-au-lait spots on the skin. The tumors are usually benign, but they may cause a range of symptoms depending on their location.

Neutrons

Neutrons are subatomic particles located in the nuclei of atoms. They have a neutral charge and a mass slightly greater than that of a proton, a positively charged subatomic particle.

Nevus

A nevus is a birthmark or a mole on the skin. It is usually benign, but in rare cases, it can turn into melanoma or other skin cancers.

Nitric oxide

Nitric oxide is a naturally produced chemical in the body whose most important function is vasodilation—the relaxation of the inner muscles of blood vessels, causing them to widen and increase blood circulation.

Non–small cell lung cancer

There are several types of non–small cell lung cancer. Squamous cell carcinoma forms in the thin, flat cells lining the inside of the lungs. Large cell carcinoma begins in several different types of large cells. Adenocarcinoma begins in cells that line the alveoli and makes substances such as mucus. Less common types of non–small cell lung cancer include adenosquamous carcinoma, sarcomatoid carcinoma, salivary gland carcinoma, carcinoid tumor, and unclassified carcinoma. Smoking is the major and most important risk factor for non–small cell lung cancer.

Novichok nerve agent

Novichok nerve agent belongs to a class of organophosphate acetylcholinesterase inhibitors. Novichok acts by preventing the normal breakdown of the neurotransmitter acetylcholine.

Obesity

Obesity is the condition of having too much body fat. The weight may come from muscle, bone, fat, or body water. Obesity is different from being overweight, which means weighing too much. Both terms mean that a person's weight is greater than what is considered healthy for his or her height. Being obese increases the risk of having heart disease, diabetes, high blood pressure, and certain types of cancers. Although there are genetic, behavioral, metabolic, and hormonal influences on body weight, obesity occurs when more calories are ingested than are burned through normal daily activities and exercise. As a result, the body stores the excess calories as fat.

Occipital bone

The occipital bone is the bone that forms the back and base of the skull, and through which the spinal cord passes.

Oropharyngeal cancer

Oropharyngeal cancer is a disease in which cancer cells form in the tissues of the oropharynx, the middle part of the throat. Smoking or being infected with HPV can increase the likelihood of developing oropharyngeal cancer.

Oropharynx

The oropharynx is the part of the throat at the back of the mouth and behind the oral cavity. It includes the back third of the tongue, the soft palate at the back part of the roof of the mouth, the side and back walls of the throat, and the tonsils.

Osteomyelitis

Osteomyelitis is inflammation or swelling that occurs in bone. It can result from an infection somewhere else in the body that has spread to the bone, or it can start in the bone, often as a result of an injury.

Oxygen

Oxygen is a highly reactive element and an oxidizing agent that readily forms oxides with most elements and with other compounds. During the process of inhalation, oxygen from the air enters the lungs, where it is exchanged for carbon dioxide in the blood. The carbon dioxide, in turn, is then exhaled.

Pancreatic cancer

Pancreatic cancer is often detected late, mainly because there are no symptoms in its early stages. Pancreatic cancer spreads rapidly, and it has a poor prognosis. Later stages of pancreatic cancer are associated with symptoms, but they are non-specific, such as a lack of appetite and weight loss. Treatment of pancreatic cancer includes surgically removing the pancreas, radiation, and chemotherapy.

Pancreatic ductal carcinoma

Pancreatic ductal adenocarcinoma is a highly aggressive lethal malignancy that develops in the exocrine compartment of the pancreas. It is the most prevalent type of pancreatic cancer, accounting for more than 90 percent of all pancreatic cancer cases.

Pancreatic neuroendocrine cancer

Pancreatic neuroendocrine tumors, or islet cell tumors, are a relatively uncommon type of pancreatic cancer. They develop in the endocrine compartment of the pancreas and make up less than 2 percent of all pancreatic cancers. Pancreatic neuroendocrine tumors have a better prognosis than cancer of the exocrine pancreas, such as the more common pancreatic ductal adenocarcinoma.

Pancytopenia

Pancytopenia is a condition in which there are lower-than-normal numbers of red and white blood cells and platelets in the blood. Pancytopenia occurs when there is a problem with the blood-forming stem cells in the bone marrow. Treatment includes drugs to stimulate blood cell production in the bone marrow; blood transfusions to replace red blood cells, white blood cells, and platelets; and antibiotics to treat any infection.

Pathogen

A pathogen is any organism that can produce disease. There are five main types of pathogens: bacteria, viruses, fungi, protists, pathogens that affect plants and food crops and cause dysentery when ingested, and parasitic worms, such as flatworms and roundworms.

Pectus excavatum

Pectus excavatum is a condition in which the breastbone is sunken into the chest. In severe cases, pectus excavatum can interfere with the function of the heart and lungs.

Penile verrucous nodule

Penile verrucous nodule is a benign lesion, unlike penile verrucous carcinoma, which is cancerous. Penile verrucous nodule can arise anywhere on the penis but mostly occurs on the glans or foreskin.

Peptic ulcer

A peptic ulcer is a sore on the lining of the stomach, small intestine, or esophagus. The most common causes of peptic ulcer are an infection with the bacterium *Helicobacter pylori* and long-term use of nonsteroidal anti-inflammatory drugs, such as ibuprofen and naproxen.

Pericardium

The pericardium is a membrane or sac that surrounds the heart. A normal pericardium consists of an outer sac called the fibrous pericardium and an inner one called the serous pericardium. The two layers of the serous pericardium, visceral and parietal, are separated by the pericardial cavity, which contains twenty to sixty milliliters of a plasma ultrafiltrate. The function of the pericardium is to protect the heart and big vessels and to act as a lubricant to reduce friction between the heart and the surrounding structures.

Peripheral neuropathy

Peripheral neuropathy is a result of damage to the nerves located outside of the brain and spinal cord. A common cause of peripheral neuropathy is diabetes, but it can also result from injuries, infections, and exposure to toxins. Symptoms of peripheral neuropathy include pain, a pins-and-needles sensation, numbness, and weakness.

Peritoneum

The peritoneum is the tissue that lines the abdominal wall and covers most of the organs in the abdomen. A peritoneal fluid lubricates the surface of the peritoneum.

Peritonitis

Peritonitis is an inflammation of the membrane lining the abdominal wall and covering the abdominal organs. Peritonitis is usually infectious and often life-threatening. It is caused by leakage from the intestines, such as from a burst appendix. Symptoms usually include pain, tenderness, rigid abdominal muscles, fever, nausea, and vomiting.

Petechiae

Petechiae are small, often less than three millimeters in diameter, red or purple spots on the skin that do not blanch when pressed.

They are red because they contain red blood cells that have leaked from capillaries into the skin.

Plaque

Plaque is caused by a buildup of cholesterol deposits in blood vessels. When it occurs in coronary arteries, it can reduce the size of the lumen, decrease the flow of oxygen-rich blood to the heart, and increase the risk for a heart attack.

Plasma

Plasma is the liquid portion of blood. The main function of plasma is to transport nutrients, hormones, and proteins to various parts of the body, and waste products from cells to the liver for metabolism and to be excreted in the kidneys and lungs.

Pleural adhesions

"Pleural adhesions" refers to the formation of fibrotic bands that span the pleural space, which lies between the parietal and visceral layers of the pleura, a thin layer of tissue that covers the lungs and lines the interior wall of the chest cavity.

Polonium-210

Polonium-210 is a rare radioisotope of polonium. Polonium-210 undergoes alpha decay with a half-life of 138.376 days, the longest half-life of all naturally occurring polonium isotopes. Because polonium-210 emits alpha particles that can travel only a short distance, it cannot be detected by a whole-body or Geiger counter.

If polonium-210 enters the body by inhalation or ingestion, or through broken skin, the effect on internal organs can be fatal.

Polypharmacy

Polypharmacy is the simultaneous ingestion of several drugs, often with similar pharmacological and toxicological properties. Although each drug may be taken at therapeutic doses, their combination increases the likelihood of toxic effects, such as central nervous system and respiratory depression, and possibly death.

Postmortem redistribution

Postmortem redistribution refers to the changes that occur in drug concentrations in the blood after death. It involves the redistribution of drugs into blood from the lungs, liver, and heart.

Potassium cyanide

Potassium cyanide releases hydrogen cyanide gas, a highly toxic chemical that interferes with the body's ability to utilize oxygen. Exposure to potassium cyanide can be rapidly fatal. It particularly affects those organ systems most sensitive to low oxygen levels— the brain, the lungs, and the cardiovascular system, including the heart and blood vessels.

Prussian blue

Prussian blue is a dark blue pigment produced by oxidation of ferrous ferrocyanide salts. Prussian blue is used to treat thallium poisoning by binding thallium, the combination of which is then excreted from the body.

Pseudotubercles

Pseudotubercles are nodules, histologically similar to tuberculous granuloma, that are due to an infection by a microorganism other than *Mycobacterium tuberculosis*.

Psychological autopsy

A psychological autopsy is an in-depth reconstruction of an unclear suicide death. A trained mental health expert reviews all available evidence, including suicide notes, and interviews family members, friends, and others who are able to provide relevant information about the victim and the behaviors and events that led up to the death, after which a conclusion is made as to whether the cause of death was suicide or accidental.

Pylorus

The pylorus is that part of the stomach that connects to the duodenum, the first part of the small intestine. It is a valve that opens and closes during digestion, allowing partly digested food and other stomach contents to pass from the stomach to the small intestine.

Quinsy

Quinsy, one of the most common head and neck bacterial infections in adults, is an accumulation of pus due to an infection behind the tonsils. Symptoms of quinsy include fever, throat pain, trouble opening the mouth, and a voice change. Swollen tissues can block the airways. The first steps in the management of quinsy are treatments with broad-spectrum antibiotics that cover aerobic and anaerobic bacteria. Steroids may be used to alleviate the symptoms of pain and swelling and to reduce recovery period. Oxygen is often provided, and intubation may be necessary because of blockage of the airways.

Regulation D violation

Regulation D imposes reserve requirements on certain deposits and other liabilities of depository institutions solely for the purpose of implementing monetary policy. Regulation D violations can cause excessive transfer fees to be implemented by potentially having high-yield savings accounts converted into transactional accounts that may not earn any interest.

Respiratory depression

Respiratory depression is a breathing disorder characterized by slow and ineffective breathing. When caused by an overdose of barbiturates or opioid drugs, respiratory depression is the result of inhibition of respiratory centers in the brain.

Respiratory failure

Respiratory failure is a condition in which the blood does not have enough oxygen or has too much carbon dioxide. Symptoms of respiratory failure include shortness of breath, a bluish tint in the face and lips, and confusion.

Respiratory system

The respiratory system is a biological system that moves fresh air and oxygen into the body while removing waste gases, such as carbon dioxide. The main organ of the respiratory system is the lungs. Other respiratory organs include the nose, the trachea, and the breathing muscles—the diaphragm and the intercostal muscles. Some common problems of the respiratory system include asthma, bronchitis, emphysema, hay fever, influenza, laryngitis, and pneumonia.

Schistosomiasis

Schistosomiasis is a disease caused by parasitic worms. Although the worms that cause schistosomiasis are not found in the United States, the disease is second only to malaria as the most devastating parasitic disease. Within one to two months of infection, symptoms of schistosomiasis may develop; these include fever, chills, cough, and muscle aches. The disease can persist for years without treatment with signs and symptoms such as abdominal pain, enlarged liver, blood in the stool or blood in the urine, and problems passing urine.

Scurvy

Scurvy is a disease caused by a deficiency of vitamin C. It is characterized by swollen bleeding gums and the opening of previously healed wounds. Scurvy can lead to anemia; debility; exhaustion; spontaneous bleeding; pain in the limbs, especially in the legs; swelling in some parts of the body; and possible ulceration of the gums and loss of teeth.

Sepsis

Sepsis is a life-threatening medical emergency. It happens when an infection, most often in the lungs, urinary tract, skin, or gastrointestinal tract, causes a release of chemicals into the bloodstream, triggering inflammation throughout the body and a cascade of changes that damages multiple organ systems, leading them to fail, sometimes even resulting in death. Symptoms of sepsis include fever, difficulty breathing, low blood pressure, fast heart rate, and mental confusion. Treatment includes antibiotics and intravenous fluids.

Septic shock

Septic shock is a life-threatening condition that happens when the blood pressure drops to a dangerously low level after a bacterial infection. Most people recover from mild sepsis, but the mortality rate for septic shock is about 40 percent.

Sleep apnea

Sleep apnea is a potentially serious sleep disorder in which breathing repeatedly stops and starts. Symptoms of sleep apnea include snoring loudly and feeling tired even after a full night's sleep. Treatment often includes lifestyle changes, such as weight loss, and the use of a breathing assistance device at night, including a continuous positive airway pressure machine.

Sphenoid sinuses

Sphenoid sinuses are hollow spaces in the sphenoid bone, which is located behind the nose and between the eyes. They are lined with cells that make mucus to keep the nose from drying out.

Squamous cells

Squamous cells are thin, flat cells found in the tissue that forms the surface of the skin, the lining of the hollow organs of the body, and the linings of the respiratory and digestive tracts.

Stereotactic radiosurgery

Stereotactic radiosurgery uses precisely focused radiation beams to treat tumors in the brain, neck, lungs, liver, spine, and other parts of the body. Like other forms of radiation, it damages the DNA of cancer cells, which then lose their ability to reproduce, causing the tumors to shrink.

Stomach ulcer

Stomach ulcers occur when stomach acid damages the lining of the digestive tract. Common causes include the bacteria *Helicobacter pylori* and anti-inflammatory pain relieving drugs, such as aspirin. Upper abdominal pain is a common symptom. Treatment usually includes medication to decrease stomach acid production.

Stridular suffocates

Stridular suffocates is a blockage of the larynx or throat.

Stroke

A stroke occurs when the blood supply to a part of the brain is interrupted or reduced, preventing brain tissue from getting oxygen and nutrients, and causing brain cells to die. There are two main causes of stroke—a blocked artery or leaking or bursting of a blood vessel. A stroke is a medical emergency, and prompt treatment with tPA (clot buster) is crucial to minimize brain damage. Symptoms of stroke include trouble walking, speaking, and understanding, as well as paralysis or numbness of the face, arm, or leg.

Sudden death

Sudden death is an unexpected death caused by loss of heart function. It is the result of a malfunctioning electrical system in the heart that leads the heartbeat to become very irregular and dangerously fast. The ventricles may flutter or quiver. The greatest concern in the initial minutes is that blood flow to the brain will be drastically reduced. Death follows unless emergency treatment is immediately initiated.

Sudden unexplained death in epilepsy

Sudden unexplained death in epilepsy (SUDEP) is the sudden, unexpected death of someone with epilepsy who was otherwise healthy. No other cause of death is found at autopsy. Each year, more than one in one thousand people with epilepsy die from SUDEP. It is the leading cause of death in people with uncontrolled seizures.

Suicidal hanging

Hanging is a common mode of committing suicide and the most frequently used method of suicide in the United Kingdom. Suicidal hanging has a high rate of fatality, greater than 70 percent. Death usually occurs within a few minutes of hanging.

Suppuration

Suppuration is the discharging of pus from a wound or sore.

Tachycardia

Tachycardia is a fast heart rate, usually over one hundred beats per minute. There are many heart rhythm disorders and arrhythmias that can cause tachycardia. Common causes of tachycardia include high blood pressure, poor blood supply to the heart muscle due to coronary artery disease, heart valve disease, heart failure, heart muscle disease, tumors, and infections. Treatment ranges from medication to surgery.

Temporal and frontal regions of the brain

The temporal region of the brain plays a key role in auditory processing, including perception of sounds, assigning meaning to those sounds, and remembering and integrating sounds with sensations of taste, sight, and touch. The frontal region of the brain is important for cognitive functions and control of voluntary movement or activity and is generally where higher executive functions occur, including emotional regulation, planning, reasoning, and problem-solving.

Thallium

Thallium was discovered by Sir William Crookes in 1861. It is tasteless and odorless and has been used by murderers since it is difficult to detect. Thallium has not been produced in the United States since 1984.

Thromboembolism

A thromboembolism is an obstruction of a blood vessel by a blood clot that has become dislodged from another site in the circulatory system. The clot may plug a vessel in the lungs; the brain, causing a stroke; the gastrointestinal tract; the kidneys; or the leg.

Thrombosis

Thrombosis occurs when blood clots block veins or arteries. Symptoms include pain and swelling in one leg, chest pain, or numbness on one side of the body. Complications of thrombosis, such as stroke or heart attack, can be life-threatening.

Thyroid cartilage

The thyroid cartilage is a structure that sits in front of the larynx and above the thyroid gland. It is composed of two halves that meet in the middle at a peak called the laryngeal prominence, also called the "Adam's apple."

Tolerance

Tolerance is the body's diminished response to a drug due to adaptation after repeated use. When tolerance to a particular drug develops, higher doses are needed to achieve the same desired effect.

Torsades de pointes

Torsades de pointes is one of several types of life-threatening heart rhythm disturbances or arrhythmias. In torsades de pointes, the heart's ventricles beat faster and are out of sync with the beating of the upper chambers, called the atria. Symptoms of torsades de pointes include heart palpitations, dizziness, nausea, chest pain, cold sweats, shortness of breath, a rapid pulse, and a low blood pressure.

Tracheobronchial tree

The tracheobronchial tree is composed of the trachea and the intrapulmonary airways, including the bronchi, bronchioles, and respiratory bronchioles. The tracheobronchial tree is a system of airways that allows passage of air into the lungs, where gas exchange occurs.

Tracheotomy

Tracheotomy is the act of making an incision into the trachea to forms an opening, called a "tracheostomy." Tracheotomy is usually performed to deliver oxygen to the lungs or to bypass an obstructed upper airway.

Trismus

Trismus, commonly called "lockjaw," refers to the restriction of the range of motion of the jaws. It typically stems from a sustained tetanic spasm of the muscles of mastication or chewing.

Type 1 diabetes

Diabetes is a chronic condition in which the pancreas produces little or no insulin. People with type 1 diabetes do not produce insulin. There is no cure for type 1 diabetes, so people with type 1 diabetes must regularly inject insulin.

Type 2 diabetes

Diabetes is a chronic condition in which the pancreas produces little or no insulin. People with type 2 diabetes do not respond to insulin as well as they should. Type 2 diabetes can sometimes be reversed with diet and exercise alone. Many people with type 2 diabetes can managed the condition with medications that help the body use insulin more effectively.

Undifferentiated hepatocellular carcinoma

Undifferentiated hepatocellular carcinoma is an extremely rare liver-malignant disease accounting for less than 2 percent of all liver cancers.

Ventricular fibrillation

Ventricular fibrillation is a rapid, life-threatening heart rhythm starting in the ventricles. Since the heart does not pump adequately during ventricular fibrillation, it can lead to low blood pressure, loss of consciousness, or death. Emergency treatment of ventricular fibrillation includes defibrillation with an automated external defibrillator and cardiopulmonary resuscitation. Long-term therapy includes medications to prevent a recurrence and implantable defibrillators.

Ventricular tachycardia

Ventricular tachycardia is an arrhythmia caused by abnormal electrical signals in the ventricles. It is defined as three or more heartbeats in a row at a rate of more than one hundred beats per minute. The rapid heartbeat does not give the heart enough time to fill with blood before it contracts again, which can affect blood flow to the rest of the body. If ventricular tachycardia lasts for more than a few seconds at a time, it can become life-threatening.

Verrucous carcinoma

Verrucous carcinoma is an uncommon variant of squamous cell carcinoma. This form of cancer is often seen in people who chew tobacco or use snuff orally.

Vertigo

Vertigo, a sensation of whirling and loss of balance, is associated particularly with looking down from a great height; it may be caused by disease affecting the inner ear or the vestibular nerve.

Vitreous humor

Vitreous humor is a transparent gel-like substance that fills the space between the lens and the retina of the eye. It is composed mostly of water and a small amount of collagen, glycosaminoglycans (sugars), electrolytes (salts), and proteins.

Volvulus

Volvulus is an abnormal twisting of a portion of the gastrointestinal tract, usually the small intestine, which can impair blood flow. The area of the intestine above the obstruction continues to function and fill with food, fluid, and gas. Volvulus can lead to gangrene and death of the involved segment, as well as intestinal obstruction, perforation of the small intestine, and peritonitis, a life-threatening infection of the membrane lining the abdominal wall. Symptoms and signs of volvulus may include abdominal pain, nausea, vomiting, and blood in the stool.

Von Hippel Lindau syndrome

Von Hippel Lindau syndrome is a rare inherited disorder that causes tumors and cysts to grow in certain parts of the body, including the brain, spinal cord, eyes, inner ear, adrenal glands, pancreas, kidney, and reproductive tract.

NOTES

Introduction

[1] E. J. Wagner, "The French Connection of Sherlock Holmes," February 25, 2011, https://ejdissectingroom.wordpress.com/2011/02/25/the-french-connection-of-sherlock-holmes/; "Edmond Locard," The Forensics Library, http://aboutforensics.co.uk/edmond-locard/; H. A. Milman, "Introduction" in *Forensics: The Science Behind the Deaths of Famous People* (Bloomington, Indiana: Xlibris, 2020) pp. xi–xx.

[2] "Locard's Exchange Principle," Forensic Handbook, August 12, 2012, http://www.forensichandbook.com/locards-exchange-principle/.

[3] B. Levine, *Principles of Forensic Toxicology* (AACC Press, 2nd ed., 2003); see H. A. Milman, note 1, above.

[4] "A Simplified Guide to Toxicology," http://www.forensicsciencesimplified.org/tox/Toxicology.pdf; O. H. Drummer, "Forensic toxicology," EXS 100:579-603 (2010); see B. Levine, note 3, above.

[5] See note 4, above.

6. See note 4, above.

7. See H. A. Milman, note 1, above; see note 4, above.

8. See H. A. Milman, note 1, above.

9. M. C. Yaema and C. E. Becker, "Key Concepts in Postmortem Drug Redistribution," *Clin Toxicol* 43(4) (2005): 235–241; see H. A. Milman, note 1, above.

10. H. A. Milman, "Marilyn Monroe," in *Forensics: The Science Behind the Deaths of Famous People* (Bloomington, Indiana: Xlibris, 2020) pp. 15–34.

11. H. A. Milman, *Forensics: The Science Behind the Deaths of Famous People* (Bloomington, Indiana: Xlibris, 2020).

1. George Washington

1. W. McKenzie Wallenborn, "George Washington's Terminal Illness: A Modern Medical Analysis of the Last Illness and Death of George Washington," Washington Papers, November 5, 1997, https://washingtonpapers.org/resources/articles/illness/; "Biography of George Washington," George Washington's Mount Vernon, https://www.mountvernon.org/george-washington/biography/.

2. "George Washington's Death," https://georgewashington.org/death.jsp; "Dec. 14, 1979: The excruciating final hours of President George Washington," Public Broadcasting Service, December 14, 2014, https://www.pbs.org/newshour/health/dec-14-1799-excruciating-final-hours-president-george-washington; "The Death of George Washington, 1799," Eyewitness to History, 2001, http://www.eyewitnesstohistory.com/washington.htm; "Tobias Lear Journal," https://hsp.org/sites/default/files/Tobias%20Lear%20Journal%20Transcription%20by%20Cameron%20Kline%202018.pdf; V. V. Vadakan, "A Physician's Looks at the Death of Washington," https://www.varsitytutors.com/earlyamerica/early-america-review/volume-9/washingtons-death; G. Carlton, "The Shocking True Story of George Washington's Death, From Bloodletting to Beetles," March 23 2020, https://allthatsinteresting.

com/how-did-george-washington-die; "The Death of George Washington," https://www.mountvernon.org/library/digital/history/digital-encyclopedia/article/the-death-of-george-washington/; R. Marx, "A Medical Profile of George Washington," *American Heritage* 6(5) (1955): https://www.americanheritage.com/medical-profile-george-washngton; J. Woodruff, "Bloodletting and blisters: Solving the medical mystery of George Washington's death," Public Broadcasting Service, December 15, 2014, https://www.pbs.org/newshour/show/bloodletting-blisters-solving-medical-mystery-george-washingtons-death; see note 1, above.

3. "George Washington's Blueskin," The Presidential Pet Museum, https://www.presidentialpetmuseum.com/george-washingtons-blueskin/; K. Kovatch, "Nelson and Blueskin: The First Horses of the United States," February 16, 2015, https://www.horsenation.com/2015/02/16/nelson-and-blueskin-the-first-horses-of-the-united-states/.

4. M. Lalonde, "Did George Washington's Doctors Accidentally Torture Him to Death?" April 15, 2021, https://rare.us/rare-news/history/george-washington-death/; J. Somers, "George Washington's Tragic Death Explained," September 3, 2020, https://www.grunge.com/25722/10-things-assumed-true-american-history-arent/; see note 1, above; see "George Washington's Death," "Dec. 14, 1979: The excruciating final hours of President George Washington," "The Death of George Washington, 1799," "Tobias Lear Journal," V. V. Vadakan, G. Carlton, "The Death of George Washington," R. Marx, note 2, above.

5. D. M. Morens, "Death of a President," *N Engl J Med.* 341(24) (1999): 1845–1849; see "George Washington's Death," "Dec. 14, 1979: The excruciating final hours of President George Washington," "The Death of George Washington, 1799," "Tobias Lear Journal," W. McKenzie Wallenborn, V. V. Vadakan, G. Carlton, "The Death of George Washington," R. Marx, and "Biography of George Washington," note 2, above; see M. Lalonde, note 4, above.

6. See "George Washington's Death," "Tobias Lear Journal," W. McKenzie Wallenborn, V. V. Vadakan, G. Carlton, "The Death of George Washington," and R. Marx, note 2, above.

7. See "George Washington's Death," "The Death of George Washington, 1799," "Tobias Lear Journal," V. V. Vadakan, and G. Carlton, note 2, above.

8. See "Tobias Lear Journal," note 2, above.

9. See "Tobias Lear Journal," and R. Marx, note 2, above.

10. "George Washington: Eyewitness Account of his Death," https://doctorzebra.com/prez/z_x01death_lear_g.htm; see note 1, above; see "George Washington's Death," "Dec. 14, 1979: The excruciating final hours of President George Washington," V. V. Vadakan, "The Death of George Washington," and J. Woodruff, note 2, above; see M. Lalonde, and J. Somers, note 4, above; see DM. Morens, note 5, above; see note 9, above.

11. "James Craik," https://www.mountvernon.org/library/digitalhistory/digital-encyclopedia/article/james-craik/; see "Biography of George Washington," note 1, above; see "Dec. 14, 1979: The excruciating final hours of President George Washington" and "The Death of George Washington," note 2, above; see M. Lalonde, note 4, above; see D. M. Morens, note 5, above; see note 7, above.

12. See W. McKenzie Wallenborn, note 1, above; see "Dec. 14, 1979: The excruciating final hours of President George Washington," note 2, above; see M. Lalonde, note 4, above; see D. M. Morens, note 5, above.

13. See "Tobias Lear Journal," V. V. Vadakan, "The Death of George Washington," and R. Marx, note 2, above; see J. Somers, note 4, above; see note 12, above.

14. See "Dec. 14, 1979: The excruciating final hours of President George Washington," "Tobias Lear Journal," "The Death of George Washington," and R. Marx, note 2, above; see M. Lalonde, note 4, above; see D. M. Morens, note 5, above; see "George Washington: Eyewitness Account of his Death," note 10, above.

15. See "Tobias Lear Journal," V. V. Vadakan, and "The Death of George Washington," note 2, above; see "George Washington: Eyewitness Account of his Death," note 10, above.

16. See "Dec. 14, 1979: The excruciating final hours of President George Washington," "Tobias Lear Journal," "The Death of George Washington," and R. Marx, note 2, above; see M. Lalonde, note 4, above; see D. M. Morens, note 5, above.

17. See D. M. Morens, note 5, above; see "James Craik," note 11, above.

18. See "James Craik," note 11, above.

19. See "James Craik," note 11, above.

20. See note 18, above.

21. See "Dec. 14, 1979: The excruciating final hours of President George Washington," "Tobias Lear Journal," V. V. Vadakan, "The Death of George Washington," and R. Marx, note 2, above; see M. Lalonde, note 4, above; see D. M. Morens, note 5, above.

22. See "Dec. 14, 1979: The excruciating final hours of President George Washington," G. Carlton, and R. Marx, note 2, above; see M. Lalonde, and J. Somers, note 4, above.

23. See note 21, above.

24. See "Dec. 14, 1979: The excruciating final hours of President George Washington," G. Carlton, and "The Death of George Washington," note 2, above; see M. Lalonde, and J. Somers, note 4, above.

25. See W. McKenzie Wallenborn, note 1, above; see "Dec. 14, 1979: The excruciating final hours of President George Washington," "Tobias Lear Journal," V. V. Vadakan, "The Death of George Washington," and R. Marx, note 2, above; see D. M. Morens, note 5, above.

26. See "Dec. 14, 1979: The excruciating final hours of President George Washington," note 2, above; see D. M. Morens, note 5, above.

27. See "Tobias Lear Journal," V. V. Vadakan, and R. Marx, note 2, above; see M. Lalonde, note 4, above; see note 26, above.

28. C. B. Witt Jr., "The health and controversial death of George Washington," *ENT* (2001), 102–105; H. Mitgang, "Debate continues on Washington's death," *Chicago Tribune*, December 16, 1999, https://www.chicagotribune.com/news/

ct-xpm-1999-12-16-9912160195-story.html; see "Dec. 14, 1979: The excruciating final hours of President George Washington," and R. Marx, note 2, above; see D. M. Morens, note 5, above.

29. See W. McKenzie Wallenborn, note 1, above; see note 21, above; see "George Washington: Eyewitness Account of his Death," note 10, above; see H. Mitgang, note 28, above.

30. See "Tobias Lear Journal," "The Death of George Washington," and R. Marx, note 2, above; see note 26, above.

31. See "Tobias Lear Journal," V. V. Vadakan, G. Carlton, and R. Marx, note 2, above; see J. Somers, note 4, above; see note 26, above.

32. See "Tobias Lear Journal," note 2, above; see note 26, above.

33. See "Dec. 14, 1979: The excruciating final hours of President George Washington," "The Death of George Washington, 1799," G. Carlton, "Tobias Lear Journal," V. V. Vadakan, and "The Death of George Washington," note 2, above; see J. Somers, note 4, above; see H. Mitgang, note 28, above.

34. See "Dec. 14, 1979: The excruciating final hours of President George Washington," "Tobias Lear Journal," V. V. Vadakan, "The Death of George Washington," and R. Marx, note 2, above; see J. Somers, note 4, above.

35. See V. V. Vadakan, and "The Death of George Washington," note 2, above; see M. Lalonde, note 4, above; see note 32, above.

36. "George Washington dies," A&E Television Networks, original published date February 9, 2010, last updated December 10, 2020, https://www.history.com/this-day-in-history/george-washington-dies; see "Biography of George Washington," note 1, above; see "George Washington's Death," J. Somers, note 4, above; see note 35, above.

37. See "Dec. 14, 1979: The excruciating final hours of President George Washington," note 2, above; see "George Washington dies," note 36, above.

38. See "Tobias Lear Journal," and V. V. Vadakan, note 2, above; see "George Washington: Eyewitness Account of his Death," note 10, above.

39. See note 26, above.

40. See R. Marx and V. V. Vadakan, note 2, above; see "George Washington: Eyewitness Account of his Death," note 10, above; see note 39, above.

41. See V. V. Vadakan, and R. Marx, note 2, above.

42. See R. Marx, note 2, above; see D. M. Morens, note 5, above.

43. See H. Mitgang, note 28, above.

44. See note 43, above.

45. See V. V. Vadakan, note 2, above.

46. See note 45, above.

47. See C. B. Witt Jr., note 28, above.

48. See note 45, above.

49. J. Woodruff, "Bloodletting and blisters: Solving the medical mystery of George Washington's death," Public Broadcasting Service, December 15, 2014, https://www.pbs.org/newshour/show/bloodletting-blisters-solving-medical-mystery-george-washingtons-death.

50. "How your body replaces blood," https://www.blood.co.uk/the-donation-process/after-your-donation/how-your-body-replaces-blood/.

51. See note 50, above.

52. See note 50, above.

53. See note 50, above.

54. See H. Mitgang, note 28, above.

55. See "Dec. 14, 1979: The excruciating final hours of President George Washington," note 2, above; see J. Somers, note 4, above.

56. See C. B. Witt, Jr., note 28, above; see note 55, above.

57. N. J. Galioto, "Peritonsillar abscess," *Am Fam Physician* 95(8) (2017), 501–506; I. Mohamad and A. A. Yaroko, "Peritonsillar swelling is not always quinsy," *Malays Fam Physician.* 8(2) (2013): 53–55; see "Dec. 14, 1979: The excruciating final hours of President George Washington" and R. Marx, note 2, above; see C. B. Witt Jr., note 28, above.

58. See W. McKenzie Wallenborn, note 1, above; see D. M. Morens, note 5, above.

59. See W. McKenzie Wallenborn, note 1, above; see J. Somers, note 4, above.

60. See W. McKenzie Wallenborn, note 1, above.

61. See "Dec. 14, 1979: The excruciating final hours of President George Washington," V. V. Vadakan, and R. Marx, note 2, above; see M. Lalonde, note 4, above; see D. M. Morens, note 5, above; see "George Washington: Eyewitness Account of his Death," note 10, above; see C. B. Witt Jr., note 28, above.

62. See note 45, above.

63. See V. V. Vadakan, note 2, above; see C. B. Witt Jr., note 28, above.

64. See C. B. Witt Jr., note 28, above.

65. See V. V. Vadakan and R. Marx, note 2, above.

66. F. A. Willius and T. E. Keys, "The medical history of George Washington (1732–1799)," *Proceedings of the Staff Meetings of the Mayo Clinic* 17:14 (1942); see C. B. Witt Jr., note 28, above.

67. See note 66, above.

68. See W. McKenzie Wallenborn, note 1, above; see "Dec. 14, 1979: The excruciating final hours of President George Washington" and G. Carlton, note 2, above; see M. Lalonde and J. Somers, note 4, above; see D. M. Morens, note 5, above; see "George Washington: Eyewitness Account of his Death," note 10, above.

69. "George Washington Biography," A&E Television Networks, April 2, 2014 (last updated September 11, 2020), https://www.biography.com/us-president/george-washington; M. Mastromarino, "Biography of George Washington," Washington Papers, https://washingtonpapers.org/resources/articles/biography-of-george-washington/; see "Biography of George Washington," note 1, above; see "George Washington dies," note 36, above.

70. See "Biography of George Washington," note 1, above.

71. See "Biography of George Washington," note 1, above; see "George Washington Biography" and M. Mastromarino, note 69, above.

72. See note 71, above.

73. See "George Washington Biography," note 69, above.

74. See "Biography of George Washington," note 1, above; see M. Mastromarino, note 69, above.

75. See note 71, above.

76. See "Biography of George Washington," note 1, above; see "George Washington Biography," note 69, above.

77. See note 76, above.

78. See "Biography of George Washington" and M. Mastromarino, note 69, above.

79. See "George Washington dies," note 36, above; see "Biography of George Washington" and M. Mastromarino, note 69, above.

80. See note 76, above.

81. See note 76, above.

82. See "Biography of George Washington," note 69, above.

83. See note 82, above.

84. See note 76, above.

85. See note 76, above.

86. See note 76, above.

87. See note 83, above.

88. See note 83, above.

89. See note 83, above.

90. See "Biography of George Washington," note 1, above; see note 79, above.

91. See note 90, above.

92. "The Death of George Washington, 1799," Eyewitness to History, 2001, http://www.eyewitnesstohistory.com/washington.htm.

93. See note 71, above.

94. See note 90, above.

95. See note 83, above.

96. See J. Somers, note 4, above; see note 91, above.

97. See note 83, above.

98. See J. Somers, note 4, above.

99. See "George Washington dies," note 36, above; see "Biography of George Washington," note 69, above.

100. See note 98, above.

101. See note 47, above.

102. See note 47, above.

103. See note 47, above.

104. See "Dec. 14, 1979: The excruciating final hours of President George Washington," note 2, above.

105. See R. Marx, note 2, above.

106. G. Greenstone, "The history of bloodletting," *BCMJ* 52(1) (2010): 12–14; see C. B. Witt Jr. and H. Mitgang, note 28, above.

107. See note 105, above.

108. See R. Marx, note 2, above; see C. B. Witt, note 28, above; see "How your body replaces blood," note 50, above.

109. See note 108, above.

110. See note 105, above.

111. See note 105, above.

112. M. L. Cheatham, "The death of George Washington: an end to the controversy?" *Am Surg* 74(8) (2008): 770–774; A. Machalinski, "Hypovolemic Shock," https://www.webmd.com/a-to-z-guides/hypovolemic-shock; see W. McKenzie Wallenborn, note 1, above.

113. See D. M. Morens, note 5, above.

114. A. K. Abou-Foul, "A Lesson on Human Factors in Airway Management Learnt From the Death of George Washington," *Otolaryngol Head Neck Surg* 163(5) (2020): 1000–1002.

115. See note 113, above.

116. See note 114, above.

117. See note 105, above.

118. See note 105, above.

119. See note 105, above.

120. See note 105, above.

121. See M. L. Cheatham and Machalinski, note 112, above.

122. "A history of the pharmaceutical industry," September 1, 2020, https://pharmaphorum.com/r-d/a_history_of_the_pharmaceutical_industry/.

123. See J. Somers, note 4, above; see "A history of the pharmaceutical industry," note 122, above.

124. "Epiglottitis," Mayo Clinic, https://www.mayoclinic.org/diseases-conditions/epiglottitis/diagnosis-treatment/drc-20372231; B. Benjamin, "Acute epiglottitis," *Ann Acad Med Singap.* 20(5) (1991): 696–99.

125. See note 113, above.

126. See note 113, above.

2.   *Napoleon Bonaparte*

1. K. Fraga, "How Did Napoleon Die? Inside The French Emperor's Mysterious Demise," May 5, 2021, https://allthatsinteresting.com/how-did-napoleon-die; C. Huot, "Reopening the Case: What Killed Napoleon?" the *Washington Post*, January 20, 2003, https://www.washingtonpost.com/archive/politics/2003/01/20/reopening-the-case-what-killed-napoleon/f727fed0-aa56-4b65-9371-8d13b14820d5/; E. Munkwitz and J. L. Swanson, "A Journey to St. Helena, Home of Napoleon's Last Days," *Smithsonian Magazine*, April 2019, https://www.smithsonianmag.com/travel/journey-st-helen-home-napoleon-last-days-180971638/; A. Lugli, F. Carneiro, et al., "The gastric disease of Napoleon Bonaparte: brief report for the bicentenary of Napoleon's death on St. Helena in 1821," Virchows Arch, March 4, 2021, https://link.springer.com/article/10.1007/s00428-021-03061-1; N. Potter, "What Killed Napoleon?" ABC News, January 17, 2007, https://abcnews.go.com/Technology/story?id=2802454&page=1.

2. See E. Munkwitz, and J. L. Swanson, note 1, above.

3. See note 2, above.

4. R. E. Gosselin, "Exhuming Bonaparte," Dartmouth Medicine, https://dartmed.dartmouth.edu/spring03/html/exhuming_bonaparte.shtml; see E. Munkwitz, and J. L. Swanson, note 1, above.

5. See R. E. Gosselin, note 4, above.

6. See K. Fraga, note 1, above.

7. See note 6, above.

8. See note 5, above.

9. See note 5, above.

10. See note 5, above.

11. See note 5, above.

12. See note 5, above.

13. See note 5, above.

14. See C. Huot, note 1, above; see R. E. Gosselin, note 4, above.

15. See note 5, above.

16. See note 5, above.

17. See note 5, above.

18. A. Ribon, "Napoleon's Death; New Findings From his Autopsy," https://www.napoleon.org/en/history-of-the-two-empires/articles/napoleons-death-new-findings-from-his-autopsy/.

19. See note 5, above.

20. G. Dunea, "Francesco Antommarchi, the Malvolio of St. Helena," Hektoen International, https://hekint.org/2018/11/27/francesco-antommarchi-the-malvolio-of-st-helena/; see R. E. Gosselin, note 4, above.

21. See note 5, above.

22. M. Keynes, "The death of Napoleon," *J R Soc Med* 97(1) (2004): 507–8; N. Potter, "What Killed Napoleon?" ABC News, January 17, 2007, https://abcnews.go.com/Technology/story?id=2802454&page=1; see K. Fraga, and C. Huot, note 1, above; see R. E. Gosselin, note 4, above.

23. See M. Keynes, note 22, above.

24. See K. Fraga, note 1, above; see M. Keynes, note 22, above.

25. See note 5, above.

26. A. Ribon, "Napoleon's Death; New Findings From his Autopsy," https://www.napoleon.org/en/history-of-the-two-empires/articles/napoleons-death-new-findings-from-his-autopsy/; B. Weider, "The Assassination of Napoleon," The International Napoleonic Society, https://www.napoleon-series.org/ins/weider/c_assassination_w.html; see R. E. Gosselin, note 4, above.

27. See note 5, above.

28. See note 5, above.

29. See note 18, above.

30. See note 6, above.

31. S. Selin, "What happened to Napoleon's body?" https://shannonselin. com/2017/05/napoleons-body/; "Napoleon Bonaparte," History, A&E Television Networks, original published date November 9, 2009, last updated March 4, 2020, https://www.history.com/topics/ france/napoleon; see K. Fraga, note 1, above.

32. B. Lovejoy, "The Mysterious Deaths of 6 Historical Figures," August 22, 2019, https://www.mentalfloss.com/article/595487/ mysterious-deaths-history; "Was Napoleon Poisoned?" American Museum of Natural History, January 21, 2014, https://www.amnh. org/explore/news-blogs/on-exhibit-posts/was-napoleon-poisoned; A. Nicoud, "Napoleon poisoned with arsenic during St. Helena exile, toxicologist says," https://pnhs.psd202.org/documents/ nhoch/1551356561.pdf.

33. See note 5, above.

34. See note 5, above.

35. S. Goudarzi, "Mystery of Napoleon's Death Said Solved," January 16, 2007, https://www.livescience.com/1228-mystery-napoleon- death-solved.html; see R. E. Gosselin, note 4, above; see A. Ribon, note 26, above.

36. See K. Fraga, note 1, above; see R. E. Gosselin, note 4, above.

37. See note 6, above.

38. A. Lugli, F. Carneiro, et al., "The autopsy of Napoleon Bonaparte: Anatomo-pathological assessment for the bicentenary of the death of Napoleon I on the island of Saint Helena in 1821," *Ann Pathol* 41(4) (2021): 381–86; "Napoleon's mysterious death unmasked, UT Southwestern researcher says," https://www.eurekalert.org/news- releases/869355; see A. Lugli, F. Carneiro, et al., K. Fraga, and C. Huot, note 1, above; see R. E. Gosselin, note 4, above; see S. Selin, note 31, above.

39. See S. Selin, note 31, above; see A. Lugli, F. Carneiro, et al., note 38, above.

40. See A. Lugli, F. Carneiro, et al., note 1, above; see note 39, above.

41. See note 40, above.

42. "Post Mortem on Napoleon Bonaparte," Royal College of Physicians of Edinburgh, https://www.rcpe.ac.uk/heritage/post-mortem-napoleon-bonaparte.

43. See N. Potter, note 1, above.

44. A. Lugli, A. K. Lugli, et al., "Napoleon's autopsy: new perspectives," *Hum Pathol* 36(4) (2005): 320–24; "Napoleon's mysterious death unmasked, UT Southwestern researcher says," https://www.eurekalert.org/news-releases/869355; see K. Fraga, note 1, above.

45. A. Lugli, M. Clemenza, et al., "The Medical Mystery of Napoleon Bonaparte, An Interdisciplinary Exposé," *Adv Anat Pathol* 18(2) (2011): 152–58.

46. See S. Selin, note 31, above.

47. See note 46, above.

48. See R. E. Gosselin, note 4, above; see A. Ribon, note 26, above; see note 45, above.

49. See R. E. Gosselin, note 4, above; see A. Ribon, note 26, above.

50. See note 49, above.

51. See note 49, above.

52. See note 18, above.

53. See A. Lugli, F. Carneiro, et al., note 1, above; see R. E. Gosselin, note 4, above; see A. Ribon, note 26, above; see "Napoleon's mysterious death unmasked, UT Southwestern researcher says," note 44, above; see note 45, above.

54. G. Dunea, "Francesco Antommarchi, the Malvolio of St. Helena," Hektoen International, https://hekint.org/2018/11/27/francesco-antommarchi-the-malvolio-of-st-helena/; A. Lugli, I. Zlobec, et al., "Napoleon Bonaparte's gastric cancer: a clinicopathologic approach to staging, pathogenesis, and etiology," *Nature Clin Prac Gastroenterology Hepatology* 4 (2007): 52–57; see R. E. Gosselin, note 4, above; see note 45, above.

55. D. Marchetti, F. Cittadini, et al., "Did poisoning play a role in Napoleon's death? A systematic review," *Clin Toxicol* 59(7) (2021): 658–72; see A. Lugli, F. Carneiro, et al., note 1, above; see R. E. Gosselin, note 4, above; see "Post Mortem on Napoleon Bonaparte," note 42, above; see "Napoleon's mysterious death unmasked, UT Southwestern researcher says," note 44, above.

56. S. Goudarzi, "Mystery of Napoleon's Death Said Solved," January 16, 2007, https://www.livescience.com/1228-mystery-napolcon-death-solved.html; T. Chamberlain, "Napoleon Death Mystery Solved, Experts Say," National Geographic, January 17, 2007, https://www.nationalgeographic.com/science/article/napolean-death-mystery-solved-news; see note 55, above.

57. See "Napoleon's mysterious death unmasked, UT Southwestern researcher says," note 44, above; see S. Goudarzi, note 56, above.

58. See S. Goudarzi, and T. Chamberlain, note 56, above.

59. See "Napoleon's mysterious death unmasked, UT Southwestern researcher says," note 44, above; see A. Lugli, I. Zlobec, et al., note 54, above.

60. See note 46, above.

61. See N. Potter, A. Lugli, F. Carneiro, et al., note 1, above; see A. Lugli, A. K. Lugli, et al., and "Napoleon's mysterious death unmasked, UT Southwestern researcher says," note 44, above; see Chamberlain, note 56, above.

62. G. Dunea, "Francesco Antommarchi, the Malvolio of St. Helena," Hektoen International, https://hekint.org/2018/11/27/francesco-antommarchi-the-malvolio-of-st-helena/; see A. Lugli, F. Carneiro, et al., note 1, above; see R. E. Gosselin, note 4, above; see M. Keynes, note 22, above; see A. Lugli, F. Carneiro, et al., note 38, above; see A. Lugli, A. K. Lugli, et al., and "Napoleon's mysterious death unmasked, UT Southwestern researcher says," note 44, above; see note 45, above.

63. See K. Fraga, note 1, above; see G. Dunea, note 62, above.

64. See note 63, above.

65. See N. Potter, note 1, above; see B. Lovejoy, note 32, above.

66. D. Marchetti, F. Cittadini, et al., "Did poisoning play a role in Napoleon's death? A systematic review," *Clin Toxicol* 59(7) (2021): 658–72; R. Dotinga, "Stomach Cancer Was Napoleon's Waterloo: Study," January 19, 2007, https://consumer.healthday.com/gastrointestinal-information-15/stomach-trouble-news-638/stomach-cancer-was-napoleon-s-waterloo-study-601181.html; see A. Lugli, F. Carneiro, et al., note 1, above; see A. Lugli, F. Carneiro, et al., note 38, above; see A. Lugli, A. K. Lugli, et al., and "Napoleon's mysterious death unmasked, UT Southwestern researcher says," note 44, above; see note 45, above; see A. Lugli, I. Zlobec, et al., note 54, above; see S. Goudarzi, and T. Chamberlain, note 56, above; see note 65, above.

67. "Napoleon Biography," A&E Television Networks, original published date April 2, 2014, last updated March 31, 2021, https://www.biography.com/dictator/napoleon; see K. Fraga, note 1, above; see "Napoleon Bonaparte," note 31, above; see "Napoleon's mysterious death unmasked, UT Southwestern researcher says," note 44, above.

68. See "Napoleon Bonaparte," note 31, above.

69. See "Napoleon Bonaparte," note 31, above; see "Napoleon Biography," note 67, above.

70. See note 69, above.

71. See note 69, above.

72. See note 69, above.

73. See note 6, above.

74. See K. Fraga, note 1, above; see note 69, above.

75. See note 74, above.

76. See note 69, above.

77. See note 68, above.

78. See note 69, above.

79. See "Napoleon Biography," note 67, above.

80. See note 68, above.

81. See note 74, above.

82. See K. Fraga, note 1, above; see "Napoleon Bonaparte," note 31, above.

83. See note 82, above.

84. See note 74, above.

85. See note 68, above.

86. See note 69, above.

87. "Arsenic," World Health Organization, https://www.who.int/news-room/fact-sheets/detail/arsenic; see C. Huot, note 1, above; see R. E. Gosselin, note 4, above.

88. "Arsenic Toxicity: How Does Arsenic Induce Pathogenic Change?" US Agency for Toxic Substances and Disease Registry, https://www.atsdr.cdc.gov/csem/arsenic/arsenic_pathogen.html.

89. M. F. Hughes, "Arsenic toxicity and potential mechanisms of action," *Toxicol Lett* 133(1) (2002): 1–16; see note 88, above.

90. S. Forshufvud, H. Smith, et al., "Napoleon's Illness 1816-1821 in the Light of Activation Analyses of Hairs from Various Dates," *Arch Toxicol* 27(20) (1964): 210–19; H. Smith, S. Forshufvud, et al., "Distribution of Arsenic in Napoleon's Hair," *Nature* 194 (1962), 725–26; see R. E. Gosselin, note 4, above; see M. Keynes, note 22, above; see note 45, above.

91. See note 5, above.

92. P. Kintz, M. Ginet, et al., "Multi-Element Screening by ICP-MS of Two Specimens of Napoleon's Hair," *J Anal Toxicol* 30 (2006): 621–23.

93. See K. Fraga, A. Lugli, F. Carneiro, et al., note 1, above; see M. Keynes, note 22, above; see B. Lovejoy and "Was Napoleon Poisoned?" note 32, above.

94. See A. Lugli, F. Carneiro, et al., note 1, above; see M. Keynes, note 22, above; see B. Lovejoy and "Was Napoleon Poisoned?" note 32, above.

95. See K. Fraga, and C. Huot, note 1, above; see note 45, above.

96. See note 95, above.

97. See R. E. Gosselin, note 4, above; see note 45, above.

98. See C. Huot, note 1, above.

99. W. J. Broad, "Hair Analysis Deflates Napoleon Poisoning Theories," the *New York Times*, June 10, 2008, https://www.nytimes.com/2008/06/10/science/10napo.html; "Napoleon Death: Arsenic Poisoning Ruled Out," February 12, 2008, https://www.livescience.com/2292-napoleon-death-arsenic-poisoning-ruled.html; see B. Lovejoy and "Was Napoleon Poisoned?" note 32, above; see note 45, above.

100. See W. J. Broad and "Napoleon Death: Arsenic Poisoning Ruled Out," note 99, above.

101. "Arsenic, Hair," Mayo Clinic Laboratories, https://neuroplogy.testcatalog.org/show/ASHA.

102. S. A. Katz, "On the Use of Hair Analysis for Assessing Arsenic Intoxication," *Int J Environ Res Public Health* 16(6) (2019): 977–89.

103. See note 102, above.

104. See note 102, above.

105. See note 102, above.

106. F. Mari, E. Bertol, et al., "Channeling the emperor: what really killed Napoleon?" *J Royal Soc Med* 97 (2004): 397-99.

107. See note 106, above.

108. See note 106, above.

109. See note 106, above.

110. "Stomach Cancer," Cleveland Clinic, https://my.clevelandclinic.org/health/diseases/15812-stomach-cancer; "Stomach Cancer Risk Factors," American Cancer Society, https://www.cancer.org/cancer/stomach-cancer/causes-risks-prevention/risk-factors.html; see "Napoleon's mysterious death unmasked, UT Southwestern researcher says," note 44, above.

111. See "Napoleon's mysterious death unmasked, UT Southwestern researcher says," note 44, above.

112. See note 111, above.

113. See "Napoleon's mysterious death unmasked, UT Southwestern researcher says," note 44, above; see A. Lugli, I. Zlobec, et al., note 54, above; see T. Chamberlain, note 56; see R. Dotinga, note 66, above.

114. See note 113, above.

115. See "Napoleon's mysterious death unmasked, UT Southwestern researcher says," note 44, above; see R. Dotinga, note 66, above.

116. See B. Lovejoy, note 32, above; see S. Goudarzi, note 35, above; see note 113, above.

117. "15th Report on Carcinogens," US National Toxicology Program, https://ntp.niehs.nih.gov/whatwestudy/assessments/cancer/roc/index.html#toc1.

118. "Arsenic and Inorganic Arsenic Compounds," US National Toxicology Program, *Report on Carcinogens*, 14th edition, https://ntp.niehs.nih.gov/ntp/roc/content/profiles//arsenic.pdf.

119. See note 118, above.

120. See W. J. Broad, and Napoleon Death: Arsenic Poisoning Ruled Out," note 99, above.

3.   Grigori Rasputin

1. "World War I," History, original published date October 29, 2009, last updated April 8, 2021, https://www.history.com/topics/world-war-i/world-war-i-history.

2. See note 1, above.

3. See note 1, above.

4. J. Simkin, "The Life and Death of Rasputin," original published date September 1997, last updated January 2020, https://spartacus-educational.com/EXAMrussia5.htm; "Grigori Rasputin," https://spartacus-educational.com/RUSrasputin.htm; R. Cavendish, "The Murder of Grigori Rasputin," History Today, https://www.historytoday.com/archive/months-past/murder-grigori-rasputin.

5. "Rasputin proved to be a hard man to kill," the *Irish Times*, July 15, 1996, https://www.irishtimes.com/news/rasputin-proved-to-be-a-hard-man-to-kill-1.67169; see "Grigori Rasputin," note 4, above.

6. See J. Simkin and "Grigori Rasputin," note 4, above.

7. See J. Simkin, note 4, above.

8. See note 4, above.

9. P. Reynolds, "The murder of Rasputin," December 30, 2016, https://blog.nationalarchives.gov.uk/murder-rasputin/; see "Grigori Rasputin," note 4, above; see "Rasputin proved to be a hard man to kill," note 5, above.

10. A. Krechetnikov, "How was Russian mystic Rasputin murdered?" BBC, December 31, 2016, https://www.bbc.com/news/world-europe-38469903.

11. See R. Cavendish, note 4, above.

12. C. Harris, "The Murder of Rasputin, 100 Years Later," Smithsonian Magazine, December 27, 2016, https://www.smithsonianmag.com/history/murder-rasputin-100-years-later-180961572/; see J. Simkin, and "Grigori Rasputin," note 4, above.

13. A. Hudson, "The Death of Rasputin," September 16, 2014, https://skeptoid.com/episodes/4432?gclid=Cj0KCQjwpreJBhDvARIsAF1_BU2OtfbxRgDRy56B-PXLsL20NZQvCsRCJ2EgYKEmyLej7bMPl2QKyGYaAlGnEALw_wcB; C. Conger, "How did Rasputin really die?" History, https://history.howstuffworks.com/history-vs-myth/rasputin2.htm; "5 Myths and Truths About Rasputin," *Time*, https://time.com/4606775/5-myths-rasputin/; Prince Felix Yussupov, "Lost Splendor," 1953, https://www.alexanderpalace.org/lostsplendor/index.html; see "Grigori Rasputin," note 4, above.

14. See "Grigori Rasputin," note 4, above; see A. Hudson, C. Conger, and "5 Myths and Truths About Rasputin," note 13, above.

15. See A. Hudson, note 13, above.

16. See "Grigori Rasputin," note 4, above.

17. See C. Harris, note 12, above; see Prince Felix Yussupov, note 13, above.

18. "Stanislaus de Lazovert," https://spartacus-educational.com/RUSlazovert.htm; see J. Simkin and "Grigori Rasputin," note 4, above.

19. See note 18, above.

20. A. Milne, "Poisoned, Shot, And Left To Bleed Out: The Grisly Story of Grigori Rasputin's Death," original published date July 11, 2021, last updated July 29, 2021, https://allthatsinteresting.com/

rasputin-deth; see "Rasputin proved to be a hard man to kill," note 5, above; see P. Reynolds, note 9, above; see note 10, above.

21. See C. Harris, note 12, above; see A. Milne, note 20, above.

22. See Prince Felix Yussupov, note 13, above.

23. See "Grigori Rasputin," note 4, above; see note 22, above.

24. See "Rasputin proved to be a hard man to kill," note 5, above; see note 22, above.

25. See J. Simkin, note 4, above; see note 10, above; see C. Harris, note 12, above; see C. Conger note 13, above; see note 24, above.

26. See note 22, above.

27. See note 10, above; see note 22, above.

28. See "Grigori Rasputin," note 4, above; see P. Reynolds, note 9, above; see note 10, above; see note 22, above.

29. See note 22, above.

30. See note 22, above.

31. K. Harkup, "Poisoned, shot and beaten: why cyanide alone may have failed to kill Rasputin," the *Guardian*, January 13, 2017, https://www.theguardian.com/science/blog/2017/jan/13/poisoned-shot-and-beaten-why-cyanide-may-have-failed-to-kill-rasputin; see P. Reynolds, note 9, above; see note 10, above; see Anote 15, above; see note 22, above.

32. See A. Milne, note 20, above; see note 22, above.

33. See "Grigori Rasputin," note 4, above; see "Rasputin proved to be a hard man to kill," note 5, above; see C. Harris, note 12, above; see C. Conger note 13, above; see A. Milne, note 20, above; see note 31, above.

34. See note 22, above.

35. See J. Simkins and "Grigori Rasputin," note 4, above; see "Rasputin proved to be a hard man to kill," note 5, above; see P. Reynolds, note 9, above; see C. Harris, note 12, above; see C. Conger, note 13, above; see note 15, above; see A. Milne, note 20, above; see note 22, above; see K. Harkup, note 31, above.

36. See C. Harris, note 12, above.

37. See note 23, above.

38. See note 16, above.

39. See J. Simkin and "Grigori Rasputin," note 4, above; see "Rasputin proved to be a hard man to kill," note 5, above; see C. Harris, note 12, above; see A. Milne, note 20, above; see note 31, above.

40. See "Grigori Rasputin," note 4, above; see "Rasputin proved to be a hard man to kill," note 5, above; see note 22, above.

41. See J. Simkin and "Grigori Rasputin," note 4, above; see "Rasputin proved to be a hard man to kill," note 5, above; see C. Conger, note 13, above; see A. Milne, note 20, above; see note 31, above.

42. See note 41, above.

43. See "Rasputin proved to be a hard man to kill," note 5, above; see C. Conger, note 13, above; see note 15, above; see A. Milne, note 20, above.

44. See note 24, above.

45. "Stanislaus de Lazovert," https://spartacus-educational.com/RUSlazovert.htm; see note 22, above.

46. See J. Simkin and "Grigori Rasputin," note 4, above; see P. Reynolds, note 9, above; see "5 Myths and Truths About Rasputin," note 13, above; see note 15, above; see A. Milne, note 20, above; see note 22, above; see K. Harkup, note 31, above.

47. See note 22, above.

48. See P. Reynolds, note 9, above.

49. See "Grigori Rasputin," note 4, above; see note 44, above; see note 48, above.

50. See note 49, above.

51. See "Grigori Rasputin," note 4, above; see note 48, above.

52. See note 6, above.

53. See note 16, above.

54. See note 16, above.

55. See note 16, above.

56. See note 7, above.

57. See note 10, above; see note 48, above.

58. See note 15, above; see note 53, above.

59. See note 15, above; see note 48, above; see note 52, above.

60. See note 51, above; see note 56, above.

61. See note 60, above.

62. See note 60, above.

63. See note 15, above; see note 60, above.

64. See note 15, above; see note 52, above.

65. See note 16, above.

66. See note 7, above.

67. G. Milton, "Who Killed Rasputin? The secret role of MI6," March 10, 2014, https://cvhf.org.uk/history-hub/who-killed-rasputin-the-secret-role-of-mi6/; see note 6, above.

68. See C. Conger, note 13, above.

69. "Spy secrets revealed in history of MI6," the *Guardian*, September 21, 2010, https://www.theguardian.com/world/2010/sep/21/spy-secrets-history-mi6; see note 6, above.

70. See note 6, above.

71. See note 22, above.

72. See note 64, above.

73. See note 58, above.

74. N. Martyris, "Fact or Fiction? Even When It Comes to Food, It's Hard to Tell with Rasputin," National Public Radio, January 31, 2007, https://www.npr.org/sections/thesalt/2017/01/31/510802220/fact-or-fiction-even-when-it-comes-to-food-its-hard-to-tell-with-rasputin; see note 36, above.

75. See N. Martyris, note 74, above.

76. See note 22, above.

77. "Cyanide," Johns Hopkins Center for Health Security, https://www.centerforhealthsecurity.org/our-work/publications/cyanide-fact-sheet; F. Dillon, "Rasputin's Death," *Brit J Med* (July 14, 1934), 88, https://www.bmj.com/content/2/3836/88.4.

78. D. Templeton, "Cyanide has a long history in manufacturing and in murder," *Pittsburgh Post-Gazette*, February 4, 2015, https://www.post-gazette.com/news/health/2015/02/04/Cyanide-has-a-notable-history-of-famous-poisonings-along-

with-many-used-in-mining-metal-work-and-manufacturing/stories/201501230172.

79. See "Cyanide," note 77, above.

80. See note 7, above; see note 15, above.

81. See note 6, above.

82. "Rasputin Biography," A&E Networks, original published date April 27, 2017, last updated December 13, 2019, https://www.biography.com/political-figure/rasputin; see note 4, above; see C. Harris, note 12, above.

83. See note 6, above; see "Rasputin Biography," note 82, above.

84. See note 83, above.

85. See note 16, above.

86. See note 16, above.

87. See R. Cavendish, note 4, above; see C. Harris, note 12, above; see note 83, above.

88. See note 16, above.

89. See note 5, above.

90. See R. Cavendish, note 4, above; see "Rasputin proved to be a hard man to kill," note 5, above; see A. Milne, note 20, above.

91. See note 5, above.

92. See "5 Myths and Truths About Rasputin," note 13, above; see note 15, above; see note 83, above.

93. See note 15, above; see note 68, above; see note 87, above.

94. See R. Cavendish, note 4, above; see note 5, above.

95. See "Rasputin proved to be a hard man to kill," note 5, above.

96. See note 95, above.

97. See note 5, above; see note 15, above.

98. See note 15, above; see note 83, above.

99. See R. Cavendish, note 4, above; see note 95, above.

100. J. L. Marshall and V. R. Marshall, "Rediscovery of the Elements, Carl Wilhelm Scheele," the *Hexagon*, 8–13 (2005), https://chemistry.unt.edu/sites/default/files/users/owj0001/scheele.pdf.

101. See note 100, above.

102. "Arsenic, Cyanide and Strychnine—the Golden Age of Victorian Poisoners," September 18, 2014, https://britishlibrary.typepad.co.uk/untoldlives/2014/09/arsenic-cyanide-and-strychnine-the-golden-age-of-victorian-poisoners.html; S. I. Baskin, "Cyanide Poisoning," chapter 10 in *Textbook of Military Medicine: Medical Aspects of Chemical and Biological Warfare* (United States Department of the Army, Office of the Surgeon General, 2001) 271–86; K. Sasikala, V. Fernz, et al., "A Retrospective Descriptive Study on Death Due to Cyanide Poisoning Over a Period of 20 Years in Government Medical College, Thiruvananthapuram," *J Evid Based Med Health* 8(30) (2021): 2697–701.

103. See K. Sasikala, V. Fernz, et al., note 102, above.

104. See S. I. Baskin, note 102, above; see note 103, above.

105. See note 104, above.

106. See note 103, above.

107. See note 78, above; see note 103, above.

108. D. Blum, "A Cyanide Murder in Chicago," https://wired.com/2013/01/a-cyanide-murder-in-chicago/; see note 78, above; see note 29, above, see S. I. Baskin, note 103, above.

109. See note 22, above.

110. F. Dillon, "Rasputin's Death," *Brit J Med* (July 14, 1934) 88, https://www.bmj.com/content/2/3836/88.4.

111. G. A. Wilkes, "Response to 'Cyanide Poisoning: Rasputin's Death,'" *Brit J Med* (July 28, 1934), 184, https://www.ncbi.nlm.nih.gov/pmc/articles/p.m.C2447691/pdf/brmedj07163-0032c.pdf.

112. See note 111, above.

113. R. J. Brocklehurst, "Response to 'Cyanide Poisoning: Rasputin's Death,'" *Brit J Med* (July 28, 1934), 184, https://www.ncbi.nlm.nih.gov/pmc/articles/p.m.C2447691/pdf/brmedj07163-0032c.pdf.

114. See note 113, above.

115. See note 113, above.

4. *Umberto "Albert" Anastasia*

1. "Homicide of Umberto 'Albert' Anastasia," http://www.autopsyfiles. org/reports/Other/anastasia,%20albert_report.pdf.

2. See note 1, above.

3. "The Death of Albert Anastasia: Park Central Sheraton Hotel Barbershop 870 7th Avenue," Infamous New York, https:// infamousnewyork.com/2017/04/17/the-death-of-albert-anastasia-park-central-sheraton-hotel-870-7th-avenue/; see note 1, above.

4. See note 3, above.

5. "Mobster Albert Anastasia is murdered at a barbershop in 1957," *New York Daily News*, October 24, 2015, https://www.nydailynews. com/new-york/nyc-crime/albert-anastasia-dies-55-gun-shots-1957-article-1.2404077; see note 1, above.

6. See "Mobster Albert Anastasia is murdered at a barbershop in 1957," note 5, above.

7. "Albert Anastasia Biography," https://www.imdb.com/name/ nm1374388/bio#trivia; see note 1, above; see "Mobster Albert Anastasia is murdered at a barbershop in 1957," note 5, above.

8. "Albert Anastasia Biography," National Crime Syndicate, https:// www.nationalcrimesyndicate.com/albert-anastasia-biography/; see "The Death of Albert Anastasia: Park Central Sheraton Hotel Barbershop 870 7th Avenue," note 3, above; see note 6, above.

9. "How Did Albert Anastasia Get Killed?—Death Photos," National Crime Syndicate, https://www.nationalcrimesyndicate.com/albert-anastasia-death/; see "Albert Anastasia Biography," note 7, above; see note 8, above.

10. T. Hunt, "King of the Brooklyn Docks: Albert Anastasia," The American Mafia, 2005, http://mafiahistory.us/a009/f_ albertanastasia.html; "Albert Anastasia Biography," https://www. thefamouspeople.com/profiles/albert-anastasia-10905.php; see note 3, above; see note 6, above; see "Albert Anastasia Biography," note 8, above; see "How Did Albert Anastasia Get Killed?—Death Photos," note 9, above.

11. See "The Death of Albert Anastasia: Park Central Sheraton Hotel Barbershop 870 7th Avenue," note 3, above; see T. Hunt, note 10, above.

12. See "The Death of Albert Anastasia: Park Central Sheraton Hotel Barbershop 870 7th Avenue," note 3, above; see note 7, above; see "Albert Anastasia Biography," note 8, above; see "How Did Albert Anastasia Get Killed?—Death Photos," note 9, above.

13. See "The Death of Albert Anastasia: Park Central Sheraton Hotel Barbershop 870 7th Avenue," note 3, above; see note 6, above; see "Albert Anastasia Biography," note 7, above; see "Albert Anastasia Biography," note 8, above; see T. Hunt, note 10, above.

14. See note 6, above; see T. Hunt, note 10, above.

15. See note 14, above.

16. See "How Did Albert Anastasia Get Killed?—Death Photos," note 9, above; see note 14, above.

17. See note 14, above.

18. See note 6, above.

19. See note 6, above.

20. See note 1, above; see note 6, above.

21. See "The Death of Albert Anastasia: Park Central Sheraton Hotel Barbershop 870 7th Avenue," note 3, above; see "How Did Albert Anastasia Get Killed?—Death Photos," note 9, above.

22. See note 6, above.

23. See note 5, above.

24. See note 5, above.

25. See note 6, above.

26. See note 6, above.

27. See note 6, above.

28. See note 1, above.

29. See note 1, above.

30. See note 1, above.

31. See note 1, above.

32. See note 1, above.

33. See note 1, above.

34. See note 6, above.

35. "Gunshot Wound Head Trauma," American Association of Neurological Surgeons, https://www.aans.org/en/Patients/Neurosurgical-Conditions-and-Treatments/Gunshot-Wound-Head-Trauma.

36. "Albert Anastasia—Murder Inc. FBI Files," https://paperlessarchives.com/anastasia.html; see "Albert Anastasia Biography," note 7, above; see "Albert Anastasia Biography," note 8, above; see T. Hunt, note 10, above.

37. See T. Hunt and "Albert Anastasia Biography," note 10, above.

38. See "Albert Anastasia—Murder Inc. FBI Files," note 36, above; see note 37, above.

39. See T. Hunt, note 10, above.

40. See "Albert Anastasia Biography," note 8, above; see note 38, above.

41. See note 39, above.

42. See note 39, above.

43. See "Albert Anastasia Biography," note 8, above; see note 37, above.

44. See note 40, above.

45. See note 38, above.

46. See "Albert Anastasia—Murder Inc. FBI Files," note 36, above; see note 39, above.

47. See note 46, above.

48. See "How Did Albert Anastasia Get Killed?—Death Photos," note 9, above; see note 40, above.

49. See note 48, above.

50. See "Albert Anastasia Biography," note 8, above; see note 39, above.

51. See note 39, above.

52. "Albert Anastasia Biography," note 10, above.

53. See note 43, above.

54. See note 39, above.

55. See note 40, above.

56. See note 40, above.

57. See "Albert Anastasia Biography," note 7, above; see note 39, above.

58. See "Albert Anastasia Biography," note 7, above; see note 40, above.

59. See "Albert Anastasia Biography," note 7, above.

60. See note 46, above.

61. See note 37, above.

62. See note 40, above.

63. See "Albert Anastasia Biography," note 7, above; see note 48, above.

64. See note 63, above.

65. See note 63, above.

66. See note 39, above.

67. See note 40, above.

68. See "Albert Anastasia Biography," note 8, above; see "How Did Albert Anastasia Get Killed?—Death Photos," note 9, above; see note 57, above.

69. See note 57, above.

70. See note 57, above.

71. See Albert Anastasia—Murder Inc. FBI Files," note 36, above.

72. See note 39, above.

73. See "Albert Anastasia Biography," note 8, above; see "How Did Albert Anastasia Get Killed? Death Photos," note 9, above; see note 71, above.

74. See note 71, above.

75. See note 71, above.

76. See "Albert Anastasia Biography," note 7, above.

77. "Comedian Buys Home; Buddy Hackett New Owner of Anastasia House in Fort Lee," the *New York Times*, August 30, 1958, https://www.nytimes.com/1958/08/30/archives/comedian-buys-home-buddy-hackett-new-owner-of-anastasia-house-in.html.

78. "Mafia kingpin's hilltop mansion sells for $6.9 million," *Jackson Observer*, December 29, 2017. https://web.archive.org/web/20171230114500/http://jacksonobserver.com/mafia-kngpins-hilltop-mansion-sells-for-6-9million/; Zillow, https://www.zillow.com/homedetails/75-Bluff-Rd-Fort-Lee-NJ-07024/37905832_zpid/; "Live like the mob! American mafia founder Albert Anastasia's hilltop New Jersey mansion that reportedly had a SLAUGHTER ROOM sells for $6.9million," the *Daily Mail*, original published date

November 14, 2017, last updated November 15, 2017, https://www.
dailymail.co.uk/news/article-5083447/Mafia-kngpin-s-hilltop-
mansion-sells-6-9million.html.

79. "Al's Barber Beats Appeal," the *New York Daily News*, November 30, 1967, https://www.newspapers.com/clip/33716109/1957-arthur-grasso-barber-for/.

80. See note 79, above.

81. See note 52, above.

5.   *Charles Whitman*

1. S. Harrison, "From the Archives: 1966 airline strike over," *Los Angeles Times*, August 19, 2019, https://www.latimes.com/california/story/2019-08-18/from-the-archives-1966-airline-strike-over.

2. See note 1, above.

3. See note 1, above.

4. See note 1, above.

5. "Charles Whitman Biography," https://criminalminds.fandom.com/wiki/Charles_Whitman; "Charles Whitman Biography," https://military.wikia.org/wiki/Charles_Whitman; A. Hannaford, "The Mysterious Vanishing Brains," the *Atlantic*, December 2, 2014, https://www.theatlantic.com/health/archive/2014/12/the-mysterious-vanishing-brains/382869/.

6. See "Charles Whitman Biography," note 5, above.

7. See note 6, above.

8. "Biographical Notes," The Biography Project, https://www.popsubculture.com/pop/bio_project/charles_whitman.html; "Texas Tower shooting of 1966," Britannica Online Encyclopedia, https://www.britannica.com/event/Texas-Tower-shooting-of-1966; "Charles Joseph Whitman" and several documents reproduced from the collections of the Austin History Center, including a typed letter from Chares J. Whitman dated July 31, 1966, a handwritten letter from Charles J. Whitman dated August 1, 1966, a letter from Charlie to Pat dated August 1, 1966, a letter from Charlie to Johnnie dated

August 1, 1966, "Thoughts to Start the Day" dated August 1, 1966, a supplementary offense report from Officer Billy Speed dated August 1, 1966, a letter from John Connally to Police Chief R. A. Miles dated August 5, 1966, a list of "Governor's Committee and Invited Consultants," a "Report to the Governor" dated September 8, 1966, a report of Allen Crum dated August 2, 1966, an intelligence report from Howard W. Smith dated August 2, 1966, a report of Dr. Maurice D. Heatly dated March 29, 1966, and a report of J. Myers Cole dated August 15, 1966, https://murderpedia.org/male.W/w/whitman-charles.htm; see "Charles Whitman Biography," note 5, above.

9. See "Biographical Notes," note 8, above.

10. G. Jones, "AP Was there: 1966 University of Texas clock tower shooting," Associated Press, July 31, 2016, https://apnews.com/article/91cd1ab6a70e47ef850de78413acb8d5; G. M. Lavergne, "University of Texas Tower Shooting (1966)," Texas State Historical Association, https://www.tshaonline.org/handbook/entries/university-of-texas-tower-shooting-1966; G. Jones, "AP Releases 1966 Story on University of Texas Clock Tower Shooting," NBC Dallas-Fort Worth, original published date July 31, 2016, last updated August 1, 2016, https://www.nbcdfw.com/news/local/ap-releases-1966-story-on-university-of-texas-clock-tower-shooting/2018649/; A. Barr, "Whitman, Charles Joseph (1941–1966)," Texas State Historical Association, https://www.tshaonline.org/handbook/entries/whitman-charles-joseph; "Charles Whitman Biography," A&E Television Networks, original published date April 2, 2014, last updated April 2, 2021, https://www.biography.com/political-figure/charles-whitman; "Austin (Tex.). Police Department Records of the Charles Whitman Mass Murder Case," Austin History Center, https://legacy.lib.utexas.edu/taro/aushc/00489/00489-P.html; "An ex-Marine goes on a killing spree at the University of Texas," A&E Television Networks, original published date November 13, 2009, last updated August 6, 2020, https://www.history.com/this-day-in-history/

an-ex-marine-goes-on-a-killing-spree-at-the-university-of-texas; "Ex-marine Charles Whitman shoots at victims from the University of Texas tower in 1966," *New York Daily News*, original published date August 1, 2016, last updated August 2, 1966, https://www. nydailynews.com/news/national/ex-marine-charles-whitman-snipes-victims-tower-1966-article-1.2733926; see "Charles Whitman Biography," note 5, above; see note 6, above. See "Texas Tower shooting of 1966" and "Charles Joseph Whitman" and several documents, note 8, above.

11. See "Charles Whitman Biography," note 5, above; see "Charles Joseph Whitman" and several documents, note 8, above; see "Charles Whitman Biography," note 10, above.

12. See note 6, above; see note 8, above; see G. Jones, A. Barr, G. M. Lavergne, "Charles Whitman Biography," "Austin (Tex.). Police Department Records of the Charles Whitman Mass Murder Case," and "An ex-Marine goes on a killing spree at the University of Texas," note 10, above.

13. See "Charles Joseph Whitman" and several documents, note 8, above.

14. See "Charles Whitman Biography," note 10, above; see note 13, above.

15. See note 9, above; see G. M. Lavergne, note 10, above; see note 13, above.

16. See "Charles Whitman Biography," note 5, above; see note 6, above.

17. See note 16, above.

18. See G. Jones, A. Barr, G. M. Lavergne, "Texas Tower shooting of 1966," "Ex-marine Charles Whitman shoots at victims from the University of Texas tower in 1966," "An ex-Marine goes on a killing spree at the University of Texas," and G. Jones, note 10, above; see note 11, above.

19. See note 16, above.

20. See "Charles Whitman Biography," note 5, above; see G. M. Lavergne and "Ex-marine Charles Whitman shoots at victims from the University of Texas tower in 1966," note 10, above.

21. See A. Barr, "Texas Tower shooting of 1966," and "An ex-Marine goes on a killing spree at the University of Texas," note 10, above; see note 20, above.

22. See note 21, above.

23. See "Charles Whitman Biography," note 5, above.

24. See G. Jones, "Texas Tower shooting of 1966," and "Austin (Tex.). Police Department Records of the Charles Whitman Mass Murder Case," note 10, above; see note 20, above.

25. C. Bowden, "The Tower Tragedy," *Esquire*, January 29, 2007, https://www.esquire.com/news-politics/a1697/esq0299-fe-ameria-rev/; see G. M. Lavergne, G. Jones, "Texas Tower shooting of 1966," and "Ex-marine Charles Whitman shoots at victims from the University of Texas tower in 1966," note 10, above.

26. M. Abadi, "A policeman who helped end one of the deadliest school shootings in US history relives the massacre," *Insider*, August 1, 2016, https://www.businessinsider.com/policeman-relives-texas-tower-shooting-50th-anniversary-2016-7; see G. M. Lavergne, A. Barr, "Texas Tower shooting of 1966," "Ex-marine Charles Whitman shoots at victims from the University of Texas tower in 1966," and "Charles Joseph Whitman" and several documents, note 10, above; see C. Bowden, note 25, above.

27. See note 6, above; see "Charles Joseph Whitman" and several documents, note 8, above.

28. "Autopsy report—Charles J. Whitman," http://www.autopsyfiles.org/reports/Other/whitman,%20charles_report.pdf.

29. A. Hannaford, "The Mysterious Vanishing Brains," the *Atlantic*, December 2, 2014, https://www.theatlantic.com/health/archive/2014/12/the-mysterious-vanishing-brains/382869/.

30. See note 29, above.

31. See note 29, above.

32. See note 29, above.

33. See note 28, above.

34. See note 28, above.

35. See note 28, above.

36. See note 28, above.

37. See note 28, above.

38. See note 28, above.

39. See note 28, above.

40. See note 28, above.

41. See note 28, above.

42. See note 13, above.

43. See note 28, above.

44. See note 28, above.

45. S. Madhusoodanan, M. B. Ting, et al., "Psychiatric aspects of brain tumors: A review," *World J Psychiatr* 5(3) (2015): 273–85; see note 28, above.

46. See note 28, above.

47. H. A. Milman, "Robin Williams," in *Forensics: The Science Behind the Deaths of Famous People* (Bloomington, Indiana: Xlibris, 2020), 211–22; see note 28, above.

48. See note 13, above.

49. E. C. Holland, "Glioblastoma Multiforme: The terminator," PNAS 97(12): 6242–6244 (2000).

50. See note 13, above.

51. See note 13, above.

52. See note 13, above.

53. See note 13, above.

54. V. C. Prabhu, "Glioblastoma Multiforme," American Association of Neurological Surgeons, https://www.aans.org/en/Patients/Neurosurgical-Conditions-and-Treatments/Glioblastoma-Multiforme; D. Krex, B. Klink, et al., "Long-term survival with glioblastoma multiforme," Brain 130(10) (2007): 2596–606; F. W. Boele, A. G. Rooney, et al., "Psychiatric symptoms in glioma patients from diagnosis to management," *Neuropsychiatr Dis Treat* 11 (2015): 1413–20; see note 13, above; see note 49, above.

55. See note 54, above.

56. See note 13, above.

57. See note 13, above.

58. See note 13, above.

59. E. Frederick, "Experts still disagree on role of Tower shooter's brain tumor," the *Daily Texan*, July 30, 2016, https://thedailytexan.com/2016/07/30/experts-still-disagree-on-role-of-tower-shooters-brain-tumor/; "Astrocytoma," Mayo Clinic, https://www.mayoclinic.org/diseases-conditions/astrocytoma/cdc-20350132; see V. C. Prabhu, note 54, above.

60. See E. Frederick, note 59, above.

61. See note 60, above.

62. See note 60, above.

63. See note 13, above.

64. See note 13, above.

65. See note 13, above.

66. S. Madhusoodanan, M. B. Ting, et al., "Psychiatric aspects of brain tumors: A review," *World J Psychiatr* 5(3) (2015), 273–85.

67. See note 66, above.

68. See note 66, above.

69. "Charles Whitman Biography," https://www.thefamouspeople.com/profiles/charles-whitman-5239.php; see note 6, above; see "Biographical Notes," note 8, above; see A. Barr, "Charles Whitman Biography," and "Austin (Tex.). Police Department Records of the Charles Whitman Mass Murder Case," note 10, above; see note 11, above.

70. See note 13, above.

71. See note 13, above; see note 16, above.

72. "Charles Whitman Biography;" See A. Barr, and "Austin (Tex.). Police Department Records of the Charles Whitman Mass Murder Case," note 10, above; see "Charles Whitman Biography," note 69, above; see note 71, above.

73. See note 9, above; see "Charles Whitman Biography," note 10, above; see note 16, above.

74. See note 6, above.

75. See "Austin (Tex.). Police Department Records of the Charles Whitman Mass Murder Case," note 10, above; see note 16, above;

see C. Bowden, note 25, above; see "Charles Whitman Biography," note 69, above.

76. See note 27, above; see "Charles Whitman Biography," note 72, above.

77. See "Texas Tower shooting of 1966," note 8, above; see A. Barr, and "Austin (Tex.). Police Department Records of the Charles Whitman Mass Murder Case," note 10, above; see "Charles Whitman Biography," note 69, above; see note 71, above.

78. See "Texas Tower shooting of 1966," note 8, above; see "Austin (Tex.). Police Department Records of the Charles Whitman Mass Murder Case," and "Charles Whitman Biography," note 10, above; see note 13, above; see "Charles Whitman Biography," note 69, above; see "Charles Whitman Biography," note 72, above.

79. See note 6, above; see A. Barr, and "Austin (Tex.). Police Department Records of the Charles Whitman Mass Murder Case," note 10, above; see note 13, above; see "Charles Whitman Biography," note 69, above.

80. See A. Barr, and "Austin (Tex.). Police Department Records of the Charles Whitman Mass Murder Case," note 10, above; see note 13, above; see note 16, above.

81. See "Austin (Tex.). Police Department Records of the Charles Whitman Mass Murder Case," note 10, above; see note 13, above; see note 16, above.

82. See "Texas Tower shooting of 1966," note 5, above; see A. Barr, note 10, above; see note 13, above; see note 16, above; see "Charles Whitman Biography," note 69, above.

83. See note 13, above; see note 75, above.

84. See note 13, above.

85. See "Texas Tower shooting of 1966," note 8, above; see A. Barr, and "Austin (Tex.). Police Department Records of the Charles Whitman Mass Murder Case," note 10, above; see note 13, above.

86. See note 13, above; see "Charles Whitman Biography," note 69, above.

564

87. See "Texas Tower shooting of 1966," note 8, above; see "Austin (Tex.). Police Department Records of the Charles Whitman Mass Murder Case," note 10, above; see note 14, above; see "Charles Whitman Biography," note 69, above.

88. N. Thompson, "My Brain Made Me Do It," *Legal Affairs*, January/February 2006, https://www.legalaffairs.org/issues/January-February-2006/feature_thompson_janfeb06.msp.

89. "Background and History of the Insanity Defense," https://www.findlaw.com/criminal/criminal-procedure/the-insanity-defense-history-and-background.html; S. Feuerstein, F. Fortunati, et al., "The Insanity Defense," *Psychiatry* 2(9) (2005): 24–25.

90. See note 89, above.

91. R. Sorrentino, M. Musselman, et al., "Battered Woman Syndrome: Is It Enough for a Not Guilty by Reason of Insanity Plea?" *Psychiatric Times*, July 2019; see note 88, above; see "Background and History of the Insanity Defense," note 89, above.

92. J. Koebler, "Criminal Minds: Use of Neuroscience as a Defense Skyrockets," *US News & World Report*, November 9, 2012, https://www.usnews.com/news/articles/2012/11/09/criminal-minds-use-of-neuroscience-as-a-defense-skyrockets.

93. See note 92, above.

94. M. Martin, "Brain Tumor Defense for Jewish Center Bomb Threat Suspect Recalls 1991 Murder Trial," National Public Radio, March 25, 2017, https://www.npr.org/2017/03/25/521517166/lawyers-brain-tumor-defense-for-jewish-center-bomb-threat-suspect-recalls-1991-m; People v. Weinstein, 591 N.Y.S.2d 715, 156 Misc.2d 34 (1992) v; N. Hensley, "Family: Man, 80, charged in killing has brain tumor," Associated Press News, September 8, 2018, https://apnews.com/article/6b29ee934c244fb49a43436de0d47451; see note 88, above; see note 92, above.

95. See note 92, above.

96. See note 92, above.

97. See note 92, above.

98. M. Johnson, "How Responsible are Killers with Brain Damage?" *Scientific American*, January 30, 2018, https://www. scientificamerican.com/article/how-responsible-are-killers-with-brain-damage/.

99. See note 98, above.

100. See note 98, above.

101. See note 8, above; see G. M. Lavergne, note 10, above.

102. See G. M. Lavergne, note 10, above.

103. See note 101, above.

104. See note 13, above.

105. See note 13, above.

6.   Brian Jones

1. "Brian Jones: Sympathy for the Devil," Rolling Stone, August 9, 1969, https://www.rollingstone.com/music/music-news/brian-jones-sympathy-for-the-devil-182761/; "Brian Jones Biography," https://peoplepill.com/people/brian-jones-6/; "From the archive, 8 July 1969: Jones drowned while 'drunk and drugged,'" the *Guardian*, July 8, 2011, https://theguardian.com/theguardian/2011/jul/08/archive-brian-jones-death-1969; "Brian Jones Biography," https://findadeath.com/brian-jones/.

2. See note 1, above.

3. See "From the archive, 8 July 1969: Jones drowned while 'drunk and drugged,'" note 1, above.

4. See note 3, above.

5. See note 3, above.

6. "1969: Brian Jones died of 'drink and drugs,'" BBC, http://news.bbc.co.uk/onthisday/hi/dates/stories/july/7/newsid_4785000/4785320.stm; see note 3, above.

7. See "1969: Brian Jones died of 'drink and drugs,'" note 6, above.

8. See note 3, above.

9. "Brian Jones Biography," https://findadeath.com/brian-jones/; see note 3, above.

10. See note 3, above.

11. "Brian Jones Biography," https://www.thefamouspeople.com/ profiles/brian-jones-4678.php; see "Brian Jones: Sympathy for the Devil," "Brian Jones Biography," and "From the archive, 8 July 1969: Jones drowned while 'drunk and drugged,'" note 1, above; see "1969: Brian Jones died of 'drink and drugs,'" note 6, above.

12. See "Brian Jones: Sympathy for the Devil," and "From the archive, 8 July 1969: Jones drowned while 'drunk and drugged,'" note 1, above.

13. See note 12, above.

14. See "Brian Jones: Sympathy for the Devil," and "Brian Jones Biography," note 1, above; see "Brian Jones Biography," and "1969: Brian Jones died of 'drink and drugs,'" note 10, above.

15. J. Aswad, "'Life and Death of Brian Jones' Documentary Digs Deep Into the Rolling Stones Co-Founder's Demise," *Variety*, June 19, 2020, https://variety.com/2020/music/news/rolling-stones-life-death-of-brian-jones-documentary-1234643158/; "Brian Jones Biography," https://www.imdb.com/name/nm0427627/bio; G. Grundy, "The life and death of Brian," the *Guardian*, June 6, 2009, https://www.theguardian.com/books/2009/jun/07/brian-jones-laura-jackson-rolling-stones; see "Brian Jones Biography," note 11, above.

16. "Autopsy Report and Death Certificate—Brian Jones," http://www.rockmine.com/giveaway/LegDoc07/BJonesPM.htm.

17. See note 16, above.

18. See note 16, above.

19. See note 16, above.

20. See note 16, above.

21. D. K. Molina and V. M. DiMaio, "Normal organ weights in men: part I—the heart," *Am J Forensic Med Pathol* 33(4) (2012): 362–67; see note 16, above.

22. See note 16, above.

23. See note 16, above.

24. See note 16, above.

25. See note 16, above.

26. D. K. Molina and V. M. DiMaio, "Normal organ weights in men: part II—the brain, lungs, liver, spleen, and kidneys," *Am J Forensic Med Pathol* 33(4) (2012): 368–72.

27. See note 16, above; see note 26, above.

28. See note 27, above.

29. See note 16, above.

30. See note 16, above.

31. See note 16, above.

32. See note 16, above.

33. See note 16, above.

34. See note 16, above.

35. See "Brian Jones: Sympathy for the Devil" and "Brian Jones Biography," note 1, above.

36. See "Brian Jones Biography," note 1, above.

37. See note 35, above; see "Brian Jones Biography," note 11, above.

38. See note 37, above.

39. See note 37, above.

40. See note 35, above.

41. See note 37, above.

42. See note 35, above.

43. See "Brian Jones Biography" and "Brian Jones Biography," note 11, above.

44. See note 43, above.

45. See note 36, above.

46. See note 43, above.

47. See note 35, above.

48. See note 37, above.

49. See "Brian Jones: Sympathy for the Devil," note 1, above.

50. See note 49, above.

51. See "Brian Jones Biography," note 11, above; see note 49, above.

52. See note 49, above.

53. See note 49, above.

54. See note 49, above.

55. See note 36, above.

56. See "Brian Jones Biography," note 11, above.

57. See note 36, above.

58. See note 36, above.

59. See note 37, above.

60. See note 49, above.

61. See note 36, above.

62. See note 36, above.

63. See note 43, above.

64. See note 36, above.

65. See note 36, above.

66. See note 36, above.

67. E. Meisfjord, "The Tragic Death of the Rolling Stones' Brian Jones," Grunge, July 9, 2020, https://www.grunge.com/224864/the-tragic-death-of-the-rolling-stones-brian-jones/; see note 51, above.

68. See note 36, above.

69. See note 16, above.

70. See "Brian Jones Biography," note 1, above; see "1969: Brian Jones died of 'drink and drugs,'" note 6, above; see E. Meisfjord, note 67, above.

71. See note 36, above.

72. S. Nolasco, "The 'Curious Life and Death Of' Rolling Stones' Brian Jones: Murder conspiracy theory examined in new series," Fox News, September 5, 2020, https://www.foxnews.com/entertainment/curious-life-death-rolling-stones-brian-jones-murder-conspiracy-theory-examined-new-series; see note 36, above.

73. L. Rohter, "Ignobly Fading Away From the Rolling Stones," the *New York Times*, November 16, 2014, https://www.nytimes.com/2014/11/17/arts/brian-jones-the-making-of-the-rolling-stones-a-biography.html.

74. See 1969: Brian Jones died of 'drink and drugs,'" note 11, above.

75. A. Ghuran, L. R. van der Wieken, et al., "Cardiovascular complications of recreational drugs," *BMJ* 323(7311) (2001): 464–66.

76. "Illegal Drugs and Heart Disease," https://www.heart.org/en/health-topics/consumer-healthcare/what-is-cardiovascular-disease/illegal-drugs-and-heart-disease; see note 75, above.

77. See note 76, above.

78. H. A. Milman, "Whitney Houston," in *Forensics: The Science Behind the Deaths of Famous People* (Bloomington, Indiana: Xlibris, 2020) 187–202.

79. See note 78, above.

80. See note 78, above.

81. See note 78, above.

82. See "Brian Jones Biography," note 11, above.

83. H. A. Milman, *Forensics: The Science Behind the Deaths of Famous People* (Bloomington, Indiana: Xlibris, 2020), 185.

7. Sonny Liston

1. W. Griffee, "The boxer, the mob and a death still haunting after 50 years: Sonny Liston was the 'scariest' opponent Muhammad Ali ever fought, but his troubled life came to a tragic end amid rumors of heroin use, the criminal underworld and conspiracy," *Daily Mail*, August 2, 2020, https://www.dailymail.co.uk/sport/boxing/article-8474151/The-boxer-mob-death-haunting-50-years-tale-Sonny-Liston.html; G. Evans, "Sonny Liston: The mysterious death that haunts boxing," BBC, July 15, 2019, https://www.bbc.com/sport/boxing/48974341.

2. See note 1, above.

3. "Sonny Liston Biography," https://peoplepill.com/people/sonny-liston; "Sonny Liston Biography," https://totallyhistory.com/sonny-liston/; "Sonny Liston Biography," A&E Television Networks, original published dated April 2, 2014, last updated April 23, 2021, https://www.biography.com/athlete/sonny-liston; E. Gustkey, "19 Years Later: Liston Death Remains Mystery to His Friends," *Los Angeles Times*, February 22, 1989, https://www.latimes.com/archives/la-xpm-1989-02-22-sp-140-story.html; "Sonny Liston

Biography," https://unsolved.com/gallery/sonny-liston/; see note 1, above.

4.   See note 1, above; see "Sonny Liston Biography," note 3, above.

5.   See W. Griffee, note 1, above.

6.   See note 1, above.

7.   E. Gustkey, "Sonny Liston Remains a Mystery," the *Washington Post*, February 25, 1989, https://www.washingtonpost.com/archive/sports/1989/02/25/sonny-liston-remains-a-mystery/c5d578ec-9449-471a-bb00-b4ffdda6771f/; see note 1, above; see "Sonny Liston Biography," and E. Gustkey, note 3, above.

8.   See note 4, above.

9.   See E. Gustkey, note 3, above; see note 5, above.

10.   See "Sonny Liston Biography," "Sonny Liston Biography," and "Sonny Liston Biography," note 3, above; see E. Gustkey, note 7, above; see note 9, above.

11.   See "Sonny Liston Biography," note 3, above.

12.   See note 11, above.

13.   See G. Evans, note 1, above.

14.   "Sonny Liston Autopsy Report," https://www.boxingforum24.com/threads/sonny-liston-autopsy-report.285886/; see note 11, above.

15.   See note 12, above.

16.   See note 12, above.

17.   See "Sonny Liston Biography," note 3, above; see note 4, above.

18.   See "Sonny Liston Biography," note 3, above; see note 4, above; see "Sonny Liston Autopsy Report," note 14, above.

19.   "Sonny Liston Biography," https://www.thefamouspeople.com/profiles/sonny-liston-8953.php; M. Puma, "Liston was trouble in and out of ring," ESPN, https://www.espn.com/classic/biography/s/Liston_Sonny.html#:~:text=The%20 6%2Dfoot%2D1%C2%BD%2C,had%20ties%20to%20 organized%20crime; see "Sonny Liston Biography," "Sonny Liston Biography," and E. Gustkey, note 3, above; see note 5, above; see "Sonny Liston Autopsy Report," note 14, above.

20.   See note 5, above.

21. "Sonny Liston Biography," American National Biography, February 2000, https://www.anb.org/view/10.1093/anb/9780198606697.001.0001/anb-9780198606697-e-1900640;jsessionid=2058D30440B8928630C4EDEEB90EB3FA; see "Sonny Liston Biography," "Sonny Liston Biography," and "Sonny Liston Biography," note 1, above; see note 5, above.

22. See note 11, above.

23. See "Sonny Liston Biography," note 3, above; see note 11, above; see M. Puma, note 19, above; see note 21, above.

24. See note 1, above.

25. See note 23, above.

26. See G. Evans, note 1, above; see "Sonny Liston Biography," note 3, above; see note 5, above; see "Sonny Liston Biography" and "Sonny Liston Biography," note 19, above.

27. See G. Evans, note 1, above; see note 23, above.

28. "Sonny Liston Biography," https://www.imdb.com/name/nm0514288/bio; see note 1, above; see "Sonny Liston Biography" and "Sonny Liston Biography," note 3, above; see "Sonny Liston Biography," and M. Puma, note 19, above; see "Sonny Liston Biography," note 21, above.

29. See note 1, above.

30. See note 1, above; see "Sonny Liston Biography," note 28, above.

31. See "Sonny Liston Biography," and "Sonny Liston Biography," note 3, above; see note 11, above.

32. See "Sonny Liston Biography," note 3, above; see note 11, above; see Sonny Liston Biography" and M. Puma, note 19, above; see "Sonny Liston Biography," note 21, above.

33. See "Sonny Liston Biography," note 19, above; see "Sonny Liston Biography," note 21, above.

34. See note 33, above.

35. See "Sonny Liston Biography," note 6, above; see note 32, above.

36. See "Sonny Liston Biography," note 3, above; see note 11, above; see "Sonny Liston Biography," note 19, above.

37. See "Sonny Liston Biography," note 3, above; see note 11, above; see "Sonny Liston Biography," note 19, above.

38. M. Cox, "The One Heavyweight You Would Not Want To Face," https://coxcorner.tripod.com/most_feared.html; see note 11, above; see M. Puma, note 19, above.

39. See note 11, above.

40. See G. Evans, note 1, above; see "Sonny Liston Biography," note 3, above; see M. Puma, note 19, above; see "Sonny Liston Biography," note 28, above; see note 35, above.

41. See note 11, above.

42. See note 36, above.

43. See "Sonny Liston Biography," note 21, above.

44. See note 11, above.

45. See note 1, above; see M. Puma, note 19, above.

46. See note 11, above; see "Sonny Liston Biography," note 19, above.

47. See note 11, above.

48. See note 11, above.

49. See note 11, above.

50. See note 1, above; see note 35, above.

51. See note 43, above.

52. See note 13, above; see note 50, above.

53. See note 1, above.

54. See note 45, above.

55. See G. Evans, note 1, above; see note 11, above.

56. See note 4, above; see M. Puma, note 19, above; see note 33, above.

57. See M. Puma, and "Sonny Liston Biography," note 19, above; see note 55, above.

58. See "Sonny Liston Biography," note 19, above; see note 36, above; see note 45, above.

59. "What is heart failure?" American Heart Association, https://www.heart.org/en/health-topics/heart-failure/what-is-heart-failure; "Heart Failure," Mayo Clinic, https://www.mayoclinic.org/diseases-conditions/heart-failure/symptoms-causes/syc-20373142.

60. See "Heart Failure," note 59, above.

61. See "What is heart failure?" note 59, above.
62. See note 59, above.
63. See note 60, above.
64. See note 60, above.
65. See note 58, above.
66. See note 5, above.
67. See note 7, above.
68. See "Sonny Liston Biography," note 3, above; see note 4, above; see "Sonny Liston Autopsy Report," note 14, above.
69. See G. Evans, note 1, above; see M. Puma, note 19, above; see "Sonny Liston Biography," note 28, above; see note 43, above.
70. See G. Evans, note 1, above.
71. See note 1, above.
72. See note 1, above; see note 11, above.
73. See note 72, above.
74. See note 70, above.
75. See M. Puma, note 19, above.
76. See note 75, above.
77. See note 5, above.
78. See note 70, above.
79. See note 70, above.
80. See note 45, above; see note 51, above; see note 70, above.

8. Bruce Lee

1. "Bruce Lee Biography," https://findadeath.com/bruce-lee/; R. Chang, "Bruce Lee: The Mystery Surrounding the Martial Artist's Death," June 7, 2020, https://www.biography.com/news/bruce-lee-death-mystery; "Bruce Lee Biography," https://www.thefamouspeople.com/profiles/bruce-lee-938.php.
2. See "Bruce Lee Biography," note 1, above.
3. See "Bruce Lee Biography," note 1, above; see note 2, above.
4. See note 3, above.
5. See note 3, above.

6. "Bruce Lee," https://brucelee.com/bruce-lee; N. Dozome, "Enter the Forensic Pathologist," https://dozome.medium.com/enter-the-forensic-pathologist-ea32ff171448; see note 1, above.

7. "Bruce Lee Biography," A&E Television Networks, original published date April 2, 2014, last updated May 24, 2021, https://www.biography.com/actor/bruce-lee; K. Serena, "The Mysterious Circumstances Surrounding Bruce Lee's Death," original published date March 22, 2018, last updated February 2, 2021, https://allthatsinteresting.com/bruce-lees-death; see note 6, above.

8. See note 1, above; see "Bruce Lee," note 6, above; see K. Serena, note 7, above.

9. E. Watling, "How Did Bruce Lee Die?" *Newsweek*, January 15, 2019, https://www.newsweek.com/how-did-bruce-lee-die-1289822; "Bruce Lee Biography," A&E Television Networks, original published date April 2, 2014, last updated May 24, 2021, https://www.biography.com/actor/bruce-lee.

10. See note 9, above.

11. See "Bruce Lee Biography," and R. Chang, note 1, above.

12. See note 2, above.

13. M. Polly, "The Last Days of Bruce Lee," May 29, 2018, https://www.theringer.com/movies/2018/5/29/17400010/bruce-lee-death-a-life-matthew-polly; M. Polly, "How Did Bruce Lee Die?" History, original published date July 20, 2018, last updated July 21, 2019, https://www.history.com/news/bruce-lee-death-mystery-solved-sweat-glands; see R. Chang, note 1, above; see E. Watling, note 9, above.

14. See note 2, above; see M. Polly and M. Polly, note 13, above.

15. See R. Chang, note 1, above.

16. "Bruce Lee," https://brucelee.com/bruce-lee; N. Dozome, "Enter the Forensic Pathologist," https://dozome.medium.com/enter-the-forensic-pathologist-ea32ff171448; see note 14, above.

17. "Bruce Lee Biography," https://www.imdb.com/name/nm0000045/bio; see note 2, above; see K. Serena, note 7, above; see note 16, above.

18. See M. Polly and R. Chang, note 13, above.

19. See note 16, above; see K. Serena, note 7, above; see "Bruce Lee Biography," note 17, above.

20. See "Bruce Lee Biography" and R. Chang, note 1, above; see M. Polly, note 13, above; see K. Serena, "Bruce Lee," N. Dozome, and "Bruce Lee Biography," note 17, above.

21. See note 8, above; see M. Polly and M. Polly, note 13, above; see N. Dozome, note 16, above; see "Bruce Lee Biography," note 17, above.

22. See note 2, above; see "Bruce Lee Biography," note 7, above; see M. Polly, note 13, above.

23. See M. Polly, note 13, above.

24. See "Bruce Lee," note 6, above; see note 23, above.

25. See note 23, above.

26. See "Bruce Lee Biography," note 17, above.

27. J. Randerson, "Epilepsy could solve mystery of kung fu legend's death," the *Guardian*, February 24, 2006, https://www.theguardian.com/science/2006/feb/25/film.filmnews; see E. Watling, note 9, above; see M. Polly and M. Polly, note 13, above; see K. Serena, note 7, above; see "Bruce Lee," note 17, above.

28. See note 23, above.

29. See note 24, above.

30. See note 24, above.

31. See note 23, above.

32. See note 23, above.

33. See "Bruce Lee," note 6, above; see note 24, above.

34. See note 23, above.

35. See note 2, above; see M. Polly, note 13, above; see K. Serena, note 17, above; see note 24, above; see J. Randerson, note 27, above.

36. "Cerebral Edema (Brain Swelling)," https://brainfoundation.org.au/images/stories/applicant_essays/2012_essays/Cerebral_Oedema_-_Turner.pdf; S. M. Nehring, P. Tadi, et al., "Cerebral Edema," July 8, 2021, https://www.ncbi.nlm.nih.gov/books/NBK537272/.

37. B. Roybal, "Brain Swelling," https://webmd.com/brain/brain-swelling-brain-edema-intracranial-pressure; see note 36, above.

38. See "Cerebral Edema (Brain Swelling)," note 36, above.

39. See B. Roybal, note 37, above.

40. See note 39, above.

41. See E. Watling, note 9, above; see N. Dozome, note 16, above; see note 24, above.

42. See E. Watling, note 9, above; see N. Dozome, note 16, above.

43. See note 2, above; see note 23, above.

44. See note 23, above.

45. See note 23, above.

46. See "Bruce Lee," and N. Dozome, note 6, above; see M. Polly, note 13, above.

47. See N. Dozome, note 6, above; see note 9, above; see M. Polly, note 13, above; see note 23, above.

48. See N. Dozome, note 6, above; see note 23, above.

49. See N. Dozome, note 6, above; see note 9, above; see M. Polly, note 13, above.

50. See N. Dozome, note 6, above.

51. See note 50, above.

52. See note 50, above.

53. See note 49, above.

54. See note 50, above.

55. See note 50, above.

56. See R. Chang, note 1, above; see "Bruce Lee," note 6, above; see note 50, above.

57. "Reye's Syndrome," Mayo Clinic, https://www.mayoclinic.org/diseases-conditions/reyes-syndrome/symptoms-causes/syc-20377255; "Equagesic," product information, https://www.accessdata.fda.gov/drugsatfda_docs/label/2021/011702s040lbl.pdf.

58. S. Shah and W. T. Kimberly, "The Modern Approach to Treating Brain Swelling in the Neuro ICU," *Semin Neurol* 36(6) (2016): 602–7.

59. See R. Chang, note 1, above; see note 50, above.

60. See R. Chang, note 1, above; see E. Watling, note 9, above.

61. "Sudden Unexpected Death in Epilepsy (SUDEP)," US Centers for Disease Control and Prevention, https://www.cdc.gov/epilepsy/about/sudep/index.htm.

62. See note 60, above.

63. See R. Chang, note 1, above; see E. Watling, note 9, above; see M. Polly, note 13, above.

64. Anhidrosis (Inability to sweat), International Hyperhidrosis Society, https://www.sweathelp.org/where-do-you-sweat/other-sweating/anhidrosis-no-sweating.html.

65. See M. Polly, note 13, above.

66. See note 65, above.

67. See note 50, above; see note 63, above.

68. E. J. Walter and M. Carraretto, "The neurological and cognitive consequences of hyperthermia," *Crit Care 20* (2016): 199.

69. See note 65, above.

70. See note 1, above; see note 9, above; see "Bruce Lee," note 6, above; see note 25, above.

71. See note 3, above; see "Bruce Lee Biography," note 7, above; see note 25, above.

72. See note 3, above; see "Bruce Lee," note 6, above; see E. Watling, note 9, above; see note 25, above.

73. See note 3, above; see "Bruce Lee Biography," note 7, above.

74. See note 2, above; see note 25, above.

75. See "Bruce Lee," note 6, above; see "Bruce Lee Biography," note 7, above.

76. See note 3, above; see note 25, above.

77. See note 3, above.

78. See R. Chang, note 1, above; see "Bruce Lee," note 6, above; see note 71, above.

79. See note 2, above; see note 25, above; see note 75, above.

80. See note 2, above; see "Bruce Lee," note 6, above.

81. See note 1, above; see "Bruce Lee," note 6, above.

82. See "Bruce Lee Biography," note 7, above; see E. Watling, note 9, above; see note 25, above; see note 81, above.

83. See "Bruce Lee Biography," note 7, above; see note 81, above.

84. See note 2, above; see "Bruce Lee," note 6, above; see note 25, above.

85. See note 2, above.

86. See note 1, above; see "Bruce Lee Biography," note 7, above.

87. See note 76, above.

88. See note 73, above.

89. See note 79, above.

90. See note 3, above; see "Bruce Lee," note 6, above; see E. Watling, note 9, above.

91. See note 25, above.

92. See "Bruce Lee," note 6, above; see note 76, above.

93. See note 82, above.

94. See note 83, above.

95. See J. Randerson, note 27, above.

96. See note 2, above.

97. See note 1, above; see note 23, above.

98. See note 25, above.

99. See E. Watling, note 9, above; see note 25, above.

100. See note 25, above.

101. See note 25, above.

102. See "Bruce Lee Biography," note 17, above.

9. Jim Jones

1. D. Chiu, "Jonestown: 13 Things You Should Know About Cult Massacre," *Rolling Stone*, original published date November 2017, last updated May 29, 2020, https://www.rollingstone.com/feature/jonestown-13-things-you-should-know-about-cult-massacre-121974/.

2. R. Lindsey, "Jim Jones—From Poverty to Power of Life and Death," the *New York Times*, November 26, 1978, https://www.nytimes.com/1978/11/26/archives/jim-jonesfrom-poverty-to-power-of-life-and-death-arrested-for-lewd.html; see note 1, above.

3. J. O. Conroy, "An apocalyptic cult, 900 dead: remembering the Jonestown massacre, 40 years on," the *Guardian*, November 17, 2018, https://www.theguardian.com/world/2018/nov/17/an-apocalyptic-cult-900-dead-remembering-the-jonestown-massacre-40-years-on.

4. See note 1, above.

5. "The Peoples Temple in Guyana," Public Broadcasting Service, https://www.pbs.org/wgbh/americanexperience/features/jonestown-guyana/; "Jim Jones Biography," A&E Television Networks, original published date April 2, 2014, last updated September 15, 2020, https://www.biography.com/crime-figure/jim-jones.

6. See note 5, above.

7. "Jonestown," A&E Television Networks, original published date October 18, 2010, last updated January 13, 2021, https://www.history.com/topics/crime/jonestown; see note 3, above; "The Peoples Temple in Guyana," note 5, above.

8. See note 7, above.

9. See "The Peoples Temple in Guyana," note 5, above; see "Jonestown," note 7, above.

10. See "The Peoples Temple in Guyana," note 5, above.

11. See note 10, above.

12. See note 3, above.

13. J. Polk, "Jones plotted cyanide deaths years before Jonestown," CNN, November 12, 2008, https://www.cnn.com/2008/US/11/12/jonestown.cyanide/index.html.

14. "Jim Jones," Public Broadcasting Service, https://www.pbs.org/wgbh/americanexperience/features/jonestown-bio-jones/.

15. "Jonestown," https://www.fbi.gov/history/famous-cases/jonestown; see Jim Jones Biography," note 5, above; see note 7, above.

16. See note 1, above; see note 3, above; see "Jonestown," note 7, above.

17. "Jim Jones," Encyclopedia.com, https://www.encyclopedia.com/people/philosophy-and-religion/protestant-christianity-biographies/jim-jones; see "Jim Jones Biography," note 5, above; see "Jonestown," note 15, above; see note 16, above.

18. "Jim Jones Biography," https://www.imdb.com/name/nm0428385/bio; see note 13, above; see note 16, above; see "Jonestown," note 15, above; see "Jim Jones," note 17, above.

19. See note 18, above.

20. See "Jim Jones Biography," note 5, above; see "Jonestown," note 7, above; see "Jonestown," note 15, above; see J. Polk, note 18, above.

21. See "Jim Jones Biography," note 18, above.

22. L. Barcella, A&E Television Networks, "How Jim Jones Used Drugs to Run Jonestown and Control Members of the Peoples Temple," https://www.aetv.com/real-crime/jim-jones-drugs-jonestown-control-peoples-temple; L. Piva, "Jonestown: The Life and Death of Peoples Temple: A Commentary on Religious Movements Turning Sinister," https://onlineacademiccommunity.uvic.ca/sociologyofreligion/2017/12/31/jonestown-the-life-and-death-of-peoples-temple-a-commentary-on-religious-movements-turning-sinister/; see note 1, above; see "Jim Jones Biography," note 5, above.

23. See note 10, above.

24. See J. Polk, note 18, above.

25. See note 1, above.

26. See note 1, above.

27. See note 3, above; see "Jonestown," note 15, above.

28. C. Gorney, "Jonestown's Haunted Son," the *Washington Post*, November 7, 1983, https://www.washingtonpost.com/archive/lifestyle/1983/11/07/jonestowns-haunted-son/f9369588-008b-497a-9ad3-b303dc01a8df/.

29. See "Jonestown," note 15, above.

30. See note 29, above.

31. See note 1, above.

32. See note 1, above.

33. See note 1, above.

34. See note 1, above; see note 3, above.

35. See note 1, above.

36. A. Valiente and M. Delarosa, "40 Years after the Jonestown massacre: Jim Jones' Surviving Sons on what they think of their

father, the Peoples Temple today," ABC News, https://abcnews. go.com/US/40-years-jonestown-massacre-jim-jones-surviving-sons/story?id=57997006; S. Nolasco, "Jim Jones' sons recall Jonestown massacre, describe cult leader's drug addiction in new do," Fox News, November 16, 2018, https://www.foxnews.com/ entertainment/jim-jones-sons-recall-jonestown-massacre-describe-cult-leaders-drug-addiction-in-new-doc.

[37] See note 36, above.

[38] See "Jonestown", note 15, above; see "Jim Jones Biography," note 5, above; see note 34, above.

[39] See note 13, above.

[40] "Autopsy report—Jim Jones," https://jonestown.sdsu.edu/ wpcontent/uploads/2013/10/JimJones.pdf.

[41] "Autopsies in the United States," https://jonestown.sdsu.edu/?page_ id=13661; see note 40, above.

[42] R. B. Brannon and W. M. Morlang, "Jonestown Tragedy Revisited: The Role of Dentistry," *J Forensic Sci* 47(1) (2002): 3–7; D. R. Jones, "Secondary disaster victims: the emotional effects of recovering and identifying human remains," *Am J Psychiatry* 142(3) (1985): 303–7.

[43] See note 42, above.

[44] See note 40, above; see R. B. Brannon and W. M. Morlang, note 42, above.

[45] See note 40, above.

[46] See note 40, above.

[47] R. L. Thompson, W. W. Manders, et al., "Postmortem Findings of the Victims of the Jonestown Tragedy," *J Forensic Sciences* 32(2) (1987): 433–43; E-P Soriano, M-V Diniz, et al., "The post-mortem pink teeth phenomenon: a case report," *Med Oral Patol Oral Cir Bucal* 14(7) (2009): E337–E339; see R. B. Brannon and W. M. Morlang, note 42, above.

[48] See note 41, above.

[49] See note 40, above.

[50] See note 40, above.

51. See note 40, above; see R. L. Thompson, W. W. Manders, et al., note 47, above.

52. See note 52, above.

53. See note 40, above.

54. See note 40, above.

55. See note 40, above.

56. See note 40, above.

57. See note 40, above.

58. See note 40, above.

59. See note 40, above.

60. K. Sasikala, V. Fernz, et al., "A Retrospective Descriptive Study on Death Due to Cyanide Poisoning Over a Period of 20 Years in Government Medical College, Thiruvananthapuram," *J Evid Based Med Health* 8(30) (2021): 2697–2701.

61. See note 40, above.

62. See note 40, above.

63. See note 40, above.

64. See note 40, above.

65. See note 40, above.

66. See note 10, above.

67. See note 10, above.

68. See S. Nolasco, note 36, above.

69. See note 68, above.

70. See "Autopsies in the United States," note 41, above; see note 68, above.

71. "Autopsy report—Laurence Eugene Schacht," https://jonestown. sdsu.edu/wp-content/uploads/2013/10/LawrenceSchacht.pdf; "Autopsy report—Maria Katsaris," https://jonestown.sdsu.edu/ wp-content/uploads/2013/10/MariaKatsaris.pdf; "Autopsy report— Carolyn Layton Moore," https://jonestown.sdsu.edu/wp-content/ uploads/2013/10/CarolynMooreLayton.pdf; J. L. McAllister, R. J. Roby, et al., "Stability of Cyanide in Cadavers and in Postmortem Stored Tissue Specimens: A Review," *J Analytical Toxicol* 32(8):

612–20 (2008); see note 41, above; see R. L. Thompson, W. W. Manders, et al., note 47, above.

72. See note 41, above; see note 70, above; see "Autopsy report—Laurence Eugene Schacht," "Autopsy report—Maria Katsaris," and "Autopsy report—Carolyn Layton Moore," note 71, above.

73. A. Pick-Jones, "Jim Jones and the History of Peoples Temple," https://jonestown.sdsu.edu/?page_id=33190.

74. "Autopsy report—Ann Elizabeth Moore," https://jonestown.sdsu.edu/wp-content/uploads/2013/10/AnnElizabethMoore.pdf.

75. See note 73, above; see "Autopsy report—Ann Elizabeth Moore," note 74, above.

76. See note 75, above.

77. See note 1, above; see note 73, above.

78. See note 40, above.

79. See note 40, above.

80. See note 51, above.

81. See R. Lindsey, note 2, above; see "Jim Jones Biography," note 5, above; see "Jim Jones," note 17, above; see "Jim Jones Biography," note 18, above.

82. See R. Lindsey, note 2, above.

83. "Jim Jones," https://www.thefamouspeople.com/profiles/james-warren-jones-1841.php; see R. Lindsey, note 2, above; see "Jim Jones Biography," note 5, above; see "Jim Jones Biography," note 18, above.

84. "Jim Jones Biography: Religious Cult Leader Responsible for Mass Suicide," Biographics, May 30, 2018, https://biographics.org/jim-jones-biography-religious-cult-leader-responsible-for-a-mass-suicide/; see "Jim Jones Biography," note 5, above.

85. See note 84, above.

86. See "Jim Jones Biography: Religious Cult Leader Responsible for Mass Suicide," note 84, above.

87. D. Carpenter, "Countdown to Armageddon: The Reverend Jim Jones," https://indianahistory.org/stories/countdown-to-armageddon-the-reverend-jim-jones-and-indiana/; E. Paul, "The Radicalization of

Jim Jones's People's Temple," https://onlineacademiccommunity. uvic.ca/sociologyofreligion/tag/jim-jones/; see note 1, above; see "Jim Jones Biography," note 18, above; see "Jim Jones Biography: Religious Cult Leader Responsible for Mass Suicide," note 84, above.

88. See note 1, above.

89. See note 14, above; see "Jim Jones," note 18, above; see note 82, above; see note 84, above.

90. See note 82, above.

91. See "Jim Jones," note 18, above; see note 82, above; see note 84, above.

92. See note 14, above; see note 82, above; see "Jim Jones," note 83, above; see note 84, above.

93. See note 82, above; see note 84, above.

94. See note 82, above.

95. See "Jim Jones Biography," note 5, above; see "Jim Jones Biography," note 18, above; see "Jim Jones," note 83, above.

96. See note 14, above; see "Jim Jones," note 17, above; see "Jim Jones Biography," note 18, above; see note 82, above; see "Jim Jones Biography," note 87, above.

97. See A. Valiente and M. Delarosa, note 36, above.

98. See D. Carpenter, note 87, above.

99. See note 98, above.

100. See note 82, above.

101. See note 82, above.

102. See note 82, above.

103. See note 98, above.

104. "Jim Jones," https://www.britannica.com/biography/Jim-Jones; see "Jim Jones," note 17, above; see note 82, above; see "Jim Jones," note 83, above.

105. See note 82, above.

106. See "Jim Jones Biography," note 18, above; see "Jim Jones," note 83, above; see "Jim Jones Biography: Religious Cult Leader Responsible for Mass Suicide," note 84, above.

107. See note 98, above.

108. See note 98, above.

109. See note 5, above; see A. Valiente and M. Delarosa, note 36, above; see note 82, above; see "Jim Jones," note 83, above.

110. See "Jim Jones Biography," note 18, above; see note 82, above; see "Jim Jones," note 83, above; see "Jim Jones," note 104, above.

111. See note 82, above.

112. See note 82, above.

113. See note 82, above.

114. See note 82, above.

115. J. Rothenberg Gritz, "Drinking the Kool-Aid: A Survivor Remembers Jim Jones," the *Atlantic*, November 18, 2011, https://www.theatlantic.com/national/archive/2011/11/drinking-the-kool-aid-a-survivor-remembers-jim-jones/248723/.

116. See note 82, above.

117. See "Jonestown," note 7, above.

118. See "Jim Jones Biography," note 18, above; see note 82, above.

119. See Jim Jones Biography: Religious Cult Leader Responsible for Mass Suicide," note 84, above.

120. See note 42, above; see note 119, above.

121. See note 42, above.

122. See note 119, above.

123. See "Jim Jones Biography," note 5, above; see "Jim Jones," note 83, above; see note 118, above.

124. J. T. Richardson, "People's Temple and Jonestown: A Corrective Comparison and Critique," *J for the Scientific Study* 19 (3) (1980): 239–55.

125. See L. Piva, note 22, above.

126. See note 69, above.

127. See note 125, above.

128. See note 125, above.

129. "Jonestown," History, original published date October 18, 2010, last updated November 20, 2019, https://www.history.com/topics/crime/jonestown; see note 125, above.

130. See note 98, above.

131. See note 28, above.

132. See note 28, above; see note 73, above.

133. See note 97, above.

134. See note 28, above; see "Jonestown," note 129, above.

135. See note 28, above.

136. See note 97, above.

137. See note 69, above; see note 73, above; see note 97, above.

138. See note 97, above; see "Jonestown," note 129, above.

139. See note 97, above.

140. See note 82, above.

141. See note 73, above; see "Jonestown," note 129, above.

142. See note 97, above.

143. See note 115, above.

144. See note 115, above.

145. See "Jim Jones Biography," note 18, above.

146. See note 98, above.

147. See note 73, above.

148. See note 73, above.

149. J. I. Lasaga, "Death in Jonestown: techniques of political control by a paranoid leader," *Suicide Life Threat Behav* 10(4) (1980): 210–13.

150. See note 73, above.

151. See note 73, above.

152. A. Black Jr., "Jonestown—two faces of suicide: a Durkheimian analysis," *Suicide Life Threat Behav* 20(4) (1990): 285–306.

153. See note 152, above.

154. See note 152, above.

155. See note 28, above.

10. David Koresh

1. M. Wilson, "How failures during the Waco siege changed everything for the FBI, ATF," *Austin-American Statesman*, original published date April 19, 2018, last updated September

25, 2018, https://www.statesman.com/news/20180419/how-failures-during-the-waco-siege-changed-everything-for-the-fbi-atf; P. Colloff, "The Fire That Time," *Texas Monthly*, April 2008, https://www.texasmonthly.com/articles/the-fire-that-time/; "Report to the Deputy Attorney General on the Events at Waco, Texas," https://www.justice.gov/archives/publications/waco/report-deputy-attorney-general-events-waco-texas.

2. "Remembering Waco," https://www.atf.gov/our-history/remembering-waco; see M. Wilson, and P. Colloff, note 1, above.

3. See P. Colloff, note 1, above.

4. See M. Wilson, and P. Colloff, note 1, above.

5. See note 3, above.

6. See note 2, above.

7. See. M. Wilson, note 1, above.

8. See "Remembering Waco," note 2, above; see note 7, above.

9. See P. Colloff, note 1, above; see note 7, above.

10. See note 7, above.

11. See note 7, above.

12. See note 3, above.

13. See note 3, above.

14. See note 3, above.

15. See note 3, above.

16. See note 2, above.

17. See note 1, above.

18. See note 4, above.

19. See "Report to the Deputy Attorney General on the Events at Waco, Texas," note 1, above; see note 5, above.

20. See note 3, above.

21. See note 3, above.

22. See note 3, above.

23. See note 3, above.

24. See note 3, above.

25. M. Pearson, S. Wilking, et al., "Survivors of 1993 Waco siege describe what happened in fire that ended the 51-day standoff,"

ABC News, January 3, 2018, https://abcnews.go.com/US/ survivors-1993-waco-siege-describe-happened-fire-ended/ story?id=52034435.

26. See note 3, above.
27. See note 3, above.
28. See note 3, above.
29. See note 3, above.
30. See note 3, above.
31. See note 3, above.
32. See note 3, above.
33. See note 3, above.
34. See note 3, above.
35. See note 3, above.
36. See note 19, above.
37. See note 3, above.
38. See note 19, above.
39. See note 3, above.
40. See note 3, above.
41. See note 3, above.
42. See note 3, above.
43. See note 3, above.
44. See "Report to the Deputy Attorney General on the Events at Waco, Texas," note 1, above; see note 7, above; see M. Pearson, S. Wilking, et al., note 44, above.
45. See note 3, above.
46. See note 3, above.
47. See "Report to the Deputy Attorney General on the Events at Waco, Texas," note 1, above; see note 7, above.
48. See "Remembering Waco," note 2, above; see note 44, above.
49. See M. Pearson, S. Wilking, et al., note 44, above.
50. See note 49, above.
51. See note 3, above; see note 49, above.
52. See "Report to the Deputy Attorney General on the Events at Waco, Texas," note 1, above; see note 49, above.

53. See note 4, above.

54. See note 3, above.

55. See note 3, above.

56. See note 1, above; see note 49, above.

57. M. Pearson, S. Wilking, et al., "Who was David Koresh: Ex-followers describe life inside apocalyptic religious sect involved in 1993 Waco siege," ABC News, January 2, 2018, https://abcnews.go.com/US/ david-koresh-followers-describe-life-inside-apocalyptic-religious/ story?id=52033937; J. C. Danforth, "Final Report to the Deputy Attorney General Concerning the 1993 Confrontation at the Mt. Carmel Complex in Waco Texas," November 8, 2000, https://upload. wikimedia.org/wikipedia/commons/8/85/Danforthreport-final.pdf; see note 56, above.

58. See note 52, above.

59. See note 3, above.

60. See note 3, above.

61. See note 3, above.

62. See "Remembering Waco," note 2, above; see note 7, above; see note 52, above.

63. See note 62, above.

64. See "Remembering Waco," note 2, above.

65. See note 7, above; see note 64, above.

66. See note 64, above.

67. See note 51, above.

68. "Autopsy—David Koresh," http://www.web-ak.com/waco/death/ map/d_list00.htm.

69. See note 68, above.

70. See note 68, above.

71. See note 68, above.

72. See note 68, above.

73. See note 68, above.

74. See note 68, above.

75. See note 68, above.

76. See note 68, above.

77. See note 68, above.

78. See note 68, above.

79. See note 68, above.

80. See note 68, above.

81. See note 68, above.

82. See note 68, above.

83. See note 68, above.

84. See note 68, above.

85. See note 68, above.

86. See note 68, above.

87. See note 68, above.

88. See note 68, above.

89. See note 68, above.

90. See note 68, above.

91. See note 68, above.

92. See note 68, above.

93. See note 68, above.

94. See note 68, above.

95. See note 68, above.

96. "Poison Facts: Medium Chemicals: Carbon Monoxide," "https://www.kansashealthsystem.com/-/media/Files/PDF/Poisons/Carbonmonoxide.pdf; see note 68, above.

97. See note 68, above.

98. See note 68, above.

99. See note 68, above.

100. See note 68, above.

101. See note 68, above.

102. See note 68, above.

103. See note 68, above.

104. T. Leopold, "Postmortem Alcohol Formation in a Severely Burned Victim," Toxicology Consultants and Assessment Specialists, LLC, November 5, 2013, https://www.investigativemedia.com/wp-content/uploads/2015/12/Postmortem-Alcohol-Formation-in-a-Severely-Burned-Victim-TCAS.pdf; S. Robertson, "Interpretation

of Measured Alcohol Levels in Fatal Aviation Accident Victims," https://www.atsb.gov.au/media/36390/Measured_alcohol_lev.pdf. See "Postmortem Alcohol Formation in a Severely Burned Victim," See note 68, above.

105. S. A. Pressley, "Autopsies verify deaths of Koresh's top acolytes," the *Washington Post*, May 12, 1993, https://www.washingtonpost.com/archive/politics/1993/05/12/autopsies-verify-deaths-of-koreshs-top-acolytes/20947603-b978-4b23-b0aa-0327ad8fffa8/; see note 64, above.

106. S. Gordon, "Tarrant Medical Examiner Remembers Branch Davidian Carnage," original published date February 28, 2018, last updated March 19, 2018, https://www.nbcdfw.com/news/local/tarrant-medical-examiner-remembers-branch-davidian-carnage/2062200/.

107. "David Koresh Biography," https://www.imdb.com/name/nm0466205/bio; "David Koresh Biography," A&E Television Networks, original published date April 2, 2014, last updated January 19, 2021, https://www.biography.com/crime-figure/david-koresh; "David Koresh Biography," https://www.thefamouspeople.com/profiles/david-koresh-35595.php; "David Koresh," https://criminalminds.fandom.com/wiki/David_Koresh; see M. Pearson, S. Wilking, et al., note 57, above.

108. See "David Koresh Biography," and "David Koresh Biography," note 107, above.

109. See "David Koresh Biography," note 107, above.

110. See M. Pearson, S. Wilking, et al., note 57, above.

111. See "David Koresh Biography," and "David Koresh," note 107, above.

112. See "David Koresh Biography," "David Koresh Biography," and "David Koresh Biography," note 107, above.

113. See "David Koresh Biography," note 107, above.

114. See note 111, above.

115. See note 111, above.

116. See M. Pearson, S. Wilking, et al., note 57, above; see "David Koresh Biography," "David Koresh Biography," and "David Koresh Biography," note 107, above.

117. See M. Pearson, S. Wilking, et al., note 57, above.

118. See note 64, above; see note 116, above.

119. See note 64, above.

120. See M. Pearson, S. Wilking, et al., note 57, above; see note 64, above; see "David Koresh," note 107, above.

121. See note 110, above; see note 108, above.

122. See note 121, above.

123. See "David Koresh Biography," note 107, above; see note 111, above.

124. See "David Koresh," note 107, above; see note 108, above.

125. See note 123, above.

126. See "David Koresh Biography," note 107, above.

127. See note 110, above.

128. See note 64, above.

129. See note 110, above.

130. See note 3, above.

131. See note 3, above.

132. See note 110, above.

133. See note 110, above.

134. See note 110, above.

135. See note 64, above.

136. See note 64, above.

137. See note 64, above.

138. See note 64, above; see "David Koresh," note 107, above; see note 112, above.

139. See "David Koresh," and "David Koresh Biography," note 107, above.

140. See note 110, above.

141. See note 110, above; see note 139, above.

142. See note 108, above.

143. See note 110, above.

144. See "David Koresh Biography," note 107, above; see note 110, above.

145. See note 110, above.
146. See note 3, above.
147. See note 3, above.
148. See note 3, above.
149. See note 3, above.
150. See note 3, above.
151. See note 3, above.
152. See note 3, above.
153. See note 3, above.
154. See note 7, above.
155. See note 7, above.
156. See note 3, above.
157. See note 7, above.
158. See note 8, above; see note 64, above.
159. See note 7, above.
160. See note 64, above; see J. C. Danforth, note 57, above.
161. See note 3, above.
162. See note 3, above.
163. See note 64, above.
164. See note 64, above.
165. See J. C. Danforth, note 57, above.
166. See note 106, above.
167. See note 106, above.
168. See note 110, above.
169. See note 110, above.
170. See note 3, above.
171. See note 3, above.
172. See note 3, above.

11.   Vince Foster

1.   D. V. Drehle and H. Schneider, "Foster's Death a Suicide," the *Washington Post*, July 1, 1994, https://www.washingtonpost.com/wp-srv/politics/special/whitewater/stories/wwtr940701.htm.

2. "Vince Foster Biography," https://www.peoplepill.com/people/vince-foster/; "Whitewater: The Foster Report. I. Introduction," the *Washington Post*, 1998, https://www.washingtonpost.com/wp-srv/politics/special/whitewater/docs/fosteri.htm; S. Schmidt, "Starr Probe Reaffirms Foster Killed Himself," the *Washington Post*, October 11, 1997, https://www.washingtonpost.com/wp-srv/politics/special/whitewater/stories/wwtr971011.htm; see D. V. Drehle and H. Schneider, note 1, above.

3. See note 1, above; see "Vince Foster Biography," and S. Schmidt, note 2, above.

4. See note 1, above.

5. R. Marcus and M. Isikoff, "Clinton Withdraws Baird's Justice Nomination," the *Washington Post*, January 22, 1993, https://www.washingtonpost.com/archive/politics/1993/01/22/clinton-withdraws-bairds-justice-nomination/567eedcf-72ba-42c9-a2d3-daccd0b8f048/; see note 1, above.

6. See note 1, above; see S. Schmidt, note 2, above.

7. See note 1, above.

8. See note 1, above.

9. See note 1, above.

10. See note 1, above.

11. See note 1, above.

12. See note 1, above.

13. "Whitewater: The Foster Report. IV. Factual Summary. A. Mr. Foster's Background and Activities on July 20, 1993," the *Washington Post*, https://www.washingtonpost.com/wp-srv/politics/special/whitewater/docs/fosteriv.htm; see note 1, above.

14. See note 6, above.

15. "Autopsy report—Vincent Walker Foster Jr.," http://www.autopsyfiles.org/reports/Celebs/foster,%20vincent_report.pdf.

16. M. Schudel, "Redoubtable N. Va. Medical Examiner James C. Beyer," the *Washington Post*, March 5, 2006, https://www.washingtonpost.com/archive/local/2006/03/04/redoubtable-nva-medical-examiner-james-c-beyer/632220f4-5c82-4d96-9ead-3663c555e36c/.

17. "Sudden Cardiac Death (Sudden Cardiac Arrest)," Cleveland Clinic, https://my.clevelandclinic.org/health/diseases/17522-sudden-cardiac-death-sudden-cardiac-arrest; see note 15, above.
18. See note 17, above.
19. See note 17, above.
20. See note 15, above.
21. See note 15, above.
22. See note 15, above.
23. See note 15, above.
24. See note 15, above.
25. See note 15, above.
26. See note 15, above.
27. See note 15, above.
28. See note 15, above.
29. See note 15, above.
30. See note 15, above.
31. See "Whitewater: The Foster Report. I. Introduction," note 2, above; see "Whitewater: The Foster Report. IV. Factual Summary. A. Mr. Foster's Background and Activities on July 20, 1993," note 13, above.
32. See note 31, above.
33. See note 15, above.
34. See note 15, above.
35. See note 15, above.
36. See "Vince Foster Biography," note 2, above; see note 15, above.
37. See "Vince Foster Biography," "Whitewater: The Foster Report. I. Introduction," and S. Schmidt, note 2, above.
38. See "Vince Foster Biography," note 2, above.
39. See note 38, above.
40. See note 38, above.
41. See note 38, above.
42. See note 38, above.
43. See note 38, above.
44. See note 38, above.

[45] See "Whitewater: The Foster Report. IV. Factual Summary. A. Mr. Foster's Background and Activities on July 20, 1993," note 31, above; see note 38, above.

[46] See note 38, above.

[47] See note 45, above.

[48] See note 45, above.

[49] See note 45, above.

[50] See note 38, above.

[51] See note 38, above.

[52] See note 38, above.

[53] See note 38, above.

[54] See note 38, above.

[55] See note 38, above.

[56] See note 38, above.

[57] See note 38, above.

[58] See note 38, above.

[59] See note 38, above.

[60] See S. Schmidt, note 2, above; see note 38, above.

[61] See note 38, above.

[62] See note 38, above.

[63] See note 38, above.

[64] See note 38, above.

[65] See note 38, above.

[66] See note 38, above.

[67] See "Whitewater: The Foster Report. I. Introduction," note 2, above.

[68] See note 67, above.

[69] See note 67, above.

[70] See note 67, above.

[71] See note 67, above.

[72] See note 67, above.

[73] See note 67, above.

[74] See S. Schmidt, note 2, above.

[75] See note 74, above.

[76] See note 1, above.

12. John Candy

1. "John Candy Biography," https://findadeath.com/john-candy/; G. Collins, "John Candy, Comedic Film Star, Is Dead of a Heart Attack at 43," the *New York Times*, March 5, 1994, https://www.nytimes.com/1994/03/05/obituaries/john-candy-comedic-film-star-is-dead-of-a-heart-attack-at-43.html; F. Wilkins, "The Tragic Death of John Candy," https://reelreviews.com/shorttakes/candyjohn.htm; "John Candy Obituary," http://www.tributes.com/obituary/read/John-Candy-837304272.

2. R. Parker, "John Candy Remembered: His Children Share New Stories About Their Late Father On the Eve of His Birthday," *Hollywood Reporter*, October 24, 2016, https://www.hollywoodreporter.com/movies/movie-features/john-candy-remembered-his-children-939218/.

3. M. Margaritoff, "Inside The Untimely Demise Of Beloved Comedian John Candy," December 17, 2020, https://allthatsinteresting.com/john-candy-death; see R. Parker, note 2, above.

4. See "John Candy Biography," and F. Wilkins, note 1, above.

5. "John Candy dies," History, A&E Television Networks, original published date November 13, 2009, last updated March 3, 2020, https://www.history.com/this-day-in-history/john-candy-dies; see F. Wilkins, note 1, above.

6. See note 4, above.

7. See "John Candy Biography," note 1, above.

8. See note 4, above.

9. "John Candy Biography," A&E Television Networks, original published date April 2, 2014, last updated May 7, 2021, https://www.biography.com/actor/john-candy; see M. Margaritoff, note 3, above; see note 4, above.

10. See "John Candy Biography," and G. Collins, note 1, above; see M. Margaritoff, note 3, above; see "John Candy Biography," note 9, above.

11. L. Sutton and G. Evans, "The day John Candy, lovable actor and comedian, died at 43 in 1994," *New York Daily News*, March 4, 2016, https://www.nydailynews.com/entertainment/movies/day-john-candy-died-43-1959-article-1.2552914; see note 7, above.

12. See L. Sutton and G. Evans, note 11, above.

13. See note 7, above.

14. P. Reeves, "Actor John Candy dies in Mexico," *Independent*, March 5, 1994, https://www.independent.co.uk/news/world/actor-john-candy-dies-mexico-1427084.html; "Death Certificate—John Candy," http://www.autopsyfiles.org/reports/deathcert/candy,%20 john_dc.pdf; see G. Collins, note 1, above; see M. Margaritoff, note 3, above; see note 11, above.

15. "John Candy Biography," https://www.famouscanadians.org/john-candy/; "John Candy Biography," https://www.imdb.com/name/ nm0001006/bio; "The Tragic Real-Life Story of John Candy," Grunge, https://www.grunge.com/231219/the-tragic-real-life-story-of-john-candy/; see G. Collins, and F. Wilkins, note 1, above; see M. Margaritoff, note 3, above; see "John Candy dies," note 5, above; see "John Candy Biography," note 9, above.

16. See F. Wilkins, note 1, above; see M. Margaritoff, note 3, above; see "John Candy Biography," note 9, above; see "John Candy Biography" and "The Tragic Real-Life Story of John Candy," note 15, above.

17. See G. Collins, note 1, above; see M. Margaritoff, note 3, above; see note 5, above; see "John Candy Biography," note 9, above.

18. See note 12, above; see P. Reeves, note 14, above; see "John Candy Biography," "John Candy Biography," and "The Tragic Real-Life Story of John Candy," note 15, above; see note 17, above.

19. See G. Collins, and F. Wilkins, note 1, above; see M. Margaritoff, note 3, above; see "John Candy Biography," note 9, above; see L. Sutton and G. Evans, note 11, above; see John Candy Biography," and "The Tragic Real-Life Story of John Candy," note 15, above.

20. See G. Collins, and F. Wilkins, note 1, above; see M. Margaritoff, note 3, above; see "John Candy Biography," note 9, above; see "John

Candy dies," "John Candy Biography," and "John Candy Biography," note 15, above.

21. See G. Collins, note 1, above.

22. See "John Candy dies," note 1, above; see "John Candy Biography," and "John Candy Biography," note 15, above; see note 21, above.

23. See note 21, above.

24. See "John Candy Biography," note 9, above; see "The Tragic Real-Life Story of John Candy," note 15, above.

25. See note 2, above.

26. See note 2, above.

27. See F. Wilkins, note 1, above.

28. See note 27, above; see M. Margaritoff, note 3, above; see L. Sutton and G. Evans, note 11, above; see "John Candy Biography," note 15, above.

29. See M. Margaritoff, note 3, above.

30. See note 29, above; see "John Candy Biography," note 15, above.

31. See "The Tragic Real-Life Story of John Candy," note 15, above.

32. "Know Your Risk for Heart Disease," US Centers for Disease Control and Prevention, https://www.cdc.gov/heartdisease/risk_factors.htm; C. Skrzynia, J. S. Berg, et al., "Genetics and Heart Failure: A Concise Guide for the Clinician," *Curr Cardiol Rev* 11(1) (2015): 10–17.

33. See "John Candy Biography," and "The Tragic Real-Life Story of John Candy," note 15, above; see note 29, above.

34. R. Sanchez, "Deadly Addiction: John Candy Smoked 'A Pack A Day' Before Heart Attack Death At 43," February 26, 2019, https://okmagazine.com/news/john-candy-smoked-pack-cigarettes-a-day-heart-attack-death/.

35. See note 5, above; see P. Reeves, note 14, above; see note 23, above; see note 30, above; see note 31, above.

36. T. M. Powell-Wiley, P. Poirier, et al., "Obesity and Cardiovascular Disease: A Scientific Statement From the American Heart Association," *Circulation* 143 (2021): e984–e1010; S. Carbone, J.

M. Canada, et al., "Obesity paradox in cardiovascular disease: where do we stand?" *Vasc Health Risk Manag* 15 (2019): 89–100.

37. H. A. Milman, "Cass Elliot" in *Forensics: The Science Behind the Deaths of Famous People* (Bloomington, Indiana: Xlibris, 2020) 55–60; see "John Candy Biography," note 9, above; see note 29, above; see note 31, above; see note 34, above.

38. See note 34, above.

39. "Smoking and Cardiovascular Disease," https://www.hopkinsmedicine.org/health/conditions-and-diseases/smoking-and-cardiovascular-disease; "Smoking and Your Heart," US National Heart, Lung, and Blood Institute, National Institutes of Health, https://www.nhlbi.nih.gov/health-topics/smoking-and-your-heart.

40. "Smoking and Cardiovascular Disease," US Centers for Disease Control and Prevention, https://www.cdc.gov/tobacco/data_statistics/sgr/50th-anniversary/pdfs/fs_smoking_CVD_508.pdf; see "Smoking and Your Heart," note 39, above.

41. See "Smoking and Cardiovascular Disease," note 39, above.

42. See note 29, above.

43. See note 31, above; see note 34, above.

44. M. Manning, "Cocaine and Heart Attack Risk: Everything You Need to Know," https://www.webmd.com/connect-to-care/addiction-treatment-recovery/cocaine/cocaine-and-heart-attack-risk; B. G. Schwartz, S. Rezkalla, et al., "Cardiovascular Effects of Cocaine," *Circulation* 122 (2010): 2558–69.

45. See note 29, above.

46. See note 31, above; see note 45, above.

47. H. A. Milman, "John Belushi," in *Forensics: The Science Behind the Deaths of Famous People* (Bloomington, Indiana: Xlibris, 2020) 85–92; see note 31, above.

48. See note 39, above.

49. See note 2, above.

50. See note 2, above.

51. See "John Candy Obituary," note 1, above.

52. See note 45, above.

13.   Kurt Cobain

1. O. Waring, "With the Lights Out: When did Kurt Cobain die and what did his suicide note say?" the *Sun*, April 6, 2021, https://www.the-sun.com/entertainment/2645136/kurt-cobain-die-suicide/; "Nirvana's Kurt Cobain was high when he shot himself," *Baltimore Sun*, April 15, 1994, https://www.baltimoresun.com/news/bs-xpm-1994-04-15-1994105028-story.html; "Kurt Cobain Biography," https://www.thefamouspeople.com/profiles/kurt-donald-cobain-2093.php; "Kurt Cobain Biography," https://www.imdb.com/name/nm0001052/bio; "Kurt Cobain Biography," A&E Television Networks, original published date April 2, 2014, last updated February 18, 2020, https://www.biography.com/musician/kurt-cobain; F. Micelotta, "Grunge rock icon Kurt Cobain dies by suicide," A&E Television Networks, original published date November 13, 2009, last updated April 6, 2021, https://www.history.com/this-day-in-history/kurt-cobain-commits-suicide.

2. See O. Waring, "Kurt Cobain Biography," and F. Micelotta, note 1, above.

3. See note 2, above.

4. See note 2, above.

5. See O. Waring, note 1, above.

6. J. Phillips, "Inside Kurt Cobain's autopsy report—lethal heroin overdose and heartbreaking note," *Daily Star*, April 5, 2021, https://www.dailystar.co.uk/showbiz/inside-kurt-cobains-autopsy-report-23844353.

7. B. Witter, "Inside Kurt Cobain's Final Days Before His Suicide," A&E Television Networks, original published date March 27, 2019, last updated June 16, 2020, https://www.biography.com/news/kurt-cobain-final-days-suicide; see note 1, above; see note 6, above.

8. See note 1, above; see B. Witter, note 7, above.

9. See note 6, above; see note 8, above.

10. See B. Witter, note 7, above.

11. See note 10, above.

12. See O. Waring, and F. Micelotta, note 1, above; see note 6, above; see note 11, above.

13. "Kurt Cobain death scene photos," CBS News, May 13, 2021, https://www.cbsnews.com/pictures/new-kurt-cobain-death-scene-photos/; see "Nirvana's Kurt Cobain was high when he shot himself," "Kurt Cobain Biography," and "Kurt Cobain Biography," note 1, above; see note 12, above.

14. C. Heller, "Kurt Cobain File Released by FBI 27 Years After His Death," NBC Chicago, original published date May 8, 2021, last updated May 10, 2021, https://www.nbcchicago.com/entertainment/entertainment-news/kurt-cobain-file-released-by-fbi-27-years-after-his-death/2506248/; M. Cieysinski,"Detective who reviewed Kurt Cobain's death file details evidence, CBS News, April 5, 2019, https://www.cbsnews.com/news/kurt-cobain-death-detective-who-reviewed-kurt-cobains-case-file-details-evidence/; see "Nirvana's Kurt Cobain was high when he shot himself," "Kurt Cobain Biography," "Kurt Cobain Biography," and Micelotta, note 1, above; see B. Witter, note 7, above.

15. See "Kurt Cobain Biography," note 1, above; see C. Heller, note 14, above.

16. See M. Cieysinski, note 14, above.

17. "Kurt Cobain Found Dead After Committing Suicide Three Days Earlier," April 8, 1994, https://worldhistoryproject.org/1994/4/8/kurt-cobain-found-dead-after-committing-suicide-three-days-earlier.

18. See note 17, above.

19. See "Nirvana's Kurt Cobain was high when he shot himself," note 1, above.

20. See note 19, above.

21. See note 19, above.

22. See note 19, above.

23. See note 10, above; see note 19, above.

24. See note 2, above; see note 6, above; see "Kurt Cobain Biography," note 7, above; see C. Heller, note 14, above.

25. See note 19, above.

26. See "Death Certificate—Kurt Cobain," note 1, above.

27. See C. Heller, note 14, above; see note 17, above.

28. See note 27, above.

29. See F. Micelotta, note 1, above; see note 10, above.

30. See M. Cieysinski, note 14, above.

31. See note 30, above.

32. R. C. Baselt, "Heroin," in *Disposition of Toxic Drugs and Chemicals in Man*, 10th ed. (Foster City, California: Biomedical Publications, 2014) 992–96.

33. See note 32, above.

34. See note 19, above.

35. See note 32, above.

36. S. Galea, J. Ahern, et al., "Drugs and firearm deaths in New York City, 1990-1998," *J Urban Health* 79(1) (2002): 70–86.

37. See note 32, above.

38. See "Kurt Cobain Biography," "Kurt Cobain Biography," and "Kurt Cobain Biography," note 1, above.

39. See "Kurt Cobain Biography," note 1, above.

40. See "Kurt Cobain Biography," and "Kurt Cobain Biography," note 1, above.

41. D. Western, "40 Kurt Cobain Quotes About Life, Depression & Love," https://wealthygorilla.com/26-inspirational-kurt-cobain-quotes/.

42. See note 38, above.

43. See note 41, above.

44. See note 40, above.

45. See note 39, above.

46. See note 40, above.

47. See note 39, above.

48. See note 39, above.

49. See note 40, above.

50. See note 38, above.

51. See note 38, above.

52. See note 38, above.

53. See note 38, above.

54. See note 5, above; see note 38, above.

55. See note 54, above.

56. See note 38, above.

57. See "Kurt Cobain Biography," note 1, above.

58. See note 57, above.

59. See "Kurt Cobain Biography" and "Kurt Cobain Biography," note 1, above.

60. See "Kurt Cobain Biography," note 1, above.

61. See note 38, above.

62. See note 40, above.

63. See note 59, above.

64. See note 39, above.

65. See note 2, above.

66. See note 2, above.

67. "Heroin Research Report: What are the long-term effects of heroin use?" US National Institutes of Health, https://www.drugabuse.gov/publications/research-reports/heroin/what-are-long-term-effects-heroin-use.

68. X. Wang, B. Li, et al., "Changes in brain gray matter in abstinent heroin addicts," *Drug Alcohol Depend* 126(3) (2012): 304–8; H. Liu, L. Li, et al., "Disrupted white matter integrity in heroin dependence: a controlled study utilizing diffusion tensor imaging," *Am J Drug Alcohol Abuse* 34(5) (2008): 562–75; see note 67, above.

69. J. A. Tamargo, A. Campa, et al., "Cognitive Impairment among People Who Use Heroin and Fentanyl: Findings from the Miami Adult Studies on HIV (MASH) Cohort," *J Psychoactive Drugs* 53(3) (2021): 215–23; B. Ma, D. Mei, et al., "Cognitive enhancers as a treatment for heroin relapse and addiction," *Pharmacol Res* 141 (2019): 378–83.

70. "91 Quotes By Kurt Cobain That Will Surely Strike The Right Chord," https://quotes.thefamouspeople.com/kurt-cobain-2093.php.

71. D. Western, "40 Kurt Cobain Quotes About Life, Depression & Love," https://wealthygorilla.com/26-inspirational-kurt-cobain-quotes/; see note 70, above.

72. See note 71, above.

73. See "Kurt Cobain Biography," note 1, above; see note 71, above.

74. See note 71, above.

75. See note 71, above.

76. See note 71, above.

77. See note 70, above.

78. See note 70, above.

79. See note 73, above.

80. See note 70, above.

81. See note 70, above.

82. See note 70, above.

83. See note 70, above.

84. See "Kurt Cobain Biography," note 1, above.

85. See note 84, above.

86. See note 84, above.

87. See "Kurt Cobain Biography," and "Kurt Cobain Biography," note 1, above.

14.   Jerry Garcia

1. A. Brown, "Obituary: Jerry Garcia," *Independent*, August 9, 1995, https://www.independent.co.uk/news/people/obituary-jerry-garcia-1595556.html.

2. See note 1, above.

3. See note 1, above.

4. C. Howe, "Exclusive: How Grateful Dead's Jerry Garcia was so stoned on heroin he drooled on his mic, drummer Bill Kreutzmann slept with 13 groupies in one night and the rockers fired 300 shots at Ronald Reagan on the TV screen, reveal new books," Daily Mail, May 1, 20015, https://www.dailymail.co.uk/news/article-3063451/How-Grateful-Dead-s-Jerry-Garcia-stoned-heroin-drooled-mic-

drummer-Bill-Kreutzmann-slept-13-groupies-one-night-rockers-fired-300-shots-Ronald-Reagan-TV-screen-reveals-new-book.html; see note 1, above.

5. D. Browne, "Bruce Hornsby Looks Back on Jerry Garcia's Last Days: 'I Miss Him So Much,'" *Rolling Stone*, August 9, 2020, https://www.rollingstone.com/music/music-features/bruce-hornsby-interview-jerry-garcia-grateful-dead-1038619/.

6. See note 5, above.

7. See note 5, above.

8. See C. Howe, note 4, above.

9. "News Account First," https://www.hoboes.com/pub/Fenario/Jerry/News/.

10. See note 9, above.

11. See note 9, above.

12. See note 9, above.

13. "Garcia died of ailing heart," https://www.upi.com/Archives/1995/08/30/Garcia-died-of-ailing-heart/8952809755200/; T. Mead, "Heroin Use Didn't Kill Jerry Garcia: His Heart just gave out, Marin coroner concludes," August 30, 1995, https://www.sfgate.com/news/article/Heroin-Use-Didn-t-Kill-Jerry-Garcia-His-heart-3025834.php.

14. "Autopsy Report—Jerry Garcia," https://www.celbrityarchive.com/Jerry-Garcia-Autopsy-p/1408.htm.

15. See note 14, above; see note 13, above.

16. See note 14, above.

17. See note 14, above.

18. See note 8, above; see T. Mead, note 13, above.

19. See note 9, above; see note 14, above.

20. "Jerry Garcia Biography," https://www.thefamouspeople.com/profiles/jerome-john-garcia-1811.php; "Jerry Garcia Biography," https://www.imdb.com/name/nm0305263/bio; see note 1, above; see note 9, above; see "Garcia died of ailing heart," note 13, above.

21. See note 1, above; see note 9, above; see "Jerry Garcia Biography," note 20, above.

22. See note 21, above.
23. See Jerry Garcia Biography" and "Jerry Garcia Biography," note 20, above.
24. See note 23, above.
25. See "Jerry Garcia Biography," note 20, above.
26. See "Jerry Garcia Biography," note 20, above.
27. See note 25, above.
28. See note 1, above.
29. See note 23, above.
30. See note 9, above; see note 26, above.
31. See note 1, above.
32. See note 21, above.
33. See note 9, above; see note 25, above.
34. See note 33, above.
35. See note 21, above.
36. See note 23, above.
37. See note 1, above; see note 9, above; see "Garcia died of ailing heart," note 13, above; see note 23, above.
38. See "Jerry Garcia Biography," note 20, above; see note 33, above.
39. See note 23, above.
40. See note 9, above.
41. See note 9, above.
42. See note 38, above.
43. See note 38, above.
44. D. Browne, "'I won't see the end of the year': Backstage at Jerry Garcia and the Grateful Dead's final shows," Salon, July 4, 2015, https://www.salon.com/2015/07/04/i_wont_see_the_end_of_the_year_backstage_at_jerry_garcia_and_the_grateful_deads_final_shows/; see note 24, above.
45. See note 8, above.
46. See note 1, above; see note 43, above.
47. See note 46, above.
48. See note 29, above.
49. See D. Browne, note 44, above.

50. See note 49, above.

51. See note 8, above.

52. See note 9, above; see note 44, above.

53. See note 49, above.

54. See "Garcia died of ailing heart," note 13, above; see "Jerry Garcia Biography," note 20, above.

55. "Smoking and Your Heart," US National Heart, Lung and Blood Institute, National Institutes of Health, https://www.nhlbi.nih.gov/health-topics/smoking-and-your-heart.

56. See note 14, above.

57. "Diabetes," Mayo Clinic, https://www.mayoclinic.org/diseases-conditions/diabetes/symptoms-causes/syc-20371444; "What is Diabetes?" US National Institute of Diabetes and Digestive and Kidney Diseases, National Institutes of Health, https://www.niddk.nih.gov/health-information/diabetes/overview/what-is-diabetes.

58. See note 57, above.

59. "What is Diabetes?" US Centers for Disease Control and Prevention, https://www.cdc.gov/diabetes/basics/diabetes.html; see note 57, above.

60. See note 59, above.

61. See note 57, above.

62. See "What is Diabetes?" note 57, above; see "What is Diabetes?" note 59, above.

63. See "Diabetes," note 57, above.

64. See note 14, above; see note 62, above; see note 63, above.

65. "Obesity and Heart Disease," Cleveland Clinic, https://my.clevelandclinic.org/health/articles/17308-obesity--heart-disease; "Three Ways Obesity Contributes to Heart Disease," Penn Medicine, March 25, 2019, https://www.pennmedicine.org/updates/blogs/metabolic-and-bariatric-surgery-blog/2019/march/obesity-and-heart-disease; "Weight: A Silent Heart Risk," Johns Hopkins Medicine, https://www.hopkinsmedicine.org/health/wellness-and-prevention/weight-a-silent-heart-risk; see note 14, above; see note 26, above.

66. "Severe Obesity Revealed as a Stand-Alone High-Risk Factor for Heart Failure," Johns Hopkins Medicine, August 22, 2016, https://www.hopkinsmedicine.org/news/media/releases/severe_obesity_revealed_as_a_stand_alone_high_risk_factor_for_heart_failure; B. Hendrick, "Obesity Increases Risk of Deadly Heart Attacks," Febraury 14, 2011, https://www.webmd.com/heart-disease/news/20110214/obesity-increases-risk-of-deadly-heart-attacks; C. Cercato and F. A. Fonseca, "Cardiovascular risk and obesity," Diabetology & Metabolic Syndrome, August 28, 2019, https://dmsjournal.biomedcentral.com/articles/10.1186/s13098-019-0468-0; see "Weight: A Silent Heart Risk," note 65, above.

67. See "Weight: A Silent Heart Risk," note 65, above; see "Severe Obesity Revealed as a Stand-Alone High-Risk Factor for Heart Failure," note 66, above.

68. See note 67, above.

69. See B. Hendrick, note 66, above.

70. M. Manning, "Cocaine and Heart Attack Risk: Everything You Need to Know," https://www.webmd.com/connect-to-care/addiction-treatment-recovery/cocaine/cocaine-and-heart-attack-risk; K. A. S. Barnes, E. O. Fasanmi, et al., "Cocaine-Induced Cardiomyopathy," *US Pharm*, 40(2) (2015): HS11–HS15; L. R. Goldfrank and R. S. Hoffman, "The cardiovascular effects of cocaine," *Ann Emerg Med* 20 (1991): 165–75; see note 1, above; see note 14, above.

71. See M. Manning, note 70, above.

72. B. G. Schwartz, S. Rezkalla, et al., "Cardiovascular Effects of Cocaine," *Circulation*, 122 (2010): 2558–69; U. Wilvert-Lampen, S. C. Zilker, et al., "Cocaine increases the endothelial release of immunoreactive endothelin and its concentrations in human plasma and urine: reversal by coincubation with sigma-receptor antagonists," *Circulation* 98 (1998): 335–90; see K. A. S. Barnes, E. O. Fasanmi, et al., note 70, above.

73. See K. A. S. Barnes, E. O. Fasanmi, et al., note 70, above; see note 71, above; see B. G. Schwartz, S. Rezkalla, et al., note 72, above.

74. "Smoking and Cardiovascular Disease," Johns Hopkins Medicine, https://www.hopkinsmedicine.org/health/conditions-and-diseases/ smoking-and-cardiovascular-disease; "Smoking and Cardiovascular Disease," US Centers for Disease Control and Prevention, https:// www.cdc.gov/tobacco/data_statistics/sgr/50th-anniversary/pdfs/fs_ smoking_CVD_508.pdf; "How Smoking Affects Heart Health," US Food and Drug Administration, https://www.fda.gov/tobacco-products/health-effects-tobacco-use/how-smoking-affects-heart-health; see "Smoking and Your Heart," note 55, above.

75. See "Smoking and Your Heart," note 55, above; see "Smoking and Cardiovascular Disease" and "How Smoking Affects Heart Health," note 74, above.

76. See "Smoking and Your Heart," note 55, above; see "Smoking and Cardiovascular Disease" and "How Smoking Affects Heart Health," note 74, above.

77. See note 26, above.

78. See note 49, above.

79. See note 49, above.

80. See note 49, above.

81. See note 49, above.

82. See note 8, above.

83. See note 8, above.

84. See note 8, above; see note 26, above.

15. Mickey Mantle

1. B. Barnes, "Mickey Mantle, Legend of Baseball, Dies at 63," *Washington Post*, August 14, 1995, https://www.washingtonpost.com/wp-serv/sports/longterm/memories/1995/95pass6.htm.

2. See note 1, above.

3. See note 1, above.

4. See note 1, above.

5. See note 1, above.

6. J. Durso, "Mickey Mantle, Great Yankee Slugger, Dies at 63," the *New York Times*, August 14, 1995, https://www.nytimes.com/1995/08/14/obituaries/mickey-mantle-great-yankee-slugger-dies-at-63.html.

7. See note 6, above.

8. "Mickey Mantle and Liver Cancer," February 11, 2018, https://www.drmirkin.com/histories-and-mysteries/mickey-mantle-tough-childhood-can-cause-disease.html; "Mickey Mantle Biography," A&E Television Networks, original published date April 2, 2014, last updated May 6, 2021, https://www.biography.com/athlete/mickey-mantle; R. Hoffer, "The Legacy of Mickey Mantle, last great player on the last great team," August 13, 2015, https://vault.si.com/vault/1995/08/21/mickey-mantle-the-legacy-of-the-last-great-player-on-the-last-great-team; see note 1, above; see note 2, above.

9. M. Mantle, "Time in a Bottle," April 18, 1994, https://vault.si.com/vault/1994/04/18/time-in-a-bottle-after-42-years-of-alcohol-abuse-a-legendary-ballplayer-describes-his-life-of-self-destructive-behavior-and-hopes-his-recovery-will-finally-make-him-a-true-role-model; see note 1, above; see note 6, above.

10. "Mickey Mantle," https://www.cs.mcgill.ca/~rwest/wikispeedia/wpcd/wp/m/Mickey_Mantle.htm; see M. Mantle, note 9, above.

11. See M. Mantle, note 9, above.

12. See note 11, above.

13. M. F. Picco and S. A. Rizza, "Hepatitis C: How common is sexual transmission?" Mayo Clinic, https://www.mayoclinic.org/diseases-conditions/hepatitis-c/expert-answers/hepatitis-c/faq-20058441; L. Jesuino de Oliveria Andrade, A. D'Oliveira Jr., et al., "Association Between Hepatitis C and Hepatocellular Carcinoma," *J Glob Infect Dis* 1(1) (2009): 33–37; see note 6, above.

14. D. Underferth, "Hepatitis C and liver cancer: What to know," https://www.mdanderson.org/publications/focused-on-health/HepatitisC-liver-cancer-What-you-need-to-know.h16Z1591413.html.

15. See note 14, above.

16. See note 13, above; see note 14, above.

17. See note 6, above.
18. See note 1, above; see note 6, above; see "Mickey Mantle Biography," note 8, above; see M. Mantle, note 9, above.
19. See note 1, above; see note 6, above.
20. "New York Yankees star Mickey Mantle dies," A&E Television Networks, original published date November 16, 2009, last updated August 13, 2019, https://www.history.com/this-day-in-history/yankee-legend-dies; see Mickey Mantle Biography," note 8, above; see "Mickey Mantle," note 10, above.
21. See Mickey Mantle Biography," note 8, above.
22. "Mickey Mantle Biography," https://www.thefamouspeople.com/profiles/mickey-mantle-8588.php; J. L. Ray, "Mickey Mantle," Society for American Baseball Research, https://sabr.org/bioproj/person/mickey-mantle/; "Mickey Mantle Biography," https://www.notablebiographies.com/Lo-Ma/Mantle-Mickey.html; see note 1, above; see note 6, above; see note 20, above.
23. See note 6, above; see "New York Yankees star Mickey Mantle dies," note 20, above; see "Mickey Mantle Biography," J. L. Ray, and "Mickey Mantle Biography," note 22, above.
24. See note 6, above; see "Mickey Mantle," note 10, above; see "New York Yankees star Mickey Mantle dies," note 20, above; see J. L. Ray, note 22, above.
25. See note 24, above.
26. See "Mickey Mantle," note 10, above; see "New York Yankees star Mickey Mantle dies," note 20, above.
27. See note 1, above; see "Mickey Mantle," note 10, above; see "Mickey Mantle Biography," and "Mickey Mantle Biography," note 22, above.
28. See note 6, above.
29. See note 1, above; see "Mickey Mantle Biography," and "Mickey Mantle Biography," note 22, above.
30. See "Mickey Mantle," note 10, above; see note 29, above.
31. See "Mickey Mantle Biography," and "Mickey Mantle Biography," note 22, above.

32. R. Hoffer, "The Legacy of Mickey Mantle, last great player on the last great team," August 13, 2015, https://vault.si.com/vault/1995/08/21/mickey-mantle-the-legacy-of-the-last-great-player-on-the-last-great-team; see note 6, above; see "Mickey Mantle Biography," note 8, above; see note 30, above.

33. See note 6, above; see "Mickey Mantle Biography," note 8, above; see "Mickey Mantle Biography," note 17, above; see "New York Yankees star Mickey Mantle dies," note 20, above; see J. L. Ray, note 22, above; see note 30, above.

34. See note 6, above; see note 29, above.

35. See J. L. Ray, note 22, above.

36. See note 35, above.

37. See "Mickey Mantle," note 10, above; see note 34, above.

38. See note 37, above.

39. See "Mickey Mantle Biography," note 22, above.

40. See "New York Yankees star Mickey Mantle dies," and "Mickey Mantle Biography," note 20, above; see note 27, above.

41. See note 18, above; see "New York Yankees star Mickey Mantle dies," note 20, above; see Mickey Mantle Biography," note 22, above.

42. See "Mickey Mantle," note 10, above.

43. See note 42, above.

44. See note 31, above.

45. See note 19, above; see note 21, above; see note 39, above.

46. See note 19, above; see note 39, above; see note 42, above.

47. See note 18, above; see "New York Yankees star Mickey Mantle dies," note 20, above; see note 39, above.

48. See note 6, above.

49. D. Falkner, "The Last Days of Mickey Mantle," *Dallas Observer*, December 14, 1995, https://www.dallasobserver.com/news/the-last-days-of-mickey-mantle-6398127; see "Mickey Mantle," note 10, above; see "Mickey Mantle Biography," note 18, above; see note 27, above.

50. See note 35, above.

51. See note 35, above.

52. See "Mickey Mantle Biography," note 22, above; see note 29, above.

53. See note 42, above.

54. See note 42, above.

55. See note 1, above; see note 35, above.

56. S. Jacobson, "Death Hits Painfully Close to Home Again for Mickey Mantle," *Los Angeles Times*, March 20, 1994, https://www.latimes. com/archives/la-xpm-1994-03-20-sp-36363-story.html; see R. Hoffer, note 8, above; see note 21, above; see note 24, above.

57. See note 6, above.

58. See note 42, above; see S. Jacobson, note 56, above.

59. See S. Jacobson, note 56, above.

60. "Hodgkin's lymphoma (Hodgkin's disease)," Mayo Clinic, https://www.mayoclinic.org/diseases-conditions/hodgkins-lymphoma/symptoms-causes/syc-20352646; "Causes Hodgkin's lymphoma," https://www.nhs.uk/conditions/hodgkin-lymphoma/causes/.

61. See note 59, above.

62. See note 59, above.

63. "Liver cancer," Mayo Clinic, https://www.mayoclinic.org/diseases-conditions/hepatocellular-carcinoma/cdc-20354552.

64. See M. F. Picco and S. A. Rizza, note 13, above.

65. See note 11, above.

66. H. J. Edenberg and T. Foroud, "Genetics and alcoholism," *Nat Rev Gastroenterol Hepatol* 10(8) (2013): 487–94.

67. See "Mickey Mantle and Liver Cancer," note 8, above; see note 21, above; see "Mickey Mantle Biography," note 22, above; see note 59, above.

68. See note 21, above.

69. See note 1, above; see note 21, above.

16. Marshall Applewhite

1. J. Sturken and J. Angier, "Heaven's Gate Investigator Saw Dozens Dead With Their Shoes On," ABC News, March 25, 2007, https://

abcnews.go.com/US/story?id=2977618&page=1; "Heaven's Gate cult members found dead," A&E Television Networks, original published date February 9, 2010, last updated March 24, 2021, https://www.history.com/this-day-in-history/heavens-gate-cult-members-found-dead; B. Drummond Ayres, Jr., "Families Learning of 39 Cultists Who Died Willingly," the *New York Times*, March 29, 1997, https://www.nytimes.com/1997/03/29/us/families-learning-of-39-cultists-who-died-willingly.html; "CNN: Heaven's Gate suicides remembered," March 25, 2011, https://www.youtube.com/watch?v=IzWpfql03q4.

2. See "CNN: Heaven's Gate suicides remembered," note 1, above.

3. M. Reimann, "Suicide, Nikes, and comet space ships: the story of the Heaven's Gate cult," October 14, 2016, https://timeline.com/the-heavens-gate-mass-suicide-7f440ab4b333; "Mass suicide involved sedatives, vodka and careful planning," CNN, March 27, 1997, http://edition.cnn.com/US/9703/27/suicide/index.html; see "CNN: Heaven's Gate suicides remembered," note 1, above.

4. C. Morello, "Castrated Men Among Cult Victims Voices Of The Dead Flood Airwaves As Families Are Notified Across U.S.," the *Spokesman-Review*, March 29, 1997, https://www.spokesman.com/stories/1997/mar/29/castrated-men-among-cult-victims-voices-of-the/; J. Wilkens, "Focus: 20 years later, Heaven's Gate lives on—via internet, scholarly debates," the *San Diego Union-Tribune*, March 18, 2017, https://www.sandiegouniontribune.com/news/local-history/sd-me-heavens-gate-20170316-story.html; J. Rivera, "In farewell video, UFO cult members welcomed death," *Baltimore Sun*, March 29, 1997, https://www.baltimoresun.com/bal-cult5-story.html; "Post mortems on all 39 of San Diego suicide group completed," *Irish Times*, May 31, 1997, https://www.irishtimes.com/news/post-mortems-on-all-39-of-san-diego-suicide-group-completed-1.57402; J. Rivera, "Death in three shifts," *Baltimore Sun*, March 28, 1997, https://www.baltimoresun.com/bal-cult3-story.html; see J. Sturken and J. Angier, and "Heaven's Gate cult members found dead," note 1, above.

5. E. Hawkins, "'It's The Cult of Cults!': Parents Lose Their Daughter To Infamous Heaven's Gate Mass Suicide," Oxygen, May 17, 2020, https://www.oxygen.com/deadly-cults/crime-news/heavens-gate-cult-gail-maeder-victim-in-mass-suicide; see J. Sturken and J. Angier, "Heaven's Gate cult members found dead," and B. Drummond Ayres Jr., note 1, above; see J. Wilkens and "Mass suicide involved sedatives, vodka and careful planning," note 3, above; see C. Morello and J. Rivera, note 4, above.

6. M. Hafford, "Heaven's Gate 20 Years Later: 10 Things You Didn't Know," Rolling Stone, March 24, 2017, https://www.rollingstone.com/feature/heavens-gate-20-years-later-10-things-you-didnt-know-114563/; see J. Sturken and J. Angier, note 1, above; see E. Hawkins, note 5, above.

7. See M. Hafford, note 6, above.

8. See note 6, above.

9. "Tests show wide range of drugs in cultists' bodies," *Deseret News*, April 5, 1997, https://www.deseret.com/1997/4/5/19304825/tests-show-wide-range-of-drugs-in-cultists-bodies; see J. Wilkens, note 3, above; see E. Hawkins and M. Hafford, note 6, above.

10. "Autopsy results of Heaven's Gate cultists released," *Chicago Tribune*, April 13, 1997, https://www.chicagotribune.com/news/ct-xpm-1997-04-13-9704130188-story.html; see B. Drummond Ayres Jr., note 1, above; see M. Reimann, note 3, above; see J. Rivera, note 4, above; see J. Rivera, note 5, above; see E. Hawkins and M. Hafford, note 6, above; see "Tests show wide range of drugs in cultists' bodies," note 9, above.

11. See B. Drummond Ayres Jr., note 1, above; see note 3, above; see C. Morello, note 4, above; see E. Hawkins and M. Hafford, note 6, above.

12. See J. Wilkens and M. Reimann, note 3, above; see E. Hawkins, note 6, above.

13. See E. Hawkins, note 2, above.

14. See note 13, above.

15. See J. Sturken and J. Angier, note 1, above.

16. See note 15, above.

17. See note 13, above.

18. "First autopsies completed in cult suicide," CNN, http://www.cnn.com/US/9703/28/mass.suicide/index.html; see "Heaven's Gate cult members found dead," note 1, above; see note 3, above; see C. Morello, J. Rivera, and J. Rivera, note 4, above.

19. See "Heaven's Gate cult members found dead," and B. Drummond Ayres Jr., note 1, above; see note 3, above; see C. Morello and J. Rivera, note 4, above.

20. See J. Rivera, note 4, above; see note 13, above.

21. See note 7, above.

22. See note 7, above.

23. See note 7, above.

24. See "Mass suicide involved sedatives, vodka and careful planning," note 3, above; see J. Rivera, note 4, above; see note 15, above.

25. See "Mass suicide involved sedatives, vodka and careful planning," note 3, above.

26. See J. Rivera and B. Drummond Ayres Jr., note 4, above; see note 15, above.

27. See J. Rivera, note 4, above; see note 15, above.

28. See note 13, above.

29. See "Autopsy results of Heaven's Gate cultists released," note 10, above.

30. "Coroner says cult leader did not have cancer," *South Coast Today*, original published date March 31, 1997, last updated January 10, 2011, https://www.southcoasttoday.com/article/19970331/news/303319975; "Autopsies completed in suicide cult as probe winds down," CNN, March 31, 1997, http://www.cnn.com/US/9703/31/suicide/index.html; see note 29, above.

31. See "Heaven's Gate cult members found dead," note 1, above; see "Mass suicide involved sedatives, vodka and careful planning," note 3, above.

32. Among Cult, Lethal Drugs and Alcohol," the *New York Times*, April 4, 1997, https://www.nytimes.com/1997/04/05/us/

among-cult-lethal-drugs-and-alcohol.html; see "Tests show wide range of drugs in cultists' bodies," note 9, above.

33. See note 32, above.

34. See "Tests show wide range of drugs in cultists' bodies," note 9, above.

35. See note 32, above.

36. See "Among Cult, Lethal Drugs and Alcohol," note 32, above; see Autopsies completed in suicide cult as probe winds down," note 30, above.

37. See note 36, above.

38. See "Mass suicide involved sedatives, vodka and careful planning," note 3, above.

39. See "Autopsies completed in suicide cult as probe winds down," note 30, above; see note 38, above.

40. See C. Morello, and J. Rivera, note 4, above.

41. See "Post mortems on all 39 of San Diego suicide group completed," note 4, above; see "Autopsy results of Heaven's Gate cultists released," note 10, above.

42. See note 41, above.

43. "Marshall Applewhite Biography," https://ww.imdb.com/name/nm0032457/bio; M. Fisher and S. A. Pressley, "Crisis of Sexuality Launched Strange Journey," the *Washington Post*, March 29, 1997, https://www.washingtonpost.com/archive/politics/1997/03/29/crisis-of-sexuality-launched-strange-journey/3709d9ff-51ee-4f50-a9cd-a45525d7ad8f/; J. Steinberg, "From Religious Childhood To Reins of a U.F.O. Cult," the *New York Times*, March 29, 1997, https://www.nytimes.com/1997/03/29/us/from-religious-childhood-to-reins-of-a-ufo-cult.html; "Marshall Applewhite," https://criminalminds.fandom.com/wiki/Marshall¬¬_Applewhite.

44. J. Holliman, "Applewhite: From young overachiever to cult leader," CNN, http://www.cnn.com/SPECIALS/1998/hgate.review/applewhite/.

45. See note 44, above.

46. See "Marshall Applewhite Biography," M. Fisher and S. A. Pressley, and J. Steinberg, note 43, above; see note 44, above.

47. See note 46, above.

48. See J. Steinberg, note 43, above.

49. See note 48, above.

50. "Marshall Applewhite Biography," A&E Television Networks, original published date April 2, 2014, last updated July 17, 2020, https://www.biography.com/crime-figure/marshall-herff-applewhite; see "Marshall Applewhite Biography," note 43, above.

51. See "Marshall Applewhite Biography," and M. Fisher and S. A. Pressley, note 43, above.

52. See M. Fisher and S. A. Pressley, and J. Steinberg, note 43, above.

53. See M. Fisher and S. A. Pressley, note 43, above; see note 50, above.

54. See "Marshall Applewhite Biography," note 43, above.

55. See M. Fisher and S. A. Pressley, note 43, above; see note 53, above.

56. "Marshall Applewhite," https://criminalminds.fandom.com/wiki/Marshall¬¬_Applewhite; see M. Fisher and S. A. Pressley, note 43, above; see note 50, above.

57. See J. Rivera, note 4, above; see note 52, above.

58. See note 52, above.

59. See note 52, above.

60. See note 45, above; see note 52, above.

61. See note 52, above; see note 53, above.

62. See J. Wilkens, note 5, above; see note 55, above.

63. See M. Fisher and S. A. Pressley, note 43, above.

64. See note 15, above; see "Marshall Applewhite Biography," note 50, above.

65. See "Heaven's Gate cult members found dead," note 1, above; see note 15, above; see note 50, above; see note 63, above.

66. See "Heaven's Gate cult members found dead," note 1, above; see J. Wilkens, and M. Reimann, note 3, above; see "J. Rivera," note 4, above; see note 15, above; see "Autopsies completed in suicide cult as probe winds down," note 36, above; see M. Fisher and S. A. Pressley, note 43, above.

67. "Marshall Applewhite," https://criminalminds.fandom.com/wiki/ Marshall¬¬_Applewhite; see "Heaven's Gate cult members found dead" and B. Drummond Ayres Jr., note 1, above; see J. Wilkens, note 3, above; see J. Rivera, note 4, above; see M. Reimann, note 10, above; see note 15, above; see "Autopsies completed in suicide cult as probe winds down," note 36, above; see M. Fisher and S. A. Pressley, note 43, above.

68. See note 63, above.

69. See note 44, above; see "Marshall Appelwhite Biography," note 50, above.

70. See J. Wilkens, note 3, above.

71. See M. Reimann, note 3, above.

72. See J. Rivera, note 4, above.

73. See note 72, above.

74. See note 34, above.

75. See note 13, above.

76. See note 13, above; see "First autopsies completed in cult suicide," note 18, above.

77. See note 13, above.

78. See note 13, above.

79. See B. Drummond Ayres Jr., note 1, above; see C. Morello, note 4, above; see note 13, above.

80. See B. Drummond Ayres Jr., note 1, above; see C. Morello and J. Rivera, note 4, above.

81. See note 80, above.

82. See J. Wilkens, note 3, above.

83. H. K. Lee, "Ex-Member Wishes He'd Taken Dose, Too / His wife stayed with cult and died," March 31, 1997, https://www.sfgate. com/news/article/Ex-Member-Wishes-He-d-Taken-Dose-Too-His-wife-2847779.php; see "Coroner says cult leader did not have cancer," note 30, above.

84. See "Coroner says cult leader did not have cancer," note 30, above.

85. See note 83, above.

86. See note 63, above.

87. See B. Drummond Ayres Jr., note 1, above; see C. Morello, note 4, above.

88. See B. Drummond Ayres Jr., note 1, above.

89. See "Coroner says cult leader did not have cancer," note 30, above.

90. See note 63, above.

91. See C. Morello, note 4, above.

92. L. Saad, "Do Americans Believe in UFOs?" Gallup, May 20, 2021, https://news.gallup.com/poll/350096/americans-believe-ufos.aspx.

93. C. Kennedy and A. Lau, "Most Americans believe in intelligent life beyond Earth; few see UFOs as a major national security threat," Pew Research Center, June 30, 2021, https://www.pewresearch.org/fact-tank/2021/06/30/most-americans-believe-in-intelligent-life-beyond-earth-few-see-ufos-as-a-major-national-security-threat/.

94. See "Post mortems on all 39 of San Diego suicide group completed," note 4, above.

95. See note 13, above.

96. See note 13, above.

97. M. Taylor, "Another Heaven's Gate Suicide / Cultist found dead in Encinitas hotel," May 7, 1997, https://www.sfgate.com/news/article/Another-Heaven-s-Gate-Suicide-Cultist-found-2841156.php.

98. See note 97, above.

99. See note 97, above.

100. See note 97, above.

101. See note 97, above.

102. See note 97, above.

103. See note 97, above.

104. See note 97, above.

105. See note 97, above.

106. "Do Not Revive," CBS News, February 20, 1998, https://www.cbsnews.com/news/do-not-revive/.

107. See note 71, above; see note 106, above.

108. See note 97, above.

109. See note 97, above.

110. See note 97, above.

17. Chris Farley

1. C. Nashawaty, "Chris Farley's sad, drug-fueled final days," Entertainment Weekly, January 8, 1998, dayshttps://ew.com/article/1998/01/09/chris-farleys-sad-drug-fueled-final-days/; C. Bertram, "Chris Farley: The Rise and Fall of a Comedy Icon," A&E Networks, original published date May 14, 2019, last updated May 14, 2020, https://www.biography.com/news/chris-farley-rise-fall-death; "The Tragic Real-Life Story of Chris Farley," Grunge, https://www.grunge.com/195294/the-tragic-real-life-story-of-chris-farley/.

2. See C. Nashawaty, and "The Tragic Real-Life Story of Chris Farley," note 1, above.

3. J. Anglis, "How Did Chris Farley Die? The Inside Story Of The Doomed Comedian's Final Days," original published date January 13, 2020, last updated March 3, 2021, https://allthatsinteresting.com/chris-farley-death; see note 1, above.

4. See C. Nashawaty, note 1, above; see J. Anglis, note 3, above.

5. See note 4, above.

6. See note 4, above.

7. See C. Bertram, note 1, above; see note 4, above.

8. See C. Bertram, note 1, above; see J. Anglis, note 3, above.

9. See note 7, above.

10. F. Wilkins, "The Death of Chris Farley," Grunge, https://reelreviews.com/shorttakes/farley.htm; see "The Tragic Real-Life Story of Chris Farley," note 1, above.

11. "Chart Review: Christopher Crosby 'Chris' Farley," http://neurosciencecme.com/chairsummit/PDF/CH007-day3-1030-gold-ob.pdf; see note 10, above.

12. See note 11, above.

13. M. Fox, "Comedian and Actor Chris Farley Found Dead in His Chicago Apartment of Unknown Causes," December 19, 1997, https://apnews.com/article/ecd894320d54f60f89b0cd371efe4a33; "Farley died from overdose of cocaine, morphine," CNN, January 2, 1998, http://edition.cnn.com/SHOWBIZ/9801/02/farley.autopsy/; S.

Mills, "Drug Overdose Killed Comedian Farley," *Chicago Tribune*, January 3, 1998, https://www.chicagotribune.com/news/ct-xpm-1998-01-03-9801030066-story.html; see C. Bertram, note 1, above; see F. Wilkins, note 10, above; see "Chart Review: Christopher Crosby 'Chris' Farley," note 11, above.

14. "Farley autopsy completed," United Press International, December 19, 1997, https://www.upi.com/Archives/1997/12/19/Farley-autopsy-completed/3613882507600/; S. Mills, "Drug Overdose Killed Comedian Farley," *Chicago Tribune*, January 3, 1998, https://www.chicagotribune.com/news/ct-xpm-1998-01-03-9801030066-story.html; see F. Wilkins, note 10, above; see "Chart Review: Christopher Crosby 'Chris' Farley," note 11, above; see M. Fox, note 13, above.

15. See F. Wilkins, note 10, above; see "Chart Review: Christopher Crosby 'Chris' Farley," note 11, above.

16. See note 15, above.

17. See note 15, above.

18. See "Farley died from overdose of cocaine, morphine," and S. Mills, note 13, above.

19. See note 18, above.

20. "Sudden Cardiac Death (Sudden Cardiac Arrest)," Cleveland Clinic, https://my.clevelandclinic.org/health/diseases/17522-sudden-cardiac-death-sudden-cardiac-arrest; "Sudden Cardiac Death (Sudden Cardiac Arrest)," Cleveland Clinic, https://my.clevelandclinic.org/health/diseases/17522-sudden-cardiac-death-sudden-cardiac-arrest.

21. "Fatty Liver Disease," https://medlineplus.gov/fattyliverdisease.html.

22. See note 21, above.

23. J. Jeter, "Chris Farley Died of Drug Overdose," *The Washington Post*, January 3, 1998, https://www.washingtonpost.com/archive/politics/1998/01/03/chris-farley-died-of-drug-overdose/3706d464-bd7b-4d2e-a889-8be618e18293/; H. A. Milman, "Errol Flynn," in *Forensics: The Science Behind the Deaths of Famous People* (Bloomington, Indiana: Xlibris, 2020), 1–14; see note 18, above.

24. R. C. Baselt, "Heroin," in *Disposition of Toxic Drugs and Chemicals in Man*, 10th ed., (Seal Beach, California: Biomedical Publications, 2014) 992–96; see "Farley died from overdose of cocaine, morphine," note 13, above.

25. See J. Anglis, note 6, above; see S. Mills, note 13, above; see note 24, above.

26. See J. Anglis, note 6, above; see S. Mills, note 13, above.

27. See note 26, above.

28. H. A. Milman, "John Belushi," in *Forensics: The Science Behind the Deaths of Famous People* (Bloomington, Indiana: Xlibris, 2020), 85–92; see J. Anglis, note 6, above; see S. Mills, note 13, above; see J. Jeter, note 23, above.

29. See J. Jeter, note 23, above.

30. See note 29, above.

31. H. A. Milman, "River Phoenix," in *Forensics: The Science Behind the Deaths of Famous People* (Bloomington, Indiana: Xlibris, 2020), 113–20; see note 29, above.

32. H. A. Milman, "Philip Seymour Hoffman," in *Forensics: The Science Behind the Deaths of Famous People* (Bloomington, Indiana: Xlibris, 2020), 203–210.

33. H. A. Milman, "Carrie Fisher," in *Forensics: The Science Behind the Deaths of Famous People* (Bloomington, Indiana: Xlibris, 2020), 247–58.

34. "Death Certificate—Chris Farley," http://www.autopsyfiles.org/reports/deathcert/farley,%20chris_dc.pdf; see F. Wilkins, note 10, above; see note 18, above; see note 29, above.

35. See F. Wilkins, note 10, above; see note 18, above; see "Death Certificate—Chris Farley," note 34, above.

36. "Chris Farley Biography," https://www.imdb.com/name/nm0000394/bio; "Chris Farley Biography," A&E Networks, original published date May 20, 2019, last updated June 22, 2020, https://www.biography.com/actor/chris-farley.

37. "Chris Farley," https://www.thefamouspeople.com/profiles/christopher-crosby-farley-1047.php; see "Chris Farley Biography," note 36, above.

38. See "Chris Farley," note 37, above.

39. See note 36, above; see note 38, above.

40. See note 39, above.

41. See "Chris Farley Biography," note 36, above.

42. See note 39, above.

43. See note 36, above.

44. I. Crouch, "The Big, Funny, Tragic Life of Chris Farley," *New Yorker*, August 10, 2015, https://www.newyorker.com/culture/cultural-comment/the-big-funny-tragic-life-of-chris-farley.

45. See note 44, above.

46. R. Tucker, "That Was Awesome!" *New York Post*, December 16, 2007, https://nypost.com/2007/12/16/that-was-awesome/.

47. See "Farley died from overdose of cocaine, morphine," note 13, above; see note 41, above.

48. See "Farley died from overdose of cocaine, morphine," note 13, above.

49. See note 29, above.

50. See note 46, above.

51. See note 46, above.

52. See note 46, above.

53. See note 46, above.

54. See note 46, above.

55. See note 46, above.

56. See note 46, above.

57. See "Chris Farley Biography," note 36, above.

58. See note 57, above.

59. See "Farley died from overdose of cocaine, morphine," note 13, above; see "Chris Farley," note 37, above.

60. See M. Fox, note 13, above.

61. See note 60, above.

62. See note 48, above.

63. See J. Anglis, note 6, above.

64. See note 57, above.

65. See note 57, above.

66. See "The Tragic Real-Life Story of Chris Farley," note 1, above.

67. See note 46, above.

68. See C. Nashawaty, note 1, above.

69. See note 68, above.

18.   *Eric Harris and Dylan Klebold*

1. "Columbine,"   https://www.niche.com/places-to-live/columbine-jefferson-co/.

2. "Columbine High School," *US News & World Report*, https://www.usnews.com/education/best-high-schools/colorado/districts/jefferson-county-school-district-no-r-1/columbine-high-school-4206.

3. "Columbine High School Shooting Details," http://www.acolumbinesite.com/event/event2.php.

4. D. Cullen, "The reluctant killer," the *Guardian*, April 24, 2009, https://www.theguardian.com/world/2009/apr/25/dave-cullen-clumbine; see note 3, above.

5. See note 3, above.

6. "The Columbine High School massacre," https://murderpedia.org/male.H/h/harris-eric.htm; "Eric Harris and Dylan Klebold," Criminal Minds, https://criminalminds.fandom.com/wiki/Eric_Harris_and_Dylan_Klebold; see note 4, above.

7. "Columbine Shooting," History, A&E Television Networks, original published date November 9, 2009, last updated March 4, 2021, https://www.history.com/topics/1990s/columbine-high-school-shootings; see note 3, above; see "The Columbine High School massacre," note 6, above.

8. See D. Cullen, note 4, above; see note 7, above.

9. See note 8, above.

10. See note 6, above.

11. See note 3, above.

12. See note 3, above.

13. "Eric Harris Biography," A&E Television Networks, original published date April 2, 2014, last updated June 18, 2020, https://www.biography.com/crime-figure/eric-harris.

14. See note 3, above; see D. Cullen, note 4, above; see "Columbine Shooting," note 7, above; see "Eric Harris and Dylan Klebold," note 10, above; see note 13, above.

15. See note 6, above.

16. See note 6, above.

17. T. Kenworthy and J. Achenbach, "Terror and Tears: Inside Columbine High," the *Washington Post*, April 21, 1999, https://www.washingtonpost.com/wp-srv/national/daily/april99/scene21.htm.

18. See note 17, above.

19. See note 4, above; see "The Columbine High School massacre," note 6, above.

20. See note 3, above.

21. "Columbine High School Shootings Fast Facts," ABC 17 News, https://abc17news.com/news/national-world/2021/05/03/columbine-high-school-shootings-fast-facts/; see "The Columbine High School massacre," and "Eric Harris and Dylan Klebold," note 6, above; see note 13, above.

22. See note 3, above; see "The Columbine High School massacre," note 6, above.

23. See "The Columbine High School massacre," note 6, above.

24. See note 22, above.

25. See note 17, above.

26. See note 17, above.

27. See note 3, above.

28. See note 3, above.

29. "Eric David Harris," http://www.acolumbinesite.com/eric.php; see note 3, above; see "Eric Harris and Dylan Klebold," note 6, above.

30. See note 22, above.

31. "Autopsy report— Dylan Klebold," http://www.acolumbinesite. com/autopsies/dylan.gif; "Autopsy report—Eric Harris," http:// www.acolumbinesite.com/autopsies/eric.gif.

32. See note 31, above.

33. See note 31, above.

34. See "Autopsy report—Eric Harris," note 31, above.

35. See note 34, above.

36. See note 34, above.

37. See note 34, above.

38. See note 34, above.

39. See note 34, above.

40. See note 34, above.

41. See note 34, above.

42. See note 34, above.

43. See note 34, above.

44. See note 34, above.

45. See note 34, above.

46. See note 34, above.

47. See note 34, above.

48. See note 34, above.

49. See note 34, above.

50. See note 34, above.

51. See note 34, above.

52. See note 34, above.

53. See note 34, above.

54. See note 34, above.

55. See note 34, above.

56. See note 34, above.

57. See note 34, above.

58. See note 34, above.

59. See note 34, above.

60. See note 34, above.

61. See note 34, above.

62. See note 31, above.

63. See "Autopsy report— Dylan Klebold," note 31, above.

64. See note 63, above.

65. See note 63, above.

66. See note 63, above.

67. See note 31, above.

68. See note 63, above.

69. See note 63, above.

70. See note 63, above.

71. See note 63, above

72. See note 63, above.

73. See note 63, above.

74. See note 63, above.

75. See note 63, above.

76. See note 63, above.

77. See note 63, above.

78. See note 63, above.

79. See note 63, above.

80. See note 63, above.

81. See note 63, above.

82. See note 63, above.

83. See note 63, above.

84. See note 63, above.

85. See note 63, above.

86. See note 63, above.

87. See note 34, above.

88. See note 34, above.

89. "Luvox; Fluvoxamine Maleate Tablets," Monograph, https://www. accessdata.fda.gov/drugsatfda_docs/label/2007/021519lbl.pdf; see note 34, above.

90. D. Ho, "Antidepressants and the FDA's Black-Box Warning: Determining a Rational Public Policy in the Absence of Sufficient Evidence," *Am Med Assoc J of Ethics* 14(6): 483–88; see "Luvox; Fluvoxamine Maleate Tablets," note 89, above.

91. "Dylan Klebold Biography," A&E Television Networks, original published date April 2, 2014, last updated June 18, 2020, https://www.biography.com/crime-figure/dylan-klebold; see D. Cullen, note 4, above; see note 23, above.

92. See note 63, above.

93. See D. Cullen, note 4, above; see "Dylan Klebold Biography," note 91, above.

94. See D. Cullen, note 4, above.

95. "Dylan Bennet Klebold," http://www.acolumbinesite.com/dylan.php.

96. "Eric David Harris," http://www.acolumbinesite.com/eric.php; "Dylan Klebold," https://peoplepill.com/people/dylan-klebold; see and Eric Harris and Dylan Klebold," note 6, above; see note 13, above; see note 23, above.

97. "Columbine High School Shooting Details," http://www.acolumbinesite.com/event/event1.php; see note 96, above.

98. See note 95, above; see note 97, above.

99. K. Simpson, P. Callahan, et al., "Life and death of a follower," the *Denver Post*, May 2, 1999, https://extras.denverpost.com/news/shot0502c.htm; see "Eric Harris and Dylan Klebold," note 6, above; see note 13, above; see note 23, above; see "Dylan Klebold," note 96, above.

100. See note 13, above; see "Dylan Klebold Biography," note 93, above; see note 95, above.

101. See "Eric Harris and Dylan Klebold," note 6, above; see note 94, above; see "Dylan Klebold," note 96, above; see K. Simpson, P. Callahan, et al., note 99, above; see note 100, above.

102. See "Eric Harris and Dylan Klebold," note 6, above; see note 95, above; see "Eric David Harris," note 96, above; see "Columbine High School Shooting Details," note 97, above.

103. See note 95, above; see "Columbine High School Shooting Details," note 97, above.

104. See note 13, above; see Dylan Klebold," note 96, above.

105. See "Dylan Klebold Biography," note 91, above.

106. See note 13, above; see note 105, above.
107. See "The Columbine High School massacre," and "Eric Harris and Dylan Klebold," note 6, above; see note 95, above; see "Dylan Klebold," note 96, above; see note 105, above.
108. See "Eric David Harris," note 96, above; see note 103, above.
109. See note 95, above.
110. See "Eric David Harris," note 96, above.
111. See "The Columbine High School massacre," and "Eric Harris and Dylan Klebold," note 6, above; see "Columbine High School Shootings Fast Facts," note 21, above; see "Columbine High School Shooting Details," note 97, above; see note 110, above.
112. See "Dylan Klebold," note 96, above; see note 106, above; see note 111, above.
113. See note 112, above.
114. See Eric Harris and Dylan Klebold," note 6, above; see note 91, above; Eric David Harris," and "Dylan Klebold," note 96, above; see "Columbine High School Shooting Details," note 97, above; see "See note 110, above.
115. D. Cullen, "The Depressive and the Psychopath," Slate, April 20, 2004, https://slate.com/news-and-politics/2004/04/at-last-we-know-why-the-columbine-killers-did-it.html.
116. See "Eric Harris and Dylan Klebold," and "The Columbine High School massacre," note 6, above; see "Columbine Shooting," note 7, above; see Dylan Klebold," note 96, above; see note 108, above.
117. See note 116, above.
118. See "Eric Harris and Dylan Klebold," note 6, above; see note 94, above; see note 103, above.
119. See note 94, above; see K. Simpson, P. Callahan, et al., note 99, above; see note 103, above.
120. See note 94, above; see "Columbine High School Shooting Details," note 97, above.
121. See note 120, above.
122. See "Columbine High School Shooting Details," note 97, above.
123. See note 122, above.

124. See note 122, above.

125. See note 122, above.

126. See note 122, above.

127. See note 3, above.

128. See note 3, above.

129. See note 3, above.

130. See note 110, above.

131. See note 110, above.

132. See note 110, above.

133. See K. Simpson, P. Callahan, et al., note 99, above.

134. See note 133, above.

135. See note 133, above.

136. See note 133, above.

137. "Eric Harris Biography," https://www.imdb.com/name/nm1286159/bio.

138. See note 133, above.

139. See note 133, above.

140. "Dylan Klebold Biography," https://www.imdb.com/name/nm1287666/bio; see note 95, above.

141. See note 95, above.

142. See note 95, above.

143. See note 95, above.

144. See note 133, above.

145. See note 133, above.

146. See note 133, above.

147. See note 95, above. See note 133, above.

148. See note 133, above.

149. See "Columbine Shooting," note 7, above.

150. See "Eric Harris and Dylan Klebold," note 6, above; see note 110, above.

151. See note 13, above; see note 95, above; see "Dylan Klebold," note 96, above; see note 110, above; see note 120, above.

152. See note 115, above.

153. See note 115, above.

154. See "Eric Harris and Dylan Klebold," note 6, above; see note 115, above.

155. See note 115, above.

156. J. Stenson, "Destined as a psychopath? Experts seek clues," NBC News, April 20, 2009, https://www.nbcnews.com/health/health-news/destined-psychopath-experts-seek-clues-flna1c9465031.

157. See "The Columbine High School massacre," note 6, above; see note 115, above.

158. See note 115, above; see note 156, above.

159. See note 110, above.

160. See note 110, above.

161. See note 110, above.

162. See note 110, above.

163. "Sandy Hook shooting: What happened?" CNN, December 12, 2012, https://www.cnn.com/interactive/2012/12/us/sandy-hook-timeline/index.html.

164. See note 163, above.

165. M. Keneally, "The 11 mas deadly school shootings that happened since Columbine," ABC News, April 19, 2019, https://abcnews.go.com/US/11-mass-deadly-school-shootings-happened-columbine/story?id=62494128.

166. A. Vigderman, "A Timeline of School Shootings Since Columbine," https://www.security.org/blog/a-timeline-of-school-shootings-since-columbine/.

167. See note 165, above.

19.   Timothy McVeigh

1. D.O. Linder, "The Oklahoma City Bombing and The Trial of Timothy McVeigh," http://law2.umkc.edu/faculty/projects/ftrials/mcveigh/mcveighaccount.html.

2. "Timothy McVeigh convicted for Oklahoma City bombing," History, A&E Television Networks, original published date July 21, 2010, last

updated June 1, 2021, https://www.history.com/this-day-in-history/ mcveigh-convicted-for-oklahoma-city-bombing; see note 1, above.

3. See note 1, above.

4. See note 1, above.

5. "Opening Statement by Prosecutor Joseph Hartzler," Oklahoma City Bombing Trial, April 24, 1997, https://famous-trials.com/ oklacity/727-hartzleropening; see note 1, above.

6. See note 1, above.

7. M. Eddy, G. Lane, et al., "Guilty on every count," the *Denver Post*, June 3, 1997, https://extras.denverpost.com/bomb/bombv1.htm; G. London; "McVeigh autopsy deal says no 'invasive procedure,'" CNN, March 19, 2001, https://www.cnn.com/2001/LAW/03/19/ mcveigh.autopsy.04/index.html; see note 2, above.

8. See note 5, above.

9. See note 5, above.

10. See note 5, above.

11. See note 1, above.

12. See note 1, above.

13. See note 5, above.

14. See note 5, above.

15. See note 1, above.

16. See note 1, above; see M. Eddy, G. Lane, et al., note 7, above.

17. See note 2, above.

18. "McVeigh Silent To The End," CBS News, May 30, 2001, https:// www.cbsnews.com/news/mcveigh-silent-to-the-end/; see note 1, above.

19. "McVeigh's Final Breath," https://www.wired.com/2001/06/ mcveighs-final-breath/; see note 1, above.

20. See note 1, above.

21. See note 1 above.

22. See "McVeigh Silent To The End," note 18, above.

23. "Eyewitnesses: McVeigh's final moments," BBC, June 11, 2001, http://news.bbc.co.uk/2/hi/americas/1383031.stm; see note 18, above.

24. G. Tejeda, "McVeigh executed for Oklahoma City bombing," United Press International, June 11, 2001, https://www.upi.com/Archives/2001/06/11/McVeigh-executed-for-Oklahoma-City-bombing/5031992232000/; see note 1, above.

25. See note 18, above.

26. See G. London, note 7, above.

27. See note 26, above.

28. See note 26, above.

29. See G. Tejeda, note 24, above.

30. "Eyewitness Accounts of McVeigh's Execution," ABC News, January 7, 2006, https://abcnews.go.com/US/story?id=90542&page=1; see "McVeigh Silent To The End," note 18, above.

31. See note 29, above.

32. "McVeigh to die from mixture of 3-drug cocktail," the *Washington Post*, April 25, 2001, https://www.washingtontimes.com/news/2001/apr/25/20010425-022139-1274r/.

33. See note 32, above.

34. See note 32, above.

35. See note 32, above.

36. See note 32, above.

37. See "Eyewitness Accounts of McVeigh's Execution," note 30, above.

38. See "McVeigh's Final Breath," note 19, above; see note 30, above.

39. See note 37, above.

40. See note 37, above.

41. See note 37, above.

42. See "McVeigh's Final Breath," note 19, above; see note 29, above; see note 37, above.

43. D. Trigoboff, "Eyewitness blues," https://www.nexttv.com/news/eyewitness-blues-97171; see note 31, above; see note 22, above; see "Eyewitnesses: McVeigh's final moments," note 23, above; see note 37, above.

44. See note 29, above.

45. See note 29, above.

46. "Timothy McVeigh Biography," https://www.imdb.com/name/nm1195540/bio; "Timothy McVeigh Biography," A&E Television Networks, original published date April 2, 2014, last updated August 14, 2019, https://www.biography.com/crime-figure/timothy-mcveigh; "Opening Statement of Defense Attorney Steven Jones in the Timothy McVeigh Trial," April 24, 1997, http://law2.umkc.edu/faculty/projects/ftrials/mcveigh/defenseopen.html.

47. "From decorated veteran to mass murderer," CNN, https://www.cnn.com/CNN/Programs/people/shows/mcveigh/profile.html; see note 1, above; see "Opening Statement of Defense Attorney Steven Jones in the Timothy McVeigh Trial," and "Timothy McVeigh Biography," note 46, above.

48. See note 1, above; see "Timothy McVeigh Biography," note 46, above.

49. See "Timothy McVeigh Biography," note 46, above; see "From decorated veteran to mass murderer," note 47, above.

50. See "Opening Statement of Defense Attorney Steven Jones in the Timothy McVeigh Trial," note 46, above; see note 49, above.

51. See note 1, above; see note 50, above.

52. See "Opening Statement by Prosecutor Joseph Hartzler," note 5, above; see note 51, above.

53. See "Timothy McVeigh convicted for Oklahoma City bombing," note 2, above; see "Opening Statement by Prosecutor Joseph Hartzler," note 5, above; see "Timothy McVeigh Biography," note 46, above; see note 50, above.

54. See "Timothy McVeigh Biography," note 46, above.

55. See "Timothy McVeigh Biography," note 46, above.

56. "From decorated veteran to mass murderer," CNN, https://www.cnn.com/CNN/Programs/people/shows/mcveigh/profile.html; A. Gumbel, "Oklahoma City bombing: 20 years later, key questions remain unanswered," the *Guardian*, April 13, 2015, https://www.theguardian.com/us-news/2015/apr/13/oklahoma-city-bombing-20-years-later-key-questions-remain-unanswered; see "Timothy

McVeigh convicted for Oklahoma City bombing," note 2, above; see "Timothy McVeigh Biography," note 46, above.

57. See note 2, above; see "Timothy McVeigh Biography," note 46, above; see "From decorated veteran to mass murderer," note 56, above.

58. See note 5, above; see "Timothy McVeigh Biography," note 46, above; see A. Gumbel, note 56, above.

59. See note 1, above.

60. See note 1, above.

61. See "Opening Statement by Prosecutor Joseph Hartzler," note 5, above.

62. See note 61, above.

63. See "From decorated veteran to mass murderer," note 47, above.

64. "National Strategy for Countering Domestic Terrorism," National Security Council, June 2021, https://www.whitehouse.gov/wp-content/uploads/2021/06/National-Strategy-for-Countering-Domestic-Terrorism.pdf.

65. See note 64, above.

66. "The War Comes Home: The Evolution of Domestic Terrorism in the United States," Center for Strategic and International Studies, October 22, 2020, https://www.csis.org/analysis/war-comes-home-evolution-domestic-terrorism-united-states.

67. See note 66, above.

68. See note 66, above.

69. S. G. Stolberg and B. M. Rosenthal, "Man Charged After White Nationalist Rally in Charlottesville Ends in Deadly Violence," the *New York Times*, August 12, 2017, https://www.nytimes.com/2017/08/12/us/charlottesville-protest-white-nationalist.html.

70. Z. Kanno-Youngs and D. E. Sanger, "Extremists Emboldened by Capitol Attack Pose Rising Threat, Homeland Security Says," the *New York Times*, originally published January 27, 2021, last updated July 1, 2021, https://www.nytimes.com/2021/01/27/us/politics/homeland-security-threat.html.

71. See note 66, above.

72. "The January 6 attack on the U.S. Capitol," American Oversight, June 24, 2021 https://www.americanoversight.org/investigation/the-january-6-attack-on-the-u-s-capitol.

73. National Terrorism Advisory System Bulletin, January 27, 2021, https://www.dhs.gov/sites/default/files/ntas/alerts/21_0127_ntas-bulletin.pdf.

74. J. E. Greve, "FBI chief calls Capitol attack 'domestic terrorism' and defends US intelligence," the *Guardian*, March 2, 201, https://www.theguardian.com/us-news/2021/mar/02/fbi-christopher-wray-capitol-attack-domestic-terrorism.

75. J. Sanborn, "Violent Extremism and Domestic Terrorism in America: The Role and Response of the Justice Department," Statement Before the House Appropriations Committee, Subcommittee on Commerce, Justice, Science, and Related Agencies, April 29, 2021, https://www.fbi.gov/news/testimony/violent-extremism-and-domestic-terrorism-in-america-the-role-and-response-of-the-department-of-justice.

76. C. Wray, "Oversight of the Federal Bureau of Investigation," Statement Before the House Judiciary Committee, June 10, 2021, https://www.fbi.gov/news/testimony/oversight-of-the-federal-bureau-of-investigation-061021.

77. See note 64, above.

78. See note 64, above.

79. R. Stein, "Ohio executes inmate using new, single-drug method for death penalty," the *Washington Post*, March 11, 2011, http://www.cnn.com/2010/CRIME/12/16/oklahoma.execution/.

80. G. Miller, "America's Long and Gruesome History of Botched Executions," May 12, 2014, https://www.wired.com/2014/05/botched-executions-austin-sarat/.

81. J. B. Zivot, "Lethal Injections: States Medicalize Execution," *University of Richmond Law Review* 49(3) (March 2, 2015) 711, https://scholarship.richmond.edu/lawreview/vol49/iss3/5/; "Baze et al. v. Rees, Commissioner Kentucky Department of Corrections, et al.," 553 U.S. 35, 47, 63, April 16, 2008, https://www.supremecourt.

gov/opinions/07pdf/07-5439.pdf; https://supreme.justia.com/cases/federal/us/553/35/.

82. See note 81, above.

83. See note 79, above; see J. B. Zivot, note 81, above.

84. See note 83, above.

85. See note 83, above.

86. D. Mims, "Death row inmate executed using pentobarbital in lethal injection," CNN, December 26, 2010, http://www.cnn.com/2010/CRIME/12/16/oklahoma.execution/; see note 79, above.

87. See note 86, above.

88. See note 79, above.

89. "Overview of Lethal Injection Protocols," Death Penalty Information Center, https://deathpenaltyinfo.org/executions/lethal-injection/overview-of-lethal-injection-protocols.

90. J. Bates, "Why the Justice Department's Plan to Use a Single Drug for Lethal Injections is Controversial," *Time*, July 29, 2019, https://time.com/5636513/pentobarbital-executions-justice-department/.

91. "Nebraska first in US to use opioid fentanyl in execution," BBC, August 14, 2018, https://www.bbc.com/news/world-us-canada-45185687; see note 89, above.

92. "Botched Executions," Death Penalty Information Center, https://deathpenaltyinfo.org/executions/botched-executions; B. Bryant, "Life and Death: How the lethal injection kills," BBC, March 5, 2018, https://www.bbc.co.uk/bbcthree/article/cd49a818-5645-4a94-832e-d22860804779; see note 39, above.

93. J. E. Stern, "The Cruel and Unusual Execution of Clayton Lockett," the *Atlantic*, June 2015, https://www.theatlantic.com/magazine/archive/2015/06/execution-clayton-lockett/392069/; see J. B. Zivot, note 82, above.

94. G. Miller, "America's Long and Gruesome History of Botched Executions," May 12, 2014, https://www.wired.com/2014/05/botched-executions-austin-sarat/; see "Botched Executions," note 92, above.

95. See G. Miller, note 94, above.

96.   See note 95, above.

97.   See note 95, above.

98.   See note 95, above.

99.   L. Segura, "Ohio's Governor Stopped an Execution Over Fears It Would Feel Like Waterboarding," the Intercept, February 7, 2019, https://theintercept.com/2019/02/07/death-penalty-lethal-injection-midazolam-ohio/; N. Caldwell, A. Chang, et al., "Gasping for Air: Autopsies Reveal Troubling Effects of Lethal Injection," National Public Radio, September 21, 2020, https://www.npr.org/2020/09/21/793177589/gasping-for-air-autopsies-reveal-troubling-effects-of-lethal-injection.

100.   See note 99, above.

101.   See note 99, above.

102.   See note 2, above; see N. Caldwell, A. Chang, et al., note 99, above.

103.   "NPR Investigation of Lethal-Injection Autopsies Finds Executed Prisoners Experience Sensations of Suffocation and Drowning," Death Penalty Information Center, September 25, 2020, https://deathpenaltyinfo.org/news/npr-investigation-of-lethal-injection-autopsies-finds-executed-prisoners-experience-sensations-of-suffocation-and-drowning.

104.   See N. Caldwell, A. Chang, et al., note 99, above.

105.   See N. Caldwell, A. Chang, et al., note 99, above; see "NPR Investigation of Lethal-Injection Autopsies Finds Executed Prisoners Experience Sensations of Suffocation and Drowning," note 103, above.

106.   See note 104, above.

20.   *George Harrison*

1.   "George Harrison," https://oralcancerfoundation.org/people/arts-entertainment/george-harrison/; "Beatle George Harrison dies," CNN, December 1, 2001, https://www.cnn.com/2001/SHOWBIZ/Music/11/30/harrison.obit/.

2. "Ex-Beatle blamed smoking for his cancer," the *Daily Mail*, https://www.dailymail.co.uk/news/article-87109/Ex-Beatle-blamed-smoking-cancer.html; "George Harrison dies," original published date November 29, 2001, last updated November 26, 2018, https://www.beatlesbible.com/2001/11/29/george-harrison-dies/; A. Dansby, "George Harrison Dead at 58," *Rolling Stone*, November 30, 2001, https://www.rollingstone.com/music/music-news/george-harrison-dead-at-58-248348/; M. Kranes, "He battled to the end desperate George hunted world for cancer cure," *New York Post*, December 1, 2001, https://nypost.com/2001/12/01/he-battled-to-the-end-desperate-george-hunted-world-for-cancer-cure/; see "George Harrison," note 1, above.

3. A. Bernstein, "Beatles' George Harrison Dies," the *Washington Post*, December 1, 2001, https://www.washingtonpost.com/archive/politics/2001/12/01/beatles-george-harrison-dies/d9854e76-af9f-497a-86a7-b62aaf9fa041/; "George Harrison Dying From Cancer," July 22, 2001, https://www.wired.com/2001/07/george-harrison-dying-from-cancer/; see note 1, above.

4. "George Harrison Biography," A&E Networks, original published date April 2, 2014, last updated April 20, 2021, https://www.biography.com/musician/george-harrison; J. Selvin, "George Harrison dies after long fight with cancer," November 30, 2001, https://www.sfgate.com/news/article/George-Harrison-dies-after-long-fight-with-cancer-2848664.php; A. Kozinn, "George Harrison, Former Beatle, Dies at 58," the *New York Times*, November 30, 2001, https://www.nytimes.com/2001/11/30/obituaries/george-harrison-former-beatle-dies-at-58.html; see "George Harrison," note 1, above; see M. Kranes, and Ex-Beatle blamed smoking for his cancer," note 2, above.

5. J. Dillon, "Cancer Claims George Harrison," Health Day, November 30, 3001, https://consumer.healthday.com/cancer-information-5/mis-cancer-news-102/cancer-claims-george-harrison-405017.html; A. Bernstein, "Beatles' George Harrison Dies," the *Washington Post*, December 1, 2001, https://www.washingtonpost.com/archive/

politics/2001/12/01/beatles-george-harrison-dies/d9854e76-af9f-497a-86a7-b62aaf9fa041/; see "George Harrison," note 1, above; see "Ex-Beatle blamed smoking for his cancer," and M. Kranes, note 2, above.

6.   D. Masko, "George Harrison died peacefully discloses widow, Olivia, and how to do it," April 9, 2012, http://www.huliq.com/10282/george-harrison-died-peacefully-discloses-widow-olivia-and-how-do-it; A. Dansby, "George Harrison Dead at 58," *Rolling Stone*, November 30, 2001, https://www.rollingstone.com/music/music-news/george-harrison-dead-at-58-248348/; see "Ex-Beatle blamed smoking for his cancer," note 2, above; see note 3, above; see "George Harrison Biography" and A. Kozinn, note 4, above; see J. Dillon, note 5, above.

7.   See "George Harrison Dying From Cancer," note 3 above; see J. Dillon, note 5, above; see D. Masko, note 6, above.

8.   See "Beatle George Harrison dies," note 1, above; see "George Harrison Dying From Cancer," note 3, above; see "George Harrison Biography" and "Ex-Beatle blamed smoking for his cancer," note 4, above.

9.   See D. Masko, note 6, above.

10.   "Death Certificate—George Harrison," http://www.autopsyfiles.org/reports/deathcert/harrison,%20george_dc.pdf; see "Ex-Beatle blamed smoking for his cancer" and M. Kranes, note 2, above; see "George Harrison Biography," note 4, above; see A. Bernstein, note 5, above.

11.   See M. Kranes, note 2, above.

12.   See "Ex-Beatle blamed smoking for his cancer" and A. Dansby, note 2, above; see "George Harrison Dying From Cancer" and A. Bernstein, note 3, above; see A. Kozinn, J. Selvin, and "George Harrison dies," note 4, above.

13.   See "Ex-Beatle blamed smoking for his cancer," note 2, above; see J. Selvin, note 4, above.

14.   See A. Dansby, note 2, above.

15. See "George Harrison dies" and M. Kranes, note 2, above; see J. Selvin and "George Harrison Biography," note 4, above; see J. Dillon, note 5, above.

16. "Franco Cavalli, UICC President," http://forms.uicc.org/templates/uicc/pdf/bod/cavalli.pdf; see "George Harrison dies" and M. Kranes, note 2, above; see A. Bernstein and "George Harrison Dying From Cancer," note 3, above; see A. Kozinn, note 4, above; see J. Dillon, note 5, above; see note 13, above.

17. See M. Kranes, note 2, above.

18. See note 16, above.

19. "Radiosurgery New York," https://www.rsny.org/; see M. Kranes, note 2, above.

20. L. Benjamin, "Beatles doctor faces Â£5m lawsuit," *Evening Standard*, April 13, 2012, https://www.standard.co.uk/hp/front/beatles-doctor-faces-aps5m-lawsuit-7285247.html; A. Goldman, "The Doctor Can't Help Himself," *New York*, December 30, 2004, https://nymag.com/nymetro/health/features/10817/; "Roberts v. Lederman," United States District Court, E.D. New York, October 4, 2004, https://casetext.com/case/roberts-v-lederman.

21. See note 20, above.

22. "Olivia vs. Dr. Gilbert Lederman," January 7, 2004, https://darksweetlady.tripod.com/lederman.html; see "Roberts v. Lederman" and A. Goldman, note 20, above.

23. See "Roberts v. Lederman," note 20, above.

24. See "Olivia vs. Dr. Gilbert Lederman," note 22, above.

25. See A. Goldman, note 20, above.

26. See note 25, above.

27. See note 9, above.

28. See note 9, above.

29. See note 9, above.

30. See "George Harrison dies," note 2, above.

31. See note 9, above.

32. "George Harrison Biography," https://www.thefamouspeople.com/ profiles/george-harrison-3425.php; see note 1, above; see "George Harrison Biography," note 4, above; see note 14, above.

33. See "George Harrison Biography," note 4, above; see "George Harrison Biography," note 21, above.

34. See note 14, above; see note 33, above.

35. See "Beatle George Harrison dies," note 1, above; see "George Harrison Biography," note 4, above.

36. See "George Harrison," note 1, above; see "George Harrison Biography," note 4, above; see J. Dillon, note 5, above.

37. See "Beatle George Harrison dies," note 1, above; see "George Harrison Biography," note 32, above.

38. See "George Harrison Biography," note 4, above; see note 37, above.

39. See note 14, above; see note 35, above.

40. See "Beatle George Harrison dies," note 1, above; see note 14, above.

41. See J. Dillon, note 5, above; see note 33, above.

42. See "George Harrison Biography," note 4, above.

43. See note 42, above.

44. See A. Bernstein, note 5, above; see note 33, above.

45. See J. Selvin, note 4, above.

46. G. Gillman, "Sybil Christopher Dies; Richard Burton's Ex-Wife Ran Nightclubs, Produced Theater," the Wrap, March 12, 2013, https:// www.thewrap.com/sybil-christopher-dies-richard-burtons-ex-wife-ran-nightclubs-produced-theater-81006/.

47. See A. Kozinn, note 4, above.

48. See note 47, above.

49. See note 47, above.

50. See J. Selvin, note 4, above; see J. Dillon, note 5, above; see A. Kozinn, note 6, above; see note 9, above; see note 14, above; see note 44, above.

51. See note 9, above.

52. See "George Harrison," note 1, above; see J. Selvin and J. Dillon, note 5, above; see note 44, above.

53. See note 1, above; see A. Kozinn, note 6, above; see note 42, above.

54. See A. Bernstein, note 5, above.

55. See "George Harrison," note 1, above.

56. "George Harrison Biography," https://www.imdb.com/name/nm0365600/bio.

57. See note 42, above.

58. See note 14, above; see note 42, above; see note 47, above.

59. See J. Dillon, note 5, above; see note 55, above; see note 58, above.

60. See A. Bernstein, note 3, above; see note 58, above.

61. See A. Kozinn, note 6, above; see note 42, above.

62. See note 54, above.

63. See A. Kozinn, note 6, above.

64. See note 63, above.

65. "Head and Neck Cancers," US National Cancer Institute, National Institutes of Health, https://www.cancer.gov/types/head-and-neck/head-neck-fact-sheet; see note 3, above.

66. "Oropharyngeal cancer," Cleveland Clinic, https://my.clevelandclinic.org/health/diseases/12180-oropharyngeal-cancer; see "Head and Neck Cancers," note 65, above.

67. D. Hashim, E. Genden, et al., "Head and neck cancer prevention: From primary prevention to impact of clinicians on reducing burden," *Ann Oncol* 39(5) (2019) 744–56; see "Head and Neck Cancers," note 65, above.

68. See "Head and Neck Cancers," note 65, above.

69. See "George Harrison Dying From Cancer," note 6, above; see note 54, above; see note 55, above.

70. "HPV and Oropharyngeal Cancer," US Centers for Disease Control and Prevention, https://www.cdc.gov/cancer/hpv/basic_info/hpv_oropharyngeal.htm; see "Oropharyngeal cancer" note 66, above; see note 68, above.

71. See note 68, above.

72. See "Ex-Beatle blamed smoking for his cancer," note 2, above; see J. Dillon, note 5, above; see note 17, above; see note 54, above; see note 55, above.

73. M. Hashibe, P. Brennan, et al., "Interaction between tobacco and alcohol use and the risk of head and neck cancer: Pooled analysis in the International Head and Neck Cancer Epidemiology Consortium," *Cancer Epidemiol Biomarkers Prev* 18(2) (2009): 541–50. See note 67, above.

74. S. Gandini, E. Botteri, et al., "Tobacco smoking and cancer: a meta-analysis," *Int J Cancer* 122(1) (2008) 155–64; M. Hashibe, P. Brennan, et al., "Alcohol drinking in never users of tobacco, cigarette smoking in never drinkers, and the risk of head and neck cancer: pooled analysis in the International Head and Neck Cancer Epidemiology Consortium," *J Natl Cancer Inst* 99(10) (2007) 777–89; L. C. Mariano, S. Warnakulasuriya, et al., "Secondhand smoke exposure and oral cancer risk: a systematic review and meta-analysis," *Tob Control* (April 26, 2021), tobaccocontrol-2020-056393. doi: 10.1136/tobaccocontrol-2020-056393; see note 68, above.

75. See "Oropharyngeal cancer," note 66, above.

76. K. A. Do, M. M. Johnson, et al., "Second primary tumors in patients with upper aerodigestive tract cancers: joint effects of smoking and alcohol (United States)," Cancer Causes Control 14(2) (2003) 131–38 (2003); A. Argiris, B. E. Brockstein, et al., "Competing causes of death and second primary tumors in patients with locoregionally advanced head cancer treated with chemotherapy," *Clin Cancer Res* 10(6) (2004): 1956–62; S. C. Chung, G. Scelo, et al., "Risk of second primary cancer among patients with head and neck cancers: A pooled analysis of 13 cancer registries," *Int J Cancer* 123(10) (2008): 2390–96 (2008); see note 68, above.

77. See "Ex-Beatle blamed smoking for his cancer," note 2, above; see "Death Certificate—George Harrison," note 10, above; see note 15, above; see note 54, above.

78. "What Is Lung Cancer?" American Cancer Society, https://www.cancer.org/cancer/lung-cancer/about/what-is.html; "Lung cancer," https://www.nhs.uk/conditions/lung-cancer/; "Lung Cancer—Non-Small Cell," American Society of Clinical Oncology, https://www.cancer.net/cancer-types/lung-cancer-non-small-cell/statistics.

79. See note 17, above; see "Lung cancer" and "Lung Cancer—Non-Small Cell," note 78, above.
80. See "Lung Cancer—Non-Small Cell," note 78, above.
81. See note 80, above.
82. See note 9, above; see note 30, above.
83. See note 9, above.
84. See note 30, above; see note 45, above; see note 54, above.

21.   *Dee Dee Ramone*

1. "Dee Dee Ramone found dead: OD suspected," CNN, June 7, 2002, http://www.cnn.com/2002/SHOWBIZ/Music/06/06/deedee.ramone/.

2. "Dee Dee Ramone Found Dead in Los Angeles," MTV, June 6, 2002, http://www.mtv.com/news/1455048/dee-dee-ramone-found-dead-in-los-angeles/.

3. J. Wilson, "Dee Dee Ramone Found Dead in L.A.," AP News, June 6, 2002, https://apnews.com/article/b76d0860ea57969865ff076747af1e62; C. Devenish, "Dee Dee Ramone Dies," *Rolling Stone*, June 6, 2002, https://www.rollingstone.com/music/music-news/dee-dee-ramone-dies-245794/; D. Campbell, "'Overdose' kills Dee Dee Ramone," the *Guardian*, June 7, 2002, https://www.theguardian.com/world/2002/jun/07/arts.artsnews; "Pioneering Punk Rocker Dee Dee Ramone Dies at Age 50," the *Washington Post*, June 7, 2002, https://www.washingtonpost.com/archive/local/2002/06/07/pioneering-punk-rocker-dee-dee-ramone-dies-at-age-50/7525189e-6529-4c2e-addf-d5b62db65015/; B. Browne, "Rocker Dee Dee Ramone of Forest Hills dies at 49," https://qns.com/2002/06/rocker-dee-dee-ramone-of-forest-hills-dies-at-49/; A. Petridis, "Dee Dee Ramone," the *Guardian*, June 8, 2002, https://www.theguardian.com/news/2002/jun/07/guardianobituaries.alexispetridis.

4. See note 2, above.

5.   "Dee Dee Ramone Biography," https://peoplepill.com/people/dee-dee-ramone.

6.   "Autopsy Report—Dee Dee Ramone," https://www.yumpu.com/fr/document/read/12286812/autopsyfilesorg-dee-dee-ramones-autopsy-report; J. Widerhorn, "19 Years Ago: Ramones Bassist Dee Dee Ramone Dies at 50," https://loudwire.com/dee-dee-ramone-dies-anniversary/; R. Cromelin, "Dee Dee Ramone, 49; One of Punk Rock's Pioneers," *Los Angeles Times*, June 7, 2002, https://www.latimes.com/archives/la-xpm-2002-jun-07-me-ramone7-story.html; G. Kaufman, "Dee Dee Ramone's Death Due to Accidental Overdose, Coroner Says," MTV, September 18, 2002, https://www.mtv.com/news/1457648/dee-dee-ramones-death-due-to-accidental-overdose-coroner-says/; "Dee Dee Ramone Biography," https://www.thefamouspeople.com/profiles/dee-dee-ramone-45858.php; see note 2, above; see J. Wilson, "Pioneering Punk Rocker Dee Dee Ramone Dies at Age 50" and B. Browne, note 3, above; see note 5, above.

7.   See J. Wilson and B. Browne, note 3, above; see "Autopsy Report—Dee Dee Ramone," note 6, above.

8.   See "Autopsy Report—Dee Dee Ramone," note 6, above.

9.   See note 2, above; see C. Devenish and B. Browne, note 3, above; see G. Kaufman, note 6, above; see note 8, above.

10.   See note 1, above; see J. Wilson, D. Campbell, and "Pioneering Punk Rocker Dee Dee Ramone Dies at Age 50," note 3, above; see note 8, above.

11.   See note 2, above; see J. Wilson, D. Campbell, and "Pioneering Punk Rocker Dee Dee Ramone Dies at Age 50," note 3, above; see J. Widerhorn, "Dee Dee Ramone Biography," and R. Cromelin, note 6, above; see note 8, above.

12.   See note 8, above.

13.   See note 8, above.

14.   See note 8, above.

15.   See note 8, above.

16.   See note 8, above.

17. See note 8, above.

18. See note 8, above.

19. See note 8, above.

20. See note 8, above.

21. See note 8, above.

22. See note 8, above.

23. See note 8, above.

24. See note 8, above.

25. See note 8, above.

26. "Coroner Confirms Overdose Killed Dee Dee Ramone," Billboard, September 18, 2002, https://www.billboard.com/articles/news/74171/coroner-confirms-overdose-killed-dee-dee-ramone; see J. Widerhorn, note 6, above.

27. "Dee Dee Ramone Biography," https://www.allmusic.com/artist/dee-dee-ramone-mn0000186299/biography; "Dee Dee Ramone Biography," https://www.imdb.com/name/nm0708493/bio; L. Tanos, "The Tragic Truth About Dee Dee Ramone's Childhood," Grunge, June 12, 2021, https://www.grunge.com/435867/the-tragic-truth-about-dee-dee-ramones-childhood/; see A. Petridis, and "Pioneering Punk Rocker Dee Dee Ramone Dies at Age 50," note 3, above; see note 5, above; see "Dee Dee Ramone Biography," note 6, above.

28. T. Hearn, "Dee Dee Ramone—Portrait of a Punk!" December 6, 2017, https://pleasekillme.com/dee-dee-ramone-portrait-of-a-punk-2/; see R. Cromelin, note 6, above; see note 27, above.

29. See L. Tanos, note 27, above; see T. Hearn, note 28, above.

30. See note 29, above.

31. See T. Hearn, note 28, above.

32. See note 31, above.

33. See note 5, above; see "Dee Dee Ramone Biography," note 6, above.

34. See note 27, above.

35. See note 31, above.

36. See "Dee Dee Ramone Biography," note 6, above; see "Dee Dee Ramone Biography," note 27, above.

37. See "Dee Dee Ramone Biography," note 6, above; see A. Petridis and "Dee Dee Ramone Biography," note 27, above.

38. See "Pioneering Punk Rocker Dee Dee Ramone Dies at Age 50," note 3, above; see note 36, above.

39. "The Ramones Biography," https://www.musicianguide.com/biographies/1608003594/The-Ramones.html; see note 1, above; see note 2, above; see B. Browne and C. Devenish, note 3, above; see note 5, above; see J. Widerhorn and R. Cromelin, note 6, above; see "Dee Dee Ramone Biography," note 27, above; see note 37, above.

40. See note L. Tanos, note 27, above.

41. See note 40, above.

42. See J. Wilson, C. Devenish, and "Pioneering Punk Rocker Dee Dee Ramone Dies at Age 50," note 3, above; see note 5, above; see "Dee Dee Ramone Biography," note 6, above.

43. See B. Browne, and A. Petridis, note 3, above.

44. See A. Petridis, and C. Devenish, note 3, above; see J. Widerhorn, note 6, above; see "Dee Dee Ramone Biography," note 27, above; see "The Ramones Biography," note 39, above.

45. See note 1, above; see J. Wilson, and "Pioneering Punk Rocker Dee Dee Ramone Dies at Age 50," note 3, above; see R. Cromelin, note 6, above; see "Dee Dee Ramone Biography," and "Dee Dee Ramone Biography," note 27, above; see note 43, above.

46. See J. Wilson, and "Pioneering Punk Rocker Dee Dee Ramone Dies at Age 50," note 3, above.

47. See note 1, above; see note 2, above; see R. Cromelin, note 6, above; see "Dee Dee Ramone Biography," note 27, above; see note 42, above; see note 43, above.

48. See note 5, above; see "Dee Dee Ramone Biography," note 27, above.

49. See note 1, above; see B. Browne, J. Wilson, C. Devenish, and "Pioneering Punk Rocker Dee Dee Ramone Dies at Age 50," note 3, above; see note 37, above.

50. See "The Ramones Biography," note 39, above.

51. See note 31, above.

52. See note 41, above.

53. See note 1, above; see note 2, above; see C. Devenish and "Pioneering Punk Rocker Dee Dee Ramone Dies at Age 50," note 3, above; see note 5, above; see R. Cromelin, note 6, above; see "Dee Dee Ramone Biography," note 27, above; see note 37, above.

54. See note 33, above.

55. See note 1, above; see J. Wilson and "Pioneering Punk Rocker Dee Dee Ramone Dies at Age 50," note 3, above; see J. Widerhorn and R. Cromelin, note 6, above; See"Dee Dee Ramone Biography," note 27, above; see note 37, above; see note 50, above.

56. See R. Cromelin, note 6, above; see "Dee Dee Ramone Biography" and "Dee Dee Ramone Biography," note 27, above; see note 33, above; see note 50, above.

57. See note 1, above; see "Dee Dee Ramone Biography," note 27, above; see note 48, above.

58. See R. Cromelin, note 6, above.

59. See note 58, above.

60. See "Dee Dee Ramone Biography," note 27, above; see note 40, above.

61. See note 58, above.

62. See note 2, above.

63. See note 2, above.

64. See note 2, above.

65. See note 2, above; see G. Kaufman, note 6, above.

66. See J. Widerhorn, note 6, above.

67. See note 50, above.

68. See A. Petridis, note 3, above; see "Dee Dee Ramone Biography," note 27, above; see note 50, above.

69. See note 50, above.

70. See A. Petridis, note 3, above.

71. See note 31, above.

22. Maurice Gibb

1. S. Candiotti, "Gibb autopsy cites twisted intestine," CNN, January 16, 2003, https://www.cnn.com/2003/SHOWBIZ/Music/01/16/gibb.autopsy/index.html; B. LaMendola and J. Needle, "Autopsy: Birth Defect Led to Gibb's Fatal Blockage," *Sun Sentinel*, January 17, 2003, https://www.sun-sentinel.com/news/fl-xpm-2003-01-17-0301161150-story.html; A. J. Tresca, "Maurice Gibb Dies at 53," https://www.verywellhealth.com/maurice-gibb-dies-at-53-1941702; "2003: Maurice Gibb dies after stomach op," BBC, http://news.bbc.co.uk/onthisday/hi/dates/stories/january/12/newsid_4071000/4071857.stm; B. Goldsborough, "Need 16 rooms on 4 floors in Lincoln Park?" *Chicago Tribune*, October 12, 2003, https://www.chicagotribune.com/news/ct-xpm-2003-10-12-0310110414-story.html.

2. See S. Candiotti, A. J. Tresca, and "2003: Maurice Gibb dies after stomach op," note 1, above.

3. See "2003: Maurice Gibb dies after stomach op," note 1, above.

4. T. Branigan, "Maurice Gibb, talented but tormented Bee Gee, dies," the *Guardian*, January 13, 2003, https://www.theguardian.com/world/2003/jan/13/arts.artsnews; see S. Candiotti and A. J. Tresca, note 1, above.

5. "Maurice Gibb in Hospital," https://www.beegees-world.com/mauricegibb_hospital.html.

6. See T. Branigan, note 4, above.

7. See note 5, above.

8. See note 6, above.

9. See note 6, above.

10. See note 6, above.

11. "Maurice Gibb Obituary," http://www.legacy.com/ns/maurice-gibb-obituary/718720.

12. See note 11, above.

13. "Autopsy report—Maurice Gibb," http://www.autopsyfiles.org/reports/Celebs/gibb,%20maurice_report.pdf.

14. See note 13, above.

15. See note 13, above.

16. See note 13, above.

17. See note 13, above.

18. See note 13, above.

19. See note 13, above.

20. See note 13, above.

21. See note 13, above.

22. See note 13, above.

23. See A. J. Tresca, note 2, above; see note 13, above.

24. See note 13, above.

25. See note 13, above.

26. See note 13, above.

27. See note 13, above.

28. See note 13, above.

29. H. A. Milman, "Errol Flynn," in *Forensics: The Science Behind the Deaths of Famous People* (Bloomington, Indiana: Xlibris, 2020) 1–14; "Cirrhosis," https://www.mayoclinic.org/diseases-conditions/cirrhosis/symptoms-causes/syc-20351487; see note 13, above.

30. See note 13, above.

31. "Volvulus," https://iffgd.org/gi-disorders/volvulus/; "Intestinal ischemia," Mayo Clinic, https://www.mayoclinic.org/diseases-conditions/intestinal-ischemia/symptoms-causes/syc-20373946; see note 13, above.

32. "Maurice Gibb Biography," A&E Television Networks, original published date April 2, 2014, last updated June 21, 2021, https://www.biography.com/musician/maurice-gibb.

33. See note 32, above.

34. See note 32, above.

35. "Maurice Gibb Biography," https://www.thefamouspeople.com/profiles/maurice-gibb-33608.php; "The Bee Gees: How Three Small-Town Brothers Became Leaders of the 70s and 80s Music Scene," https://www.biography.com/news/bee-gees-origins.

36. See note 35, above.

37. See "2003: Maurice Gibb dies after stomach op," note 2, above; see note 32, above; see note 35, above.

38. "The Bee Gees: How Three Small-Town Brothers Became Leaders of the 70s and 80s Music Scene," https://www.biography.com/news/bee-gees-origins.

39. See note 38, above.

40. See note 35, above; see "Maurice Gibb Biography," note 37, above.

41. See note 35, above.

42. See Maurice Gibb Biography," note 35, above.

43. See note 42, above.

44. See "2003: Maurice Gibb dies after stomach op," note 2, above; see note 42, above.

45. See "2003: Maurice Gibb dies after stomach op," note 2, above.

46. See, note 6, above; see note 42, above; see note 45, above.

47. "Maurice Gibb Biography," https://www.imdb.com/name/nm0316465/bio.

48. See note 11, above; see note 32, above.

49. "Fun-loving Bee Gee Maurice Gibb dead at 53," the *Badger Herald*, January 17, 2003, https://badgerherald.com/artsetc/2003/01/17/funloving-bee-gee-ma/.

50. See note 49, above.

51. See note 35, above.

52. See note 47, above.

53. See note 32, above.

54. B. Goldsborough, "Need 16 rooms on 4 floors in Lincoln Park?" *Chicago Tribune*, October 12, 2003, https://www.chicagotribune.com/news/ct-xpm-2003-10-12-0310110414-story.html; see note 49, above.

55. "Gibb Will Bestows Estate to Widow," August 18, 2003, https://apnews.com/article/8300d046a0c6c304c2e8b30076c930c7.

56. B. Husberg, K. Salehi, et al., "Congenital intestinal malrotation in adolescent and adult patients: a 12-year clinical and radiological survey," *Springerplus* 5: 245 (2016).

57. J. C. Langer, "Intestinal Rotation Abnormalities and Midgut Volvulus," *Surg Clin N Am* 97 (2017): 147–59; see B. Husberg, K. Salehi, et al., note 56, above.

58. See note 57, above.

59. See B. LaMendola and J. Needle, note 1, above.

60. See A. J. Tresca, note 2, above; see note 59, above.

61. P. Herle and T. Halder, "Intestinal malrotation in an adult patient with other congenital malformations: A case report," *Int J Surg Case Rep* 51 (2018): 364–67.

62. See note 61, above.

63. J. C. Langer, "Intestinal Rotation Abnormalities and Midgut Volvulus," *Surg Clin N Am* 97 (2017): 147–59 (2017); see B. LaMendola and J. Needle, note 1, above; see S. Candiotti, note 2, above.

64. See note 61, above; see J. C. Langer, note 63, above.

65. See J. C. Langer, note 63, above.

66. "Bee Gee's family to settle over death," the *Scotsman*, February 15, 2004, https://www.scotsman.com/news/people/bee-gees-family-settle-over-death-2509762.

67. See note 66, above.

68. See note 66, above.

69. See note 32, above.

70. "Gibb Will Bestows Estate to Widow," August 18, 2003, https://apnews.com/article/8300d046a0c6c304c2e8b30076c930c7.

71. See note 70, above.

72. "Robin Gibb Biography," https://www.imdb.com/name/nm0316471/bio.

73. See note 72, above.

74. See note 72, above.

75. "Robin Gibb, member of the Bee Gees, dies after battle with cancer," CNN, December 11, 2012, https://www.cnn.com/2012/05/20/showbiz/robin-gibb-dies/index.html.

23.　*John Ritter*

1. "John Ritter Biography," A&E Television Networks, original published date April 2, 2014, last updated March 30, 2021, https://www.biography.com/actor/john-ritter;　C.　Ornstein, "The Sad Death of John Ritter," January 24, 2008, https://www. thelifeandtimesofhollywood.com/the-sad-death-of-john-ritter/.

2. "Obituary—John Ritter," https://www.legacy.com/obituaries/ name/john-ritter-obituary?pid=1391524; "Ritter's widow and ex-wife testify in court," ABC30, March 3, 2008, https://abc7. com/archive/5996042/; "Ritter Family Files Wrongful Death Suit," AP News, September 9, 2004, https://apnews.com/ article/0e982607960789c8bbd307fb2775a646; L. Elber, "TV Sitcom Icon John Ritter Dies at 54," *Chicago Tribune*, September 12, 2003, https://www.chicagotribune.com/sns-ap-obit-ritter-story.html; "Ritter's wife gives detailed account of his death," March 3, 2008, https://www.today.com/popculture/ritters-wife-gives-detailed-account-his-death-1C9416529; S. Pal, "Jury finds John Ritter's doctors blameless in $67 million wrongful death lawsuit," March 17, 2008, https://www.diagnosticimaging.com/view/jury-finds-john-ritters-doctors-blameless-67-million-wrongful-death-lawsuit; M. Kerr, "'Three's Company' Star John Ritter Died During the Production of Another Sitcom," https://cheatsheet.com/entertainment/threes-company-star-john-ritter-died-during-production-of-another-sitcom.html/; L. Deutsch, "Closing Arguments Under way in John Ritter Death Lawsuit," ABC News, April 14, 2009, https://abcnews. go.com/Entertainment/story?id=4439736&page=1; B. Considine, "John Ritter's widow talks about wrongful death suit," February 4, 2008, https://www.today.com/popculture/john-ritters-widow-talks-about-wrongful-death-suit-2D80555805; "John Ritter Biography," https://www.thefamouspeople.com/profiles/johnathan-southworth-ritter-1958.php; see note 1, above.

3. J. Spano, "Jury clears doctors of negligence in death of actor Ritter," *Los Angeles Times*, March 15, 2008, https://www.latimes.com/

archives/la-xpm-2008-mar-15-me-ritter15-story.html; "Opening statements begin in Ritter lawsuit," the *Hollywood Reporter*, February 12, 2008, https://www.hollywoodreporter.com/business/business-news/opening-statements-begin-ritter-lawsuit-104640/; see C. Ornstein, note 1, above; see L. Deutsch and S. Pal, note 2, above.

4. See C. Ornstein, note 1, above; see B. Considine, S. Pal, and M. Kerr, note 2, above; see "Opening statements begin in Ritter lawsuit," note 3, above.

5. "Wife relates final minutes of John Ritter's life," March 4, 2008, https://www.cbc.ca/news/entertainment/wife-relates-final-minutes-of-john-ritter-s-life-1.696153; see L. Deutsch, note 2, above; see "Opening statements begin in Ritter lawsuit," note 3, above.

6. See "Ritter's wife gives detailed account of his death," note 2, above; see "Wife relates final minutes of John Ritter's life," note 5, above.

7. See "Ritter's wife gives detailed account of his death," note 2, above.

8. "John Ritter," https://www.nickiswift.com/50009/really-killed-celebrities/; see C. Ornstein, note 1, above; see B. Considine, note 2, above.

9. See C. Ornstein, note 1, above; see B. Considine, note 2, above.

10. See "John Ritter," note 8, above.

11. G. Gillenwater, "Trial over John Ritter's death begins," February 17, 2008, https://www.lawyersandsettlements.com/features/wrongful_death/wrongful-death-john-ritter.html; see "John Ritter Biography," note 1, above; see "Ritter Family Files Wrongful Death Suit," M. Kerr, "Obituary—John Ritter," L. Elber, and "John Ritter Biography," note 2, above; see "Opening statements begin in Ritter lawsuit," and J. Spano, note 3, above; see "Wife relates final minutes of John Ritter's life," note 5, above; see note 8, above.

12. See C. Ornstein, note 1, above; see note 10, above.

13. See "John Ritter Biography," note 2, above; see note 9, above.

14. See "John Ritter Biography," note 1, above; see M. Kerr and "John Ritter Biography," note 2, above.

15. "John Ritter Biography," https://www.imdb.com/name/nm0000615/bio; see M. Kerr, note 2, above.

16. See note 14, above.

17. See note 14, above.

18. See M. Kerr, note 2, above.

19. See note 14, above.

20. See note 14, above.

21. See "John Ritter Biography," note 15, above.

22. See note 14, above.

23. See note 14, above.

24. See S. Pal, note 2, above.

25. See L. Deutsch, note 2, above; see G. Gillenwater, note 11, above; see note 24, above.

26. See "Ritter's wife gives detailed account of his death," L. Deutsch, and "Ritter's widow and ex-wife testify in court," note 2, above; see note 24, above.

27. See note 7, above.

28. "Aortic dissection," Cleveland Clinic, https://my.clevelandclinic.org/health/diseases/16743-aortic-dissection; D. Juang, A. C. Braverman, et al., "Aortic Dissection," *Circulation* 118 (2008): e507–e510.

29. See D. Juang, A. C. Braverman, et al., note 28, above.

30. "Explanation of John Ritter's Death," September 12, 2003, https://www.webmd.com/heart-disease/news/20030912/explanation-of-john-ritters-death; see note 28, above.

31. See note 28, above.

32. See note 29, above.

33. See note 29, above; see "Explanation of John Ritter's Death," note 30, above.

34. See note 33, above.

35. See note 29, above.

36. See note 30, above.

37. See note 28, above.

38. See note 28, above.

39. See note 28, above.

40. See C. Ornstein, note 1, above.

41. See note 29, above.

42. See note 29, above.

43. See B. Considine, note 2, above.

44. See L. Elber and "John Ritter Biography," note 2, above.

45. See note 44, above.

24. Bobby Hatfield

1. D. Laing, "Bobby Hatfield," the *Guardian*, November 7, 2003, https://www.theguardian.com/news/2003/nov/07/guardianobituaries.artsobituaries.

2. "Billy Joel inducts The Righteous Brothers Rock and Roll Hall of Fame inductions 2003," https://www.youtube.com/watch?v=6FCNJFIZOcc; "Righteous Brother Bobby Hatfield dies," *Herald-Tribune*, November 7, 2003, https://www.heraldtribune.com/article/LK/20031107/news/605232679/SH; "Bobby Hatfield Obituary," www.legacy.com/obituaries.asp?Page=LifeStoryPrint&PersonID=157"Righteous Brothers Bobby Hatfield Died of a Heart Attack," July 7, 2011, https://www.antimusic.com/news/03/nov/item18.shtml; 5623; "Bobby Hatfield Biography," www.spectropop.com/remembers/BHobit.htm.

3. See note 1, above.

4. A. Bernstein, "Righteous Brothers' Bobby Hatfield Dies at 63," *Washington Post*, https://www.washingtonpost.com/archive/local/2003/11/07/righteous-brothers-bobby-hatfield-dies-at-63/6afdc7d6-0a8e-48db-825d-c2ffc91cf5c7/; J. Irwin, "Righteous Brothers' Bobby Hatfield Mourned," *Chicago Tribune*, November 6, 2003, https://www.chicagotribune.com/sns-ap-obit-hatfield-story.html; see note 1, above; see "Bobby Hatfield Obituary," note 2, above.

5. "Bobby Hatfield Biography," https://peoplepill.com/people/bobby-hatfield; see "Righteous Brother Bobby Hatfield dies," note 2, above.

6. See note 5, above.

7. "The Righteous Brothers perform Rock and Roll Hall of Fame inductions 2003," https://www.youtube.com/

watch?v=yLu2T85kwGU; "The Righteous Brothers accept award Rock and Roll Hall of Fame inductions 2003," https://www.youtube.com/watch?v=j0cs8VA8iFw; T. Ryan, "Still got that lovin' feeling," *Star Bulletin*, August 29, 2005, http://archives.starbulletin.com/2005/08/29/features/story3.html; see note 1, above; see "Righteous Brother Bobby Hatfield dies," "Righteous Brothers Bobby Hatfield Died of a Heart Attack," and "Bobby Hatfield Biography," note 2, above; see J. Irwin, note 4, above.

8. See "Righteous Brother Bobby Hatfield dies," note 2, above.

9. B. Sisario, "Bobby Hatfield Dies at 63; Righteous Brothers Tenor," *New York Times*, November 7, 2003, "https://www.nytimes.com/2003/11/07/arts/bobby-hatfield-dies-at-63-righteous-brothers-tenor.html/; see "Bobby Hatfield Obituary," note 2, above; see note 8, above.

10. "Bobby Hatfield," https://findadeath.com/bobby-hatfield/; see "Bobby Hatfield Obituary," note 2, above; see note 5, above; see J. Robinson, note 9, above.

11. See note 1, above; see "Bobby Hatfield Biography," note 5, above; see note 8, above; see J. Robinson, note 9, above.

12. J. Ramakers, "Bobby Lee Hatfield 11/2003," November 10, 2015, https://rockandrollparadise.com/bobby-lee-hatfield-112003/; B. Sisario, "Bobby Hatfield Dies at 63; Righteous Brothers Tenor," *New York Times*, November 7, 2003, "https://www.nytimes.com/2003/11/07/arts/bobby-hatfield-dies-at-63-righteous-brothers-tenor.html/; "Cocaine linked to death of Righteous Brother," *Tampa Bay Times*, August 27, 2005, https://www.tampabay.com/archive/2004/01/07/cocaine-linked-to-death-of-righteous-brother/; see "Bobby Hatfield Obituary" and "Righteous Brothers Bobby Hatfield Died of a Heart Attack," note 2, above; see A. Bernstein and J. Irwin, note 4, above; see "Bobby Hatfield Biography," note 5, above; see note 8, above.

13. See "Bobby Hatfield Obituary," note 2, above.

14. See "Bobby Hatfield," note 10, above.

15. "Autopsy—Bobby Hatfield," Sparrow Regional Laboratories, https://www.celebrityarchive.com/Bobby-Hatfield-Autopsy-p/1508.htm.

16. See note 14, above.

17. R. Chang, "Hatfield died of drug overdose, autopsy says," the *Baltimore Sun*, January 7, 2004, https://www.baltimoresun.com/news/bs-xpm-2004-01-07-0401070213-story.html; "Righteous Bro Hatfield Autopsy reveals," January 6, 2004, https://fanforum.glennhughes.com/forum/index.php?thread/1471-righteous-bro-hatfield-autopsy-reveals/; see T. Ryan, note 7, above; see J. Robinson, note 9, above; see "Cocaine linked to death of Righteous Brother," note 12, above.

18. See note 14, above.

19. See "Cocaine linked to death of Righteous Brother," note 12, above; see "Righteous Bro Hatfield Autopsy reveals," note 17, above.

20. See J. Robinson, note 9, above; see R. Chang, note 17, above; see note 19, above.

21. See note 19, above.

22. See note 19, above.

23. See "Bobby Hatfield Biography," note 5, above; see "Cocaine linked to death of Righteous Brother," note 12, above; see R. Chang, note 17, above.

24. "Cocaine caused death of Bobby Hatfield," the *Argus Press*, January 6, 2004, https://news.google.com/newspapers?id=ukgiAAAAIBAJ&pg=1407,379087&dq=bobby-hatfield+dead+%7C+death+%7C+died.

25. See note 24, above.

26. "Death Certificate—Bobby Hatfield," https://findadeath.com/bobby-hatfield/; "Bobby Hatfield Biography," https://www.imdb.com/name/nm0368825/bio; "Hatfield's death caused by cocaine," *Los Angeles Times*, January 7, 2004, https://www.latimes.com/archives/la-xpm-2004-jan-07-et-quick7.4-story.html; see J. Ramakers, note 12, above; see "Righteous Bro Hatfield Autopsy reveals," note 17, above; see note 23, above.

27. See R. Chang, note 17, above.

28. "Bobby Hatfield," *Independent*, November 7, 2003, https://www.independent.co.uk/news/obituaries/bobby-hatfield-37420.html; see note 1, above; see "Bobby Hatfield Biography," note 2, above; see J. Irwin and A. Bernstein, note 4, above; see note 5, above; see T. Ryan, note 7, above; see J. Ramakers and B. Sisario, note 12, above; see "Bobby Hatfield Biography," note 26, above.

29. See J. Ramakers, note 12, above.

30. See note 1, above; see "Bobby Hatfield Biography," note 5, above; see T. Ryan, note 7, above; see note 29, above.

31. See "Bobby Hatfield Biography," note 2, above; see "Bobby Hatfield Biography," note 5, above; see note 29, above.

32. See "Bobby Hatfield Obituary," note 2, above; see note 5, above; see "Bobby Hatfield Biography," note 7, above; see B. Sisario, note 12, above.

33. See note 1, above; see "Bobby Hatfield," note 28, above; see note 32, above.

34. See note 1, above; see J. Irwin, note 4, above; see T. Ryan, note 7, above; see J. Robinson, note 9, above; see note 29, above; see note 32, above.

35. See J. Robinson, note 9, above; see Bobby Hatfield," note 28, above.

36. See note 1, above; see "Bobby Hatfield Biography," note 5, above.

37. See note 1, above; see J. Irwin and A. Bernstein, note 4, above; see "Bobby Hatfield Biography," note 5, above; see T. Ryan, note 7, above; see note 9, above; see B. Sisario, note 12, above; see "Bobby Hatfield," note 28, above.

38. See "Bobby Hatfield Biography," note 7, above.

39. See note 1, above; see A. Bernstein, note 4, above; see B. Sisario, note 12, above; see Bobby Hatfield," note 28, above; see note 38, above.

40. See B. Sisario, note 12, above; see Bobby Hatfield," note 28, above.

41. See note 1, above; see "Bobby Hatfield Biography," note 5, above; see Bobby Hatfield," note 28, above.

42. See Bobby Hatfield," note 28, above.

43. See A. Bernstein, note 4, above; see note 42, above.

44. See note 42, above.

45. See J. Irwin, note 4, above; see B. Sisario, note 12, above; see note 38, above; see note 41, above.

46. See note 1, above; see A. Bernstein, note 4, above; see note 40, above.

47. See "Bobby Hatfield Biography," note 4, above; see note 38, above; see note 46, above.

48. See note 1, above; see J. Irwin and A. Bernstein, note 4, above; see note 5, above; see B. Sisario, note 12, above.

49. See note 5, above; see note 38, above; see note 46, above.

50. See note 1, above; see note 3, above; see note 5, above; see note 38, above; see note 42, above.

51. See note 1, above.

52. See B. Sisario, note 12, above; see note 38, above; see note 42, above.

53. B. G. Schwartz, S. Rezkalla, et al., "Cardiovascular Effects of Cocaine," *Circulation* (December 14, 2010) https://www.ahajournals.org/doi/full/10.1161/circulationaha.11.940569.

54. "Cocaine and Heart Attack Risk: Everything You Need to Know," https://www.webmd.com/connect-to-care/addiction-treatment-recovery/cocaine/cocaine-and-heart-attack-risk.

55. See note 54, above.

56. See note 53, above.

57. See note 53, above.

58. See note 53, above.

59. See note 53, above.

60. See note 53, above.

61. "Cardiovascular Effects of Cocaine," American College of Cardiology, June 27, 2017, https://www.acc.org/latest-in-cardiology/ten-points-to-remember/2017/06/27/13/58/the-cardiovascular-effects-of-cocaine; W. H. Frishman, A. Del Vecchio, et al., "Cardiovascular manifestations of substance abuse part 1: cocaine," *Heart Dis* 5(3) (2003), 187–201; J. L. Zimmerman, "Cocaine intoxication," *Crit care Clin* 28(4) (2012) 517–26 (2012); see note 53, above.

62. See note 53, above.

63. S. Darke, S. Kaye, et al., "Comparative cardiac pathology among deaths due to cocaine toxicity, opioid toxicant and non-drug-related causes," *Addiction* 101(12) (2006) 1771–77.

64. See note 17, above.

65. See note 53, above.

25.   *Johnny Carson*

1. "Johnny Carson makes debut as 'Tonight Show' host," A&E Television Networks, original published date November 13, 2009, last updated October 12, 2001, https://www.history.com/this-day-in-history/johnny-carson-makes-debut-tonight-show-host.

2. "Johnny Carson Quotes," https://www.brainyquote.com/quotes/johnny_carson_128070.

3. See note 2, above.

4. "Johnny Carson Biography," A&E Television Networks, original published date April 2, 2021, last updated April 14, 2021, https://www.biography.com/performer/johnny-carson.

5. See note 4, above.

6. B. Hutchison, "'Tonight Show' icon Johnny Carson dies at 69 in 2005," *New York Daily News*, original published date January 24, 2005, last updated January 23, 2017, https://www.nydailynews.com/entertainment/tv/good-night-johnnytv-icon-death-79-leaves-celebrity-pals-article-1.627409.

7. S. Kashner, "Theeeeere's Johnny!" *Vanity Fair*, January 27, 2014, https://archive.vanityfair.com/article/2014/2/theeeeeres-johnny.

8. "Johnny Carson, late-night TV legend, dies at 79," CNN, January 25, 2005, https://www.cnn.com/2005/SHOWBIZ/TV/01/23/carson.obit/index.html.

9. "Longtime host of 'Tonight Show' dies at 79," Today, February 8, 2005, https://www.today.com/popculture/longtime-host-tonight-show-dies-79-2D80555478.

10. "Johnny Carson, king of late-night TV, dies," *Lahontan Valley News*, January 22, 2005, https://www.nevadaappeal.com/news/2005/jan/22/johnny-carson-king-of-late-night-tv-dies/; see note 9, above.

11. See note 6, above.

12. See note 8, above.

13. See note 8, above.

14. "Johnny Carson Biography," https://www.imdb.com/name/nm0001992/bio.

15. See note 14, above.

16. See note 14, above.

17. See note 8, above.

18. "Johnny Carson Biography," https://peoplepill.com/people/johnny-carson-1; see note 7, above; see note 9, above; see note 14, above;

19. See note 7, above; see note 9, above; see "Johnny Carson Biography," note 18, above.

20. See note 7, above.

21. "Johnny Carson felt guilty about smoking," Today, January 26, 2005, https://www.today.com/popculture/johnny-carsen-felt-guilty-about-smoking-wbna6871828.

22. "Johnny Carson—Quitting Smoking," https://anecdotage.com/anecdotes/johnny-carson-quitting-smoking.

23. See note 22, above.

24. See note 10, above; see note 11, above; see note 14, above; see "Johnny Carson Biography," note 18, above; see note 21, above.

25. "Death certificate shows Johnny Carson died in hospital, not Malibu home," February 9, 2005, https://alt.obituaries.narkive.com/6bn2OnKK/death-certificate-shows-johnny-carson-died-in-hospital-not-malibu-home; "Johnny Carson Obituary," http://www.legacy.com/ns/johnny-carson-obituary/3075763; "Johnny Carson Biography," https://biography.yourdictionary.com/johnny-carson; "Death Certificate—Johnny Carson," https://www.findadeath.com/johnny-carson/; "Quadruple Bypass Surgery Performed on Johnny Carson," Chicago Tribune, March 25, 1999, https://www.chicagotribune.com/news/ct-xpm-1999-03-25-9903260051-story.

html; see note 1, above; see note 5, above; see note 6, above; see note 9, above; see "Johnny Carson Biography," note 18, above.

26. "Johnny Carson, 30-Year 'Tonight' Host, Dies at 79," National Public Radio, January 23, 2005, https://www.npr.org/templates/story/story. php?storyid=4463098; see note 4, above; see note 8, above; see "Death Certificate—Johnny Carson," note 25, above; see "Johnny Carson Obituary," note 25, above.

27. See note 8, above; see "Johnny Carson Obituary," note 28, above; see "Johnny Carson, 30-Year 'Tonight' Host, Dies at 79," note 26, above.

28. See note 14, above.

29. See "Johnny Carson Biography," note 18, above; see "Death Certificate—Johnny Carson," note 25, above.

30. See "Johnny Carson Biography," note 18, above.

31. See note 5, above; see note 14, above; see "Johnny Carson Biography," note 18, above.

32. See note 31, above.

33. See "Quadruple Bypass Surgery Performed on Johnny Carson," note 25, above.

34. See note 8, above; see note 29, above.

35. See "Death Certificate—Johnny Carson," note 32, above.

36. See note 35, above.

37. "More details released in death of Johnny Carson," original published date February 10, 2005, last updated February 11, 2005, https://www.wistv.com/story/2928916/more-details-released-in-death-of-johnny-carson/; "Carson died in Cedars-Sinai," United Press International, January 27, 2005, https://www.upi. com/Entertainment_News/2005/01/27/Carson-died-in-Cedars-Sinai/71621106836975/; see note 1, above; see note 6, above; see Johnny Carson, king of late-night TV, dies," note 10, above; see note 21, above; see "Johnny Carson Obituary," note 25, above; see note 34, above.

38. See note 4, above; see note 6, above; see "Johnny Carson, king of late-night TV, dies," note 10, above; see "Johnny Carson Obituary,"

note 25, above; see "Johnny Carson, 30-Year 'Tonight' Host, Dies at 79," note 26, above; see note 29, above; see "Carson died in Cedars-Sinai," and "More details released in death of Johnny Carson," note 37, above.

39. See "Johnny Carson Biography," note 18, above; see "Carson died in Cedars-Sinai," note 37, above.

40. See "Death certificate shows Johnny Carson died in hospital, not Malibu home," note 25, above.

41. See note 35, above; see "More details released in death of Johnny Carson," note 37, above; see note 40, above.

42. "Johnny Carson Biography," https://www.thefamouspeople.com/profiles/john-william-carson-1977.php; see note 1, above; see note 4, above; see note 8, above; see note 10, above; see note 14, above; see "Johnny Carson Biography," note 18, above; see "Johnny Carson Obituary" and "Johnny Carson Biography," note 25, above.

43. See note 42, above.

44. See note 42, above.

45. See note 4, above; see note 8, above; see "Johnny Carson, king of late-night TV, dies," note 10, above; see note 14, above; see "Johnny Carson Biography," note 18, above; see "Johnny Carson Obituary" and "Johnny Carson Biography," note 25, above; see "More details released in death of Johnny Carson," note 37, above; see "Johnny Carson Biography," note 42, above.

46. See note 1, above; see note 4, above; see note 8, above; see naote 14, above; see "Johnny Carson Biography," note 18, above; see "Johnny Carson Obituary," and "Johnny Carson Biography," note 25, above.

47. See note 1, above; see note 4, above; see note 8, above; see note 10, above; see note 14, above; see Johnny Carson Biography," note 18, above; see "Johnny Carson Biography," note 25, above; see "Johnny Carson Biography," note 42, above.

48. See note 14, above; see "Johnny Carson Biography," note 18, above.

49. See note 8, above; see note 10, above; see note 14, above; see "Johnny Carson Biography," note 18, above; see "Johnny Carson Obituary"

and "Johnny Carson Biography," note 25, above; see "Johnny Carson Biography," note 42, above.

50. See note 4, above; see note 8, above; see "Johnny Carson, king of late-night TV, dies," note 10, above; see note 14, above; see "Johnny Carson Biography," note 18, above; see "Johnny Carson Obituary," note 25, above.

51. See note 14, above; see "Johnny Carson Biography," note 18, above; see "Johnny Carson Obituary," note 25, above.

52. See note 1, above; see note 7, above; see note 8, above; see note 14, above; see "Johnny Carson Biography," note 18, above; see Johnny Carson Obituary," and "Johnny Carson Biography," note 25, above; see "Johnny Carson Biography," note 42, above.

53. See note 1, above; see note 10, above; see note 14, above.

54. See note 1, above; see "Johnny Carson, king of late-night TV, dies," note 10, above; see note 18, above; see "Johnny Carson Biography," note 25, above; see "Johnny Carson Biography," note 42, above.

55. See note 9, above; see "Johnny Carson Biography," note 42, above; see note 50, above.

56. See note 55, above.

57. See note 14, above.

58. "The Tonight Show Starring Johnny Carson Trivia," https://www.imdb.com/title/tt0055708/trivia; see note 1, above; see note 10, above; see note 14, above.

59. See "Johnny Carson Biography," note 18, above; see "The Tonight Show Starring Johnny Carson Trivia," note 58, above.

60. See note 7, above; see note 14, above.

61. See note 14, above.

62. See note 14, above.

63. See note 14, above.

64. See note 1, above; see "Johnny Carson, king of late-night TV, dies," note 10, above; see note 14, above; see note 30, above; see "Johnny Carson Obituary," note 25, above; see "Johnny Carson, 30-Year 'Tonight' Host, Dies at 79," note 26, above.

65. See "The Tonight Show Starring Johnny Carson Trivia," note 58, above.

66. See note 30, above; see note 65, above.

67. See note 10, above.

68. "Johnny Carson: 'King of Late Night,' A Man Unknown," National Public Radio, May 13, 2012, https://www.npr.org/2012/05/13/152496256/johnny-carson-king-of-late-night-a-man-unknown; see note 30, above; see "Johnny Carson Biography," note 42, above; see note 60, above.

69. See note 8, above.

70. See "Johnny Carson: 'King of Late Night,' A Man Unknown," note 68, above.

71. See note 30, above.

72. See note 6, above; see note 9, above; see "Johnny Carson Obituary," note 25, above; see note 35, above; see note 48, above.

73. See note 9, above; see "Johnny Carson Obituary," note 25, above; see note 35, above.

74. "Johnny Carson Dies From Common Lung Disease," January 24, 2005, https://www.webmd.com/smoking-cessation/news/20050124/johnny-carson-dies-from-common-lung-disease; "Smoking and COPD," US Centers for Disease Control and Prevention, https://www.cdc.gov/tobacco/campaign/tips/diseases/copd.html.

75. See "Smoking and COPD," note 74, above.

76. See note 74, above.

77. See Johnny Carson Dies From Common Lung Disease," note 74, above.

78. See note 77, above.

79. See note 77, above.

80. See note 77, above.

81. See note 77, above.

82. See note 74, above.

83. See note 77, above.

84. See note 6, above; see note 8, above; see note 9, above.

85. See note 84, above.

86. See note 6, above; see note 9, above.

26. *Ken Lay*

1. J. Jelter, "Enron's Ken Lay dead at 64," Market Watch, July 5, 2006, https://www.marketwatch.com/story/enron-founder-ken-lay-dies-at-64; "Kenneth Lay Biography," https://www.imdb.com/name/nm1674594/bio; "Ken Lay 1942 -," https://www.referenceforbusiness.com/biography/F-L/Lay-Ken-1942.html.

2. V. Bajaj and K. Eichenwald, "Kenneth L. Lay, 64, Enron Founder and Symbol of Corporate Excess, Dies," the *New York Times*, July 6, 2006, https://www.nytimes.com/2006/07/06/business/06lay.html; J. W. Peters and S. Romero, "Enron Founder Dies Before Sentencing," the *New York Times*, July 5, 2006, https://www.nytimes.com/2006/07/05/business/05cnd-lay.html; see J. Jelter, note 1, above.

3. "Federal Jury Convicts Former Enron Chief Executive Ken Lay, Jeff Skilling On Fraud, Conspiracy And Related Charges," Department of Justice, May 25, 2006, https://www.justice.gov/archive/opa/pr/2006/May/06_crm_328.html; see J. Jelter, note 1, above; see J. W. Peters and S. Romero, note 2, above.

4. "Autopsy report—Kenneth Lay," http://www.autopsyfiles.org/reports/Other/lay,%20kenneth_report.pdf.

5. See note 4, above.

6. See note 4, above.

7. See note 4, above.

8. See J. Jelter, note 1, above; see J. W. Peters and S. Romero, note 2, above; see note 4, above.

9. S. Horsley, "Enron Founder Kenneth Lay Dies of Heart Attack," National Public Radio, July 5, 2006, https://www.npr.org/templates/story/story.php?storyId=5534705; P. Bondarenko, "Enron scandal," Brittanica, https://www.britannica.com/event/Enron-scandal#ref1254069.

10. See note 4, above.

11. See note 4, above.

12. See note 4, above.

13. See note 4, above.

14. See note 4, above.

15. See note 4, above.

16. See note 4, above.

17. See note 4, above.

18. See note 4, above.

19. See note 4, above.

20. See note 4, above.

21. See note 4, above.

22. See note 4, above.

23. See note 4, above.

24. See note 4, above.

25. See note 4, above.

26. See note 4, above.

27. See note 4, above.

28. See note 4, above.

29. See note 4, above.

30. See note 4, above.

31. D. K. Molina and V. J. M. DiMaio, "Normal organ weights in men: part I—the heart," *Am J Forensic Med Pathol* 33(4) (2012): 362–67; N. T. Srinvasan and R. J. Schilling, "Sudden cardiac death and arrhythmias," *Arrhythm Electrophysiol Rev.* 7(2) (2018): 111–17.

32. H. A. Milman, "Elvis Presley," in *Forensics: The Science Behind the Deaths of Famous People* (Bloomington, Indiana: Xlibris, 2020) 61–72.

33. "Sudden Cardiac Death (Sudden Cardiac Arrest)," Cleveland Clinic, https://my.clevelandclinic.org/health/diseases/17522-sudden-cardiac-death-sudden-cardiac-arrest; see note 4, above.

34. See note 4, above.

35. "Heartburn or heart attack: When to worry," Mayo Clinic, https://www.mayoclinic.org/diseases-conditions/heartburn/in-depth/heartburn-gerd/art-20046483.

36. See note 35, above.

37. See note 35, above.

38. See note 4, above.

39. See note 4, above.

40. See note 4, above.

41. See note 32, above.

42. See note 32, above.

43. See note 32, above.

44. See note 4, above; see note 32, above.

45. See note 44, above.

46. See note 44, above.

47. See note 32, above.

48. See note 4, above.

49. A. Dunn and L. Brubaker Calkins, "A bittersweet legacy," *Sun-Sentinel*, https://www.sun-sentinel.com/news/fl-xpm-2006-07-06-0607051023-story.html; see J. Jelter, note 1, above; see V. Bajaj and K. Eichenwald, note 2, above.

50. D. Teather, "Kenneth Lay," https://www.theguardian.com/business/2006/jul/05/corporatefraud.enron; see J. Jelter and "Ken Lay 1942 -," note 1, above; see J. W. Peters and S. Romero, note 2, above; see A. Dunn and L. Brubaker Calkins, note 49, above.

51. See A. Dunn and L. Brubaker Calkins, note 49, above.

52. See D. Teather, note 50, above.

53. See "Ken Lay 1942 -," note 1, above.

54. See J. Jelter, note 1, above; see note 51, above; see note 53, above.

55. See J. Jelter, note 1, above; see note 51, above; see note 52, above.

56. See note 55, above.

57. See J. Jelter, note 1, above; see note 51, above.

58. See V. Bajaj and K. Eichenwald, note 2, above; see note 51, above; see note 53, above.

59. See note 52, above; see note 53, above.

60. See V. Bajaj and K. Eichenwald, note 2, above; see note 51, above; see note 52, above.

61. C. W. Thomas, "The Rise and Fall of Enron," *Journal of Accountancy*, April 1, 2002, https://www.journalofaccountancy.com/issues/2002/apr/theriseandfallofenron.html; see J. Jelter, note 1, above; see S. Horsley, note 9, above; see note 60, above.

62. See P. Bondarenko, note 9, above; see note 53, above.

63. See P. Bondarenko, note 9, above; see C. W. Thomas, note 61, above.

64. See C. W. Thomas, note 61, above.

65. See note 63, above.

66. See note 51, above.

67. See note 64, above.

68. See note 64, above.

69. See P. Bondarenko, note 9, above.

70. See note 64, above.

71. See note 53, above.

72. "Timeline: Ken Lay and the Arc of Enron," National Public Radio, https://www.npr.org/2006/07/05/5535821/timeline-ken-lay-and-the-arc-of-enron; see note 53, above; see note 64, above.

73. See note 64, above.

74. "SEC Charles Kenneth L. Lay, Enron's Former Chairman and Chief Executive Officer, with Fraud and Insider Trading," July 8, 2004, https://www.sec.gov/news/press/2004-94.htm; see J. Jelter, note 1, above; see note 53, above.

75. See note 64, above; see note 69, above; see "Timeline: Ken Lay and the Arc of Enron," note 72, above.

76. See note 51, above; see note 75, above.

77. See note 75, above.

78. See note 53, above.

79. See note 53, above.

80. See note 53, above; see "Timeline: Ken Lay and the Arc of Enron," note 72, above.

81. See note 53, above.

82. See note 53, above.

83. See note 52, above; see note 53, above.

84. See note 53, above; see "SEC Charles Kenneth L. Lay, Enron's Former Chairman and Chief Executive Officer, with Fraud and Insider Trading," note 74, above.

85. "Enron," FBI, https://www.fbi.gov/history/famous-cases/enron.

86. See J. Jelter, note 1, above; see "Federal Jury Convicts Former Enron Chief Executive Ken Lay, Jeff Skilling On Fraud, Conspiracy And Related Charges," note 3, above; see "Timeline: Ken Lay and the Arc of Enron," note 72, above.

87. See S. Horsley, note 9, above.

88. See note 87, above.

89. See note 87, above.

90. See note 87, above.

91. See note 87, above.

92. See note 87, above.

93. See note 53, above.

94. See V. Bajaj and K. Eichenwald, note 2, above.

95. "Enron Founder Kenneth Lay Dies," Wave News, July 5, 2006, https://www.wave3.com/story/5114824/enron-founder-kenneth-lay-dies/; see note 52, above; see note 57, above; see note 87, above.

96. *Wall Street* Quotes, https://www.imdb.com/title/tt0094291/quotes/qt0393950.

97. *Wall Street* Quotes, Rotten Tomatoes, https://www.rottentomatoes.com/m/wall_street/quotes/.

98. See note 94, above.

99. See note 51, above.

100. See note 51, above.

101. See "Enron Founder Kenneth Lay Dies," note 95, above.

102. See note 101, above.

103. K. Murphy, "Judge Throws Out Kenneth Lay's Conviction," the *New York Times*, October 18, 2006, https://www.nytimes.com/2006/10/18/business/18enron.html; "Ken Lay's conviction tossed out by judge," CNN, October 18, 2006, https://money.cnn.com/2006/10/17/news/newsmakers/ken_lay/index.htm.

104. See "Ken Lay's conviction tossed out by judge," note 103, above.

27. Alexander Litvinenko

1. R. Owen, "The Litvinenko Inquiry: Report into the death of Alexander Litvinenko," January 21, 2016, https://assets.publishing. service.gov.uk/government/uploads/system/uploads/attachment_ data/file/493860/The-Litvinenko-Inquiry-H-C-695-web.pdf; "Alexander Litvinenko called suspect 'a good friend', inquiry told," BBC, February 23, 2015, https://www.bbc.com/news/uk-31595540; D. Staunton, "The life and death of Alexander Litvinenko," *Irish Times*, January 21, 2016, https://www.irishtimes.com/news/ world/uk/the-life-and-death-of-alexander-litvinenko-1.2506037; "Alexander Litvinenko: Profile of murdered Russian spy," BBC, January 21, 2016, https://www.bbc.com/news/uk-19647226; G. Faulconbridge and M. Holden, "Russia was behind Litvinenko assassination, European court finds," Reuters, September 21, 2021, https://www.reuters.com/world/european-court-rules-russia-was-behind-litvinenko-killing-2021-09-21/; "Alexander Litvinenko Biography," https://www.thefamouspeople.com/profiles/alexander-litvinenko-40953.php.

2. See R. Owen and "Alexander Litvinenko: Profile of murdered Russian spy," note 1, above.

3. See R. Owen, note 1, above.

4. L. Harding, "Alexander Litvinenko: the man who solved his own murder," the *Guardian*, January 19, 2016, https://www.theguardian. com/world/2016/jan/19/alexander-litvenenko-the-man-who-solved-his-own-murder; see note 3, above.

5. "Five facts about poison victim Mario Scaramella," Reuters, January 20, 2007, https://www.reuters.com/article/us-britain-poisoning-scaramella/five-facts-about-poison-victim-mario-scaramella-idUSL0178789120061201; "Timeline: Alexander Litvinenko death case," BBC, January 27, 2015, https://www.bbc.com/news/uk-30929940; see "Alexander Litvinenko called suspect 'a good friend', inquiry told" and "Alexander Litvinenko: Profile of murdered Russian spy," note 1, above; see note 4, above.

6. See note 3, above; see "Five facts about poison victim Mario Scaramella," and "Timeline: Alexander Litvinenko death case," note 5, above.

7. See note 3, above.

8. See note 3, above.

9. See D. Staunton, note 1, above; see L. Harding, note 4, above; see note 7, above.

10. See "Timeline: Alexander Litvinenko death case," note 5, above; see note 9, above.

11. See note 4, above.

12. See note 4, above.

13. See note 3, above.

14. See note 4, above.

15. See note 4, above.

16. See "Alexander Litvinenko: Profile of murdered Russian spy," note 1, above; see note 9, above.

17. See note 4, above.

18. See note 3, above.

19. See note 4, above.

20. See note 3, above.

21. See D. Staunton, note 1, above; see note 2, above; see "Timeline: Alexander Litvinenko death case," note 5, above.

22. See note 3, above.

23. See note 3, above.

24. See note 3, above.

25. See note 3, above.

26. See note 3, above.

27. See note 21, above.

28. See note 21, above.

29. See note 3, above.

30. See note 3, above.

31. See note 3, above.

32. See note 3, above.

33. See note 3, above.

34. See note 3, above.

35. See note 3, above.

36. R. S. Hoffman, "Thallium toxicity and the role of Prussian blue in therapy," *Toxicol Rev* 22(1) (2003): 29–40; see note 10, above.

37. P. Cvjetko, I. Cvjetko, et al., "Thallium toxicity in humans," *Arh Hig Rada Toksikol* 61(1) (2010): 111–119.

38. See note 37, above.

39. "Everyday Uses of Thallium You Didn't Know About," September 17, 2018, https://noahchemicals.com/blog/everyday-uses-of-thallium-you-didnt-know-about/.

40. See note 37, above; see note 39, above.

41. See note 3, above.

42. See "Alexander Litvinenko: Profile of murdered Russian spy," note 1, above; see note 3, above; see "Timeline: Alexander Litvinenko death case," note 5, above.

43. See note 3, above.

44. See note 3, above.

45. See note 4, above.

46. See note 4, above; see "Timeline: Alexander Litvinenko death case," note 5, above.

47. See note 4, above.

48. See note 3, above.

49. See note 3, above; see "Timeline: Alexander Litvinenko death case," note 5, above.

50. See note 3, above.

51. "Poison, spies and businessmen: The Litvinenko murder case 15 years on," https://www.dw.com/en/poison-spies-and-businessmen-the-litvinenko-murder-case-15-years-on/a-59910692; M. Holden, "Litvinenko autopsy was world's most dangerous, UK inquiry hears," Reuters, https://www.reuters.com/article/us-britain-russia-litvinenko/litvinenko-autopsy-was-worlds-most-dangerous-uk-inquiry-hears-idUSKBN0L11LU20150128; see note 46, above.

52. See note 4, above.

678

53. "Russia behind Litvinenko murder, rules European rights court," BBC, September 21, 2021, https://www.bbc.com/news/world-58837572; see note 46, above; see "Poison, spies and businessmen: The Litvinenko murder case 15 years on," note 51, above.

54. See "Alexander Litvinenko: Profile of murdered Russian spy," note 1, above.

55. See note 3, above.

56. See note 3, above.

57. See note 3, above; see note 54, above.

58. See note 3, above.

59. "Litvinenko Post-Mortem "Most Dangerous Ever," Sky News, January 28, 2015, https://news.sky.com/story/litvinenko-post-mortem-most-dangerous-ever-10373601; see "Alexander Litvinenko called suspect 'a good friend', inquiry told," note 1, above; see note 54, above.

60. See note 3, above; see note 59, above.

61. See note 3, above.

62. See note 3, above.

63. See note 3, above.

64. See note 3, above.

65. See note 3, above.

66. J. Harrison, T. Fell, et al., "The polonium-210 poisoning of Mr. Alexander Litvinenko," *J Radiol Prot* 37(1) (2017): 266–78 (2017); see "Russia behind Litvinenko murder, rules European rights court," note 53, above.

67. See note 3, above; see J. Harrison, T. Fell, et al., note 66, above.

68. See note 67, above.

69. See note 3, above; see "Litvinenko Post-Mortem 'Most Dangerous Ever," note 59, above.

70. See note 68, above.

71. See note 3, above.

72. See note 68, above.

73. See note 3, above; see "Russia behind Litvinenko murder, rules European rights court," note 53, above.

74. See note 3, above.

75. See note 3, above.

76. See ntoe 68, above.

77. See note 3, above.

78. See note 3, above.

79. See note 3, above.

80. See note 3, above.

81. See note 3, above.

82. See note 3, above.

83. See note 3, above.

84. S. Neuman, "Russia Fatally Poisoned a Prominent Defector in London, a Court Concludes," National Public Radio, September 22, 2021, https://www.npr.org/2021/09/21/1039224996/russia-alexander-litvinenko-european-court-human-rights-putin; see D. Staunton and G. Faulconbridge and M. Holden, note 1, above; see note 49, above.

85. See M. Holden, note 51, above.

86. See D. Staunton and "Alexander Litvinenko Biography," note 1, above; see note 2, above.

87. See note 3, above.

88. See note 3, above.

89. See note 3, above.

90. See note 3, above.

91. See note 3, above.

92. See note 3, above.

93. See "Alexander Litvinenko Biography," note 1, above; see note 3, above.

94. See note 86, above.

95. See note 93, above.

96. See note 93, above.

97. See note 93, above.

98. See note 93, above.

99. See note 3, above.

[100.] See note 3, above.

[101.] See note 93, above.

[102.] See note 3, above.

[103.] See note 93, above.

[104.] See note 3, above.

[105.] See note 3, above.

[106.] See "Poison, spies and businessmen: The Litvinenko murder case 15 years on," note 51, above; see note 54, above; see note 93, above.

[107.] See note 3, above.

[108.] See note 3, above.

[109.] See "Poison, spies and businessmen: The Litvinenko murder case 15 years on," note 51, above; see note 93, above.

[110.] See note 93, above.

[111.] See Alexander Litvinenko Biography," note 1, above; see "Poison, spies and businessmen: The Litvinenko murder case 15 years on," note 51, above; see note 54, above.

[112.] See note 3, above; see "Poison, spies and businessmen: The Litvinenko murder case 15 years on," note 51, above; see note 54, above.

[113.] See note 3, above.

[114.] See D. Staunton, note 1, above; see note 3, above; see note 111, above.

[115.] See note 3, above.

[116.] See note 3, above.

[117.] See D. Staunton, note 1, above; see note 109, above.

[118.] S. Cotton, "Litvinenko poisoning: polonium explained," January 21, 2016, https://theconversation.com/litvinenko-poisoning-explained-53514; L. Harding, "Alexander Litvinenko and the most radioactive towel in history," the *Guardian*, March 6, 2016, https://www.theguardian.com/world/2016/mar/06/alexander-litvinenko-and-the-most-radioactive-towel-in-history.

[119.] A. Langham-Putrow, "A Matter of Elemental Facts: Polonium," September 19, 2019, https://www.continuum.umm.edu/2019/09/a-matter-of-elemental-facts-0lonium/; see note 3, above; see S. Cotton, note 118, above.

120. See S. Cotton, note 118, above.

121. See note 120, above.

122. See note 120, above.

123. See note 119, above.

124. See note 3, above.

125. See G. Faulconbridge and M. Holden, note 1, above; see "Poison, spies and businessmen: The Litvinenko murder case 15 years on," note 51, above; see note 73, above.

126. See note 3, above.

127. See G. Faulconbridge and M. Holden, note 1, above; see note 3, above.

128. See note 3, above.

129. See note 3, above.

130. See note 127, above.

131. See note 3, above.

132. See note 3, above.

133. See note 3, above.

134. See note 127, above.

135. See note 2, above.

136. See note 3, above.

137. See note 3, above.

138. See note 3, above.

139. See note 3, above.

140. See note 3, above; see L. Harding, note 118, above.

141. See L. Harding, note 4, above; see note 140, above.

142. See note 3, above; see "Poison, spies and businessmen: The Litvinenko murder case 15 years on," note 51, above.

143. See note 3, above.

144. See note 3, above.

145. "Russia was responsible for assassination of Alexander Litvinenko in the UK," European Court of Human Rights, September 21, 2021;

see "Poison, spies and businessmen: The Litvinenko murder case 15 years on," note 51, above.

146. S. Neuman, "Russia Fatally Poisoned a Prominent Defector in London, a Court Concludes," National Public Radio, September 22, 2021, https://www.npr.org/2021/09/21/1039224996/russia-alexander-litvinenko-european-court-human-rights-putin; see "Russia behind Litvinenko murder, rules European rights court," note 53, above; see note 145, above.

147. See note 3, above.

148. See note 3, above.

149. J. Daniszewski, "Lawmaker Found Shot to Death in a Moscow Park," *Los Angeles Times*, August 22, 2002, https://www.latimes.com/archives/la-xpm-2002-aug-22-fg-vlad22-story.html; see note 3, above.

150. See note 3, above.

151. See note 3, above.

152. L. Harding, "Russian FSB hit squad poisoned Alexei Navalny, report says," the *Guardian*, December 14, 2020, https://www.theguardian.com/world/2020/dec/14/russian-fsb-hit-squad-poisoned-alexei-navalny-report-says; "Hostage crisis in Moscow theater," History, A&E Television Networks, original published date November 24, 2009, last updated October 26, 2020, https://www.history.com/this-day-in-history/hostage-crisis-in-moscos-theater; B. Little, "How Opioids Were Used as Weapons During the Moscow Theater Hostage Crisis," History, https://www.history.com/news/opioid-chemical-weapons-moscow-theater-hostage-crisis; R. Nelson, "The poison-tipped umbrella: the death of Georgi Markov in 1978-archive," the *Guardian*, September 9, 2020, https://www.theguardian.com/world/from-the-archive-blog/2020/sep/09/georgi-markov-killed-poisoned-umbrella-london-1978; M. Weaver, "Poisoned umbrellas and polonium: Russian-linked UK deaths," the *Guardian*, March 6, 2018, https://www.theguardian.com/world/2018/mar-06/poisoned-umbrellas-and-polonium-russian-linked-uk-deaths; S. Kesteven and E. Stott, "How writer Georgi Markov was assassinated with

a poison-laced umbrella," May 3, 2021, https://www.abc.net.au/news/2021-05-04/georgi-markov-bulgarian-dissident-umbrella-assassination/100084600; G. Corera, "Salisbury poisoning: What did the attack mean for the UK and Russia?" BBC, March 4, 2020, https://www.bbc.com/news/uk-51722301.

28.   Evel Knievel

[1] K. Eschner, "Risk-Taker Evel Knievel Was a Big Proponent of Wearing a Helmet," *Smithsonian* magazine, November 30, 2016, https://www.smithsonianmag.com/smart-news/risk-taker-evel-knievel-was-big-proponent-wearing-helmet-180961246/.

[2] "Evel Knievel's 5 Greatest Stunts," https://www.history.co.uk/shows/evel-knievel-live/articles/evel-knievels-5-greatests-stunts; "Evel Knievel's 'last' jump," the *Week*, January 8, 2015, https://theweek.com/articles/484085/evel-knievels-last-jump; "Evel Knievel Biography," A&E Television Networks, original published date April 2, 2014, last updated July 28, 2020, https://www.biography.com/performer/evel-knievel.

[3] See "Evel Knievel's 'last' jump," note 2, above.

[4] See note 3, above.

[5] K. Dalton, "How Many Bones Did Evel Knievel Break in His Daredevil Career?" July 11, 2020, https://www.sportscasting.com/how-many-bones-did-evel-knievel-break-in-his-daredevil-career/; see note 3, above.

[6] See note 3, above.

[7] M. Carlson, "Evel Knievel," the *Guardian*, December 3, 2007, https://www.theguardian.com/news/2007/dec/03/guardianobituaries.usa1.

[8] "Evel Knievel - Wembley Stadium May 26, 1975," https://www.youtube.com/watch?v=j2ubg7Z5-x0; see note 3, above.

[9] See "Evel Knievel Biography," note 2, above; see note 8, above.

[10] C. Ross, "Evel Knievel and Wide World of Sports: A winning combination," ABC Sports, https://www.espn.com/abcsports/wwos/e_knievel.html; J. Sablich, "Evel Knievel's Last Jump:

What Made Him Finally Quit?" History, July 6, 2019, https://www.history.com/news/evel-knievel-motorcycle-jump; A. Ingram, "Freeze Frame: Evel Knievel chases Greyhound record," Hagerty, October 27, 2021, https://www.hagerty.co.uk/articles/automotive-history/freeze-frame-evel-knievel-chases-greyhound-record/; see K. Dalton, note 5, above; see note 9, above.

[11.] See note 3, above.

[12.] See note 3, above.

[13.] See note 3, above.

[14.] "Evel Knievel," May 17, 2019, https://fampeople.com/cat-evel-knievel?amp; see note 2, above; see Ross, note 10, above.

[15.] See note 3, above.

[16.] N. Frost, "What Drove Evel Knievel to Keep Battering His Body?" History, July 6, 2019, https://www.history.com/news/why-evel-knievel-continued-after-injuries-caesars-wembley-snake-river; J. Sablich, "Evel Knievel's Last Jump: What Made Him Finally Quit?" History, July 6, 2019, https://www.history.com/news/evel-knievel-motorcycle-jump; see note 3, above; see K. Dalton, note 5, above; see "Evel Knievel," note 14, above.

[17.] See note 3, above; see C. Ross, note 10, above; see J. Sablich, note 16, above.

[18.] "Daredevil Evel Knievel dies at 69," *Hollywood Reporter*, December 1, 2007, https://www.hollywoodreporter.com/business/business-news/daredevil-evel-knievel-dies-at-156183/; see "Evel Knievel's 5 Greatest Stunts," and "Evel Knievel Biography," note 2, above; see K. Dalton, note 5, above.

[19.] A. Ingram, "Freeze Frame: Evel Knievel chases Greyhound record," Hagerty, October 27, 2021, https://www.hagerty.co.uk/articles/automotive-history/freeze-frame-evel-knievel-chases-greyhound-record/; see "Evel Knievel's 5 Greatest Stunts" and "Evel Knievel Biography," note 2, above; see "Evel Knievel," note 14, above; see J. Sablich, note 16, above.

[20.] See "Evel Knievel's 5 Greatest Stunts," note 2, above.

21. R. Severo, "Evel Knievel, 69, Daredevil on a Motorcycle, Dies," the *New York Times*, December 1, 2008, https://www.nytimes.com/2007/12/01/us/01knievel.html; see note 1, above.

22. "Most broken bones in a lifetime," Guinness World Records, https://www.guinnessworldrecords.com/world-records/most-broken-bones-in-a-lifetime; "Evel Knievel Biography," https://www.imdb.com/name/nm0460773/bio; "On This Day: Fearless American stuntman Evel Knievel dies," November 29, 2020, https://thenewdaily.com.au/news/world/2020/11/29/on-this-day-evel-knievel/; "Death of a daredevil: The extraordinary, magnificent life of Evel Knievel," *Independent*, December 2, 2007, https://www.independent.co.uk/news/world/americas/death-of-a-daredevil-the-extraordinary-magnificent-life-of-evel-knievel-761793.html; see K. Dalton, note 5, above; see note 7, above; see R. Severno, note 21, above.

23. "Evel Knievel dies at 69; had long been in failing health," ESPN, original published date November 30, 2007, last updated December 2, 2007, https://www.espn.com/espn/news/story?id=3135532; see "Evel Knievel Biography," note 2, above; see "Evel Knievel," note 14, above; see "Daredevil Evel Knievel dies at 69," note 18, above; see R. Severo, note 21, above; see "Evel Knievel Biography," and "Death of a daredevil: The extraordinary, magnificent life of Evel Knievel," note 22, above.

24. See "Evel Knievel Biography," note 2, above; see "Evel Knievel," note 14, above; see "Daredevil Evel Knievel dies at 69," note 18, above; see "Death of a daredevil: The extraordinary, magnificent life of Evel Knievel," note 22, above; see "Evel Knievel dies at 69; had long been in failing health," note 23, above.

25. See "Evel Knievel," note 14, above.

26. "Evel Knievel Biography," https://peoplepill.com/people/evel-knievel; see "Evel Knievel Biography," note 2, above; see "Daredevil Evel Knievel dies at 69," note 18, above; see R. Severo, note 21, above; see "Death of a daredevil: The extraordinary, magnificent

life of Evel Knievel," note 22, above; see "Evel Knievel dies at 69; had long been in failing health," note 23, above.

27. P. Jordan, "Evel Knievel's last interview, given days before he died," March 27, 2009, https://www. strangefamousrecords.com/blogs/b-dolan-blog/evel-knievels-last-interview-given-days-before-he-died/.

28. D. Brinkley, "The Book of Evel (Knievel)," *Vanity Fair*, November 30, 2007, https://www.vanityfair.com/news/2007/11/knievel200711; see "On This Day: Fearless American stuntman Evel Knievel dies," note 22, above.

29. See note 27, above; see D. Brinkley, note 28, above.

30. See "Evel Knievel dies at 69; had long been in failing health," note 23, above.

31. See "Evel Knievel Biography," note 2, above; see "Daredevil Evel Knievel dies at 69," note 18, above; see "Evel Knievel Biography," note 26, above; see note 30, above.

32. See "Daredevil Evel Knievel dies at 69," note 18, above; see R. Severo, note 21, above; see note 25, above; see "Evel Knievel Biography," note 26, above; see note 30, above.

33. "Evel Knievel," https://evil-knievel.com; see note 7, above; see C. Ross, note 10, above; see N. Frost, note 16, above; see "Evel Knievel Biography," note 22, above; see note 25, above; see note 26, above.

34. See note 7, above; see N. Frost, note 16, above; see "Evel Knievel Biography," note 22, above; see note 25, above; see note 26, above; see "Evel Knievel," note 33, above.

35. See note 7, above; see C. Ross, note 10, above; see "Daredevil Evel Knievel dies at 69," note 18, above; see R. Severo, note 21, above; see note 25, above; see "Evel Knievel Biography," note 26, above; see note 30, above; see "Evel Knievel," note 33, above.

36. See "Evel Knievel Biography," note 2, above; see note 7, above; see N. Frost, note 16, above; see R. Severo, note 21, above.

37. See N. Frost, note 16, above; see R. Severo, note 21, above.

38. See "Death of a daredevil: The extraordinary, magnificent life of Evel Knievel," note 22, above; see "Evel Knievel Biography," note 26, above; see "Evel Knievel," note 33, above.

39. See C. Ross, note 10, above; see "Daredevil Evel Knievel dies at 69," and "Evel Knievel Biography," note 26, above; see note 30, above; see note 36, above.

40. See "Evel Knievel Biography," note 2, above; see note 7, above; see C. Ross, note 10, above; see N. Frost, note 16, above; see "Death of a daredevil: The extraordinary, magnificent life of Evel Knievel" and "Evel Knievel Biography," note 22, above; see "Evel Knievel Biography," note 26, above; see "Evel Knievel," note 33, above.

41. See note 30, above.

42. See note 30, above.

43. See note 7, above; see C. Ross, note 10, above; see N. Frost, note 16, above; see note 31, above; see "Evel Knievel," note 33, above.

44. See "Evel Knievel Biography," note 2, above; see note 7, above; see note 38, above.

45. See "Evel Knievel Biography," note 2, above; see "Daredevil Evel Knievel dies at 69," note 18, above; see note 30, above; see "Evel Knievel," note 33, above; see note 37, above.

46. See note 7, above; see N. Frost, note 16, above; see R. Severo, note 21, above; see note 25, above; see note 31, above.

47. See note 7, above; see "Evel Knievel Biography," note 26, above.

48. See "Evel Knievel Biography," note 2, above; see K. Dalton, note 5, above; see R. Severo, note 21, above; see note 47, above.

49. See "Evel Knievel Biography," note 26, above.

50. See "Evel Knievel Biography," note 2, above; see K. Dalton, note 5, above; see note 37, above; see note 49, above.

51. See note 1, above; see "Evel Knievel Biography," note 2, above; see "Evel Knievel," note 33, above; see note 49, above.

52. See R. Severo, note 21, above.

53. See "Evel Knievel Biography," note 2, above.

54. See note 7, above; see Daredevil Evel Knievel dies at 69," note 18, above; see "Evel Knievel Biography," note 22, above; see "Death of a

daredevil: The extraordinary, magnificent life of Evel Knievel," note 26, above; see note 30, above; see "Evel Knievel," note 33, above; see note 50, above.

55. See note 41, above; see note 53, above.

56. See "Evel Knievel," note 33, above; see note 53, above.

57. See "Evel Knievel," note 33, above; see note 49, above.

58. See note 57, above.

59. See K. Dalton, note 5, above; see note 57, above.

60. See note 57, above.

61. See note 57, above.

62. See note 57, above.

63. See note 27, above.

64. See note 1, above; see K. Dalton, note 5, above; see A. Ingram, note 10, above; see "Evel Knievel," note 33, above; see note 46, above.

65. "Evel Knievel and the Caesar's Palace," https://www.youtube.com/watch?v=cnPZq9rdNEI; see K. Dalton, note 5, above; see note 27, above; see "Evel Knievel," note 33, above.

66. See R. Severo, note 21, above.

67. See note 66, above.

68. See note 49, above; see note 65, above.

69. See note 7, above; see "On This Day: Fearless American stuntman Evel Knievel dies," note 22, above; see note 25, above; see note 49, above.

70. "Evel Knievel jumps snake river canyon," https://www.youtube.com/watch?v=2p1khN1xyBw; see C. Ross, note 10, above; see "On This Day: Fearless American stuntman Evel Knievel dies" and "Death of a daredevil: The extraordinary, magnificent life of Evel Knievel," note 22, above; see note 27, above; see note 46, above.

71. See note 70, above.

72. See note 27, above.

73. See note 49, above.

74. See N. Frost, note 16, above; see note 27, above; see note 53, above.

75. See note 74, above.

76. See J. Sablich, note 10, above.

77. See K. Dalton, note 5, above.

78. See note 27, above.

79. See D. Brinkley, note 28, above.

80. See note 7, above; see note 30, above.

81. See "Daredevil Evel Knievel dies at 69," note 18, above; see note 30, above; see note 76, above.

82. See note 81, above.

83. "Idiopathic Pulmonary Fibrosis," US National Heart, Lung, and Blood Institute, National Institutes of Health, https://www.nhlbi.nih.gov/health-topics/idiopathic-pulmonary-fibrosis.

84. "Idiopathic Pulmonary Fibrosis," Pulmonary Fibrosis Foundation, https://www.pulmonaryfibrosis.org/understanding-pff/types-of-pulmonary-fibrosis/idiopathic-pulmonary-fibrosis; W. Henderson, "The Two Main Types of Pulmonary Fibrosis," May 16, 2017, https://pulmonaryfibrosisnews.com/2017/05/16/two-main-types-pulmonary-fibrosis/; "Pulmonary Fibrosis," Cleveland Clinic, https://my.clevelandclinic.org/health/diseases/10959-pulmonary-fibrosis; S. Watson, "Idiopathic Pulmonary Fibrosis (IPF)," December 7, 2020, https://www.webmd.com/lung/what-is-idiopathic-pulmonary-fibrosis; L. Richeldi, H. R. Collard, et al., "Idiopathic pulmonary fibrosis," *Lancet* 389(10082) (2017): 1941–52; see note 83, above.

85. A. A. Sayf, "What is the mortality rate of idiopathic pulmonary fibrosis (IPF)? July 16, 2021, https://emedicine.medscape.com/article/301226-overview#a3; J. M. Adkins and H. R. Collard, "Idiopathic pulmonary fibrosis," *Semin Respir Crit Care Med* 33(5): 433–39 (2012); J. S. Zolak and J. A. de Andrade, "Idiopathic pulmonary fibrosis," *Immunol Allergy Clin North Am* 32(4) (2012): 473–85; see W. Henderson, "Pulmonary Fibrosis," S. Watson, and L. Richeldi, H. R. Collard, et al., note 84, above.

86. 87. See note 83, above; see "Pulmonary Fibrosis" and "Idiopathic Pulmonary Fibrosis," note 84, above.

87. See note 83, above; see "Pulmonary Fibrosis" and "Idiopathic Pulmonary Fibrosis," and S. Watson, note 84, above.

88. See S. Watson, note 84, above; see J. S. Zolak and J. A. de Andrade, note 85, above.

89. M. R. Berman, "Pulmonary Fibrosis and the End of an Era for Jerry Lewis & the Muscular Dystrophy Association," Medpage Today, August 5, 2011, https:www.medpagetoday.com/popmedicine/celebritydiagnosis/27907.

90. See note 27, above.

91. See note 27, above.

92. See note 53, above.

93. See note 33, above.

94. J. Daven, J. F. O'Conner, et al., "The Consequences of Imitative Behavior in Children: The 'Evel Knievel Syndrome,'" *Pediatrics* 57(3) (1976): 418–19.

95. See "Daredevil Evel Knievel dies at 69," note 18, above; see note 27, above; see note 55, above; see note 66, above.

96. See note 76, above.

97. See "Daredevil Evel Knievel dies at 69," note 18, above; see "Evel Knievel Biography," note 22, above; see note 30, above; see note 37, above.

98. See "Daredevil Evel Knievel dies at 69," note 18, above; see "Evel Knievel Biography," note 22, above; see note 30, above.

99. See note 98, above.

100. See note 1, above; see note 25, above.

101. See note 1, above.

102. See note 1, above.

103. See note 25, above; see note 53, above.

104. See note 25, above.

105. See note 52, above.

106. See note 25, above; see note 49, above.

107. See note 52, above.

29.   Dawn Brancheau

1. "SeaWorld," https://seaworld.com/orlando/.

2. See note 1, above.

3. T. Zimmermann, "The Killer in the Pool," July 30, 2010, https://www.outsideonline.com/outdoor-adventure/environment/killer-pool/; "Orange County Sheriff's Office Investigative Report Case Number 2010-016715," http://da15bdaf715461308003-0c725c907c2d637068751776aeee5fbf.r7.cf1.rackcdn.com/97af2028987a428cb315a357df8e7502_20brancheauorangecountysheriffreport.pdf.

4. "Dawn Brancheau Biography," https://www.thefamouspeople.com/profiles/dawn-brancheau-43343.php; see T. Zimmermann, note 3, above.

5. See note 3, above.

6. "Dawn Brancheau Biography," https://www.imdb.com/name/nm4003369/bio; see T. Zimmermann, note 3, above.

7. P. Thompson, "Swish of her ponytail made five-ton killer whale strike: Even expert trainer was vulnerable to predator's natural instinct," *Daily Mail*, February 26, 2010, https://www.dailymail.co.uk/news/article-1253881/Sea-World-killer-whale-attack-Trainer-Dawn-Brancheau-vulnerable.html; "Dawn Brancheau Obituary," www.legacy.com/ns/dawn-brancheau-obituary/140006723; "SeaWorld trainer killed by killer whale," CNN, February 25, 2010, www.cnn.com/2010/US/02/24/killer.whale.trainer.death/index.html; M. Mooney, "SeaWorld Trainer Killed by Whale Had Fractured Jaw and Dislocated Joints," ABC News, March 31, 2010, https://abcnews.go.com/GMA/seaworld-trainer-dawn-brancheau-suffered-broken-jaw-fractured/story?id=10252808; see "Dawn Brancheau Biography," note 4, above; see note 6, above.

8. See P. Thompson, note 7, above.

9. See note 8, above.

10. See T. Zimmermann, note 3, above.

11. A. Soitis, "30-minute nightmare in orca's death grip," *New York Post*, March 30, 2010, https://nypost.com/2010/03/03/30-minute-nightmare-in-orcas-death-grip/; see note 3, above.

12. See "SeaWorld trainer killed by killer whale," note 7, above; see note 10, above.
13. See note 8, above.
14. See "Orange County Sheriff's Office Investigative Report Case Number 2010-016715," note 3, above.
15. See note 8, above; see note 10, above.
16. See note 3, above.
17. See note 3, above; see "Dawn Brancheau Obituary," note 7, above; see note 8, above.
18. See note 11, above.
19. See A. Soitis, note 11, above.
20. See note 14, above.
21. See note 14, above.
22. See note 10, above.
23. See note 14, above.
24. See note 14, above.
25. See "Dawn Brancheau Obituary"and M. Mooney, note 7, above.
26. See note 14, above.
27. See note 3, above.
28. See note 14, above.
29. See note 3, above.
30. See note 10, above.
31. See note 3, above.
32. See note 18, above.
33. See "SeaWorld trainer killed by killer whale," note 7, above; see note 18, above.
34. See note 19, above.
35. "Autopsy report—Dawn Brancheau," https://pdf4pro.com/view/autopsyfiles-org-dawn-brancheau-autopsy-report-253ec1.html.
36. See note 35, above.
37. See note 35, above.
38. See note 35, above.
39. "Invisalign," https://www.invisalign.com/; see note 35, above.
40. See note 35, above.

41. See note 35, above.

42. See note 35, above.

43. See note 35, above.

44. See note 35, above.

45. See note 35, above.

46. See note 35, above.

47. D. K. Molina and V. J. M. DiMaio, "Normal Organ Weights in Women: Part I—The Heart," *Am J Forensic Med Pathol* 36(3) (2015):176–81.

48. D. K. Molina and V. J. M. DiMaio, "Normal Organ Weights in Women: Part II—The Brain, Lungs, Liver, Spleen, and Kidneys," *Am J Forensic Med Pathol* 36 (3): 182–87 (2015); see note 35, above.

49. See note 35, above.

50. See note 35, above.

51. See note 35, above.

52. See note 35, above.

53. See note 35, above.

54. See note 35, above.

55. See note 35, above.

56. See note 35, above.

57. See note 35, above.

58. See note 35, above.

59. See note 35, above.

60. See D. K. Molina and V. J. M. DiMaio, note 48, above.

61. M. Bohnert, D. Ropohl, et al., "Forensic medicine significance of the fluid content of the sphenoid sinuses," *Arch Kriminol* 209(5–6) (2002): 158–64; D. Breitmeier, M. Schultz, et al., "Aquatic fatalities—a systematic retrospective analysis," *Arch Kriminol* 226(3–4) (2010): 107–18; P. Hottmar, "Detection of fluid in paranasal sinuses as a possible diagnostic sign of death by drowning," *Arch Kriminol* 198(3–4) (1996): 89–94; see note 35, above.

62. See note 35, above.

63. See "Dawn Brancheau Biography," note 4, above; see "Dawn Brancheau Obituary," note 5, above; see "Dawn Brancheau Biography," note 6, above.

64. See note 15, above; see note 63, above.

65. See note 64, above.

66. See "SeaWorld trainer killed by killer whale," note 7, above.

67. See note 4, above; see "Dawn Brancheau Biography," note 6, above.

68. See note 67, above.

69. See "Dawn Brancheau Obituary," note 5, above; see "Dawn Brancheau Biography," note 6, above.

70. See note 4, above.

71. See "Dawn Brancheau Biography," note 7, above.

72. See note 71, above.

73. See note 71, above.

74. See "Dawn Brancheau Obituary," note 7, above; see note 15, above.

75. "A Whale of a Business," Public Broadcasting Service, https://www.pbs.org/wgbh/pages/frontline/shows/whales/etc/summary.html.

76. See note 10, above.

77. See note 10, above.

78. See note 10, above.

79. See note 10, above.

80. See note 10, above.

81. T. Zimmerman, "Tilikum, SeaWorld's Most Famous Killer Whale, Dies," https://www.outsideonline.com/outdoor-adventure/environment/tilikum-seaworlds-most-famous-killer-whale-dies/; see note 15, above.

82. See note 10, above.

83. See note 10, above.

84. See note 10, above; see T. Zimmerman, note 81, above.

85. See note 10, above.

86. See note 10, above.

87. See note 10, above.

88. See note 10, above.

89. See note 10, above.

90.   See note 10, above.

91.   See note 10, above.

92.   "SeaWorld's whale pool is no place for trainers," the *San Diego Union-Tribune*, April 21, 2010, https://www.sandiegouniontribune. com/sdut-seaworlds-whale-pool-is-no-place-for-trainers-2010apr21-story.html; See note 8, above.

93.   See note 10, above.

94.   See note 8, above.

95.   See "SeaWorld's whale pool is no place for trainers," note 92, above.

96.   E. Pilkington, "Killer whale Tilikum to be spared after drowning trainer by ponytail," the *Guardian*, February 25, 2010, https://www.theguardian.com/world/2010/feb/25/killer-whale-tilikum-drowned-trainer-hair.

97.   See note 95, above.

98.   See note 66, above.

99.   See note 95, above.

100. See note 96, above.

101. See note 96, above.

102. See note 10, above.

103. See note 66, above.

104. See note 8, above.

105. See T. Zimmerman, note 81, above.

106. "SeaWorld orca Tilikum that killed trainer dies," BBC, January 6, 2017, https://www.bbc.com/news/world-us-canada-38531967; S. Rummel, "Whale that killed Dawn Brancheau dies at SeaWorld," *Tri-County Times*, January 13, 2017, https://www.tctimes.com/news/whale-that-killed-dawn-brancheau-dies-at-seaworld/article_dacdfe7a-d9bc-11e6-aeca-cf87f69db396.html; see note 105, above.

30.   Andrew Breitbart

1.   "Brentwood Restaurant & Lounge," https://www.tripadvisor.com/Restaurant_Review-g32655-d348043-Reviews-Brentwood_Restaurant_Lounge-Los_Angeles_California.html.

2. See note 1, above.

3. D. Carr, "The Life and Death of Andrew Breitbart," The New York Times, April 13, 2012, https://www.nytimes.com/2012/04/15/business/media/the-life-and-death-of-andrew-breitbart.html; M. Belloni, "Andrew Breitbart Talked Politics in L.A. Bar an Hour Before Dying," the *Hollywood Reporter*, March 1, 2012, https://www.hollywoodreporter.com/news/general-news/andrew-breitbart-dead-la-bar-politics-296386/.

4. See M. Belloni, note 3, above.

5. See note 4, above.

6. See D. Carr, note 3, above.

7. See note 6, above.

8. See note 4, above.

9. See note 4, above.

10. T. Mak, "Breitbart's death stuns media, pols," Politico, March 1, 2012, https://www.politico.com/story/2012/03/andrew-brietbart-dead-at-43-073493; A. Dobuzinskis, "Conservative activist Andrew Breitbart dead at 43," Reuters, March 1, 2012, https://www.reuters.com/article/us-usa-politics-breitbart/conservative-activist-andrew-breitbart-dead-at-43-idUSTRE8201AV20120301; C. Beam, "Breitbart's Back," Slate, July 22, 2010, https://slate.com/news-and-politics/2010/07/a-slate-profile-of-andrew-breitbart.html; see note 6, abobve.

11. K. McVeigh, "Andrew Breitbart, conservative activist and blogger, dies aged 43," the *Guardian*, March 1, 2012, https://www.theguardian.com/world/2012/mar/01/andrew-breitbart-dies-at-43; "Autopsy report and Investigator's narrative—Andrew Breitbart," http://www.autopsyfiles.org/reports/Celebs/breitbart,%20andrew_report.pdf.

12. See "Autopsy report and Investigator's narrative—Andrew Breitbart," note 11, above.

13. E. Flock and D. Beard, "Andrew Breitbart dies: Big Journalism founder was 43," the *Washington Post*, March 1, 2012, https://www.washingtonpost.com/blogs/blogpost/post/

andrew-breitbart-dies-at-43/2012/03/01/gIQAklYPkR_blog.html; see note 4, above; see A. Dobuzinskis, note 10, above; see note 12, above.

14. See note 12, above.

15. See note 12, above.

16. See note 12, above.

17. See note 12, above.

18. See note 12, above.

19. See note 12, above.

20. See note 12, above.

21. See note 12, above.

22. See note 12, above.

23. D. K. Molina and V. J. M. DiMaio, "Normal organ weights in men: part I—the heart," *Am J Forensic Med Pathol* 33(4) (2012): 363–67 (2012); see note 12, above.

24. See note 12, above.

25. See note 23, above.

26. See note 12, above.

27. See note 12, above.

28. "Sudden Cardiac Death (Sudden Cardiac Arrest)," Cleveland Clinic, https://my.clevelandclinic.org/health/diseases/17522-sudden-cardiac-death-sudden-cardiac-arrest; see note 12, above.

29. See note 12, above.

30. See note 12, above.

31. "Heart Failure—Pathology," https://webpath.med.utah.edu/LUNGHTML/LUNG101.html.

32. See note 12, above.

33. See note 12, above.

34. See note 12, above.

35. See note 12, above.

36. "Cirrhosis," Mayo Clinic, https://www.mayoclinic.org/diseases-conditions/cirrhosis/symptoms-causes/syc-20351487.

37. See note 12, above.

38. See note 12, above.

39. See note 12, above.

40. See note 12, above.

41. See note 12, above.

42. See note 12, above.

43. See note 12, above.

44. "Andrew Breitbart Biography," https://www.thefamouspeople.com/profiles/andrew-breitbart-48783.php; C. Beam, "Breitbart's Back," Slate, July 22, 2010, https://slate.com/news-and-politics/2010/07/a-slate-profile-of-andrew-breitbart.html; see note 6, above.

45. See "Andrew Breitbart Biography," note 44, above.

46. B. Weinthal, "Comment: Andrew Breitbart, Israel and Judaism," the *Jerusalem Post*, March 4, 2012, https://www.jpost.com/Jewish-World/Jewish-Features/Comment-Andrew-Breitbart-Israel-and-Judaism.

47. See K. McVeigh, note 10, above.

48. R. Mead, "Rage Machine," the *New Yorker*, May 17, 2010, https://www.newyorker.com/magazine/2010/05/24/rage-machine; see note 45, above.

49. See C. Beam, note 44, above; see note 45, above.

50. See C. Beam, note 44, above.

51. See note 6, above; see E. Flock and D. Beard, note 13, above; see note 48, above.

52. See R. Mead, note 48, above.

53. T. Mak, "Breitbart's death stuns media, pols," Politico, March 1, 2012, https://www.politico.com/story/2012/03/andrew-brietbart-dead-at-43-073493; see note 49, above.

54. See note 52, above.

55. See A. Dobuzinskis, note 13, above; see note 52, above.

56. See note 50, above; see note 52, above.

57. See note 53, above.

58. See note 50, above.

59. See note 6, above.

60. See note 47, above.

61. See note 6, above; see note 50, above; see note 55, above.

62. J. Sappell, "Hot Links Served Up Daily," *Los Angeles Times*, August 4, 2007, https://web.archive.org/web/20080211200049/http://www.latimes.com/business/la-fi-drudge4aug04,0,4136919,full.story?coll=la-home-center.

63. See note 62, above.

64. See note 52, above.

65. See note 6, above.

66. See note 48, above.

67. See note 48, above.

68. See note 48, above.

69. See A. Dobuzinskis, note 10, above; see note 45, above.

70. See A. Dobuzinskis, note 10, above.

71. See note 6, above.

72. See note 62, above.

73. See T. Mak, note 10, above; see E. Flock and D. Beard, note 13, above; see note 70, above.

74. See note 70, above.

75. See note 70, above.

76. "Conservative blogger Andrew Breitbart died of heart failure," CNN, April 20, 2012, https://www.cnn.com/2012/04/20/politics/breitbart-autopsy/index.html.

77. See E. Flock and D. Beard, note 13, above; see note 50, above.

78. See note 6, above.

79. See note 6, above.

80. See T. Mak, note 10, above.

81. See note 6, above.

82. See note 6, above.

83. See note 80, above.

84. See note 80, above.

85. See "Sudden Cardiac Death (Sudden Cardiac Arrest)," note 28, above.

31. *Tamerlan Tsarnaev*

1. J. D. Gates, S. Arabian, et al., "The Initial Response to the Boston Marathon Bombing: Lessons Learned to Prepare for the Next Disaster," *Ann. Surg.* 260(6) (2014): 960–66; "Boston Marathon Bombing," History, original published March 28, 2014, last updated June 7, 2019, https://www.history.com/topics/21st-century/boston-marathon-bombings; "Criminal Complaint," United States of America v. Dzhokhar Tsarnaev, April 21, 2013.

2. See "Boston Marathon Bombing," note 1, above.

3. See note 2, above.

4. See note 2, above.

5. B. LoGiurato and H. Blodget, "Boston Massacre: The Full Story of How Two Deranged Young Men Terrorized An American City," Business Insider, April 29, 2013, https://www.businessinsider.com/boston-bombings-2013-4.

6. "Opening Statement by Mr. Weinreb," United States of America v. Dzhokhar A. Tsarnaev, March 4, 2015, https://s3.amazonaws.com/s3.documentcloud.org/documents/1681443/tsarnaev-dzkokhar-trial-transcript-3-4-2015.pdf; "Opening Statement by Judy Clarke," United States of America v. Dzhokhar A. Tsarnaev, March 4, 2015, https://s3.amazonaws.com/s3.documentcloud.org/documents/1681442/tsarnaev-dzkokhar-trial-transcript-3-4-2015-clarke.pdf; see "Criminal Complaint," note 1, above; see note 5, above.

7. See note 3, above.

8. See "Criminal Complaint," note 1, above; see note 2, above; see note 5, above; see "Opening Statement by Judy Clarke," note 6, above.

9. Boston Marathon Terror Attack Fast Facts," CNN, March 23, 2021, https://www.cnn.com/2013/06/03/us/boston-marathon-terror-attack-fast-facts/index.html; see "Criminal Complaint," note 1, above; see note 2, above; see note 5, above.

10. See "Opening Statement by Mr. Weinreb," note 6, above.

11. See note 10, above.

12. See note 10, above.

13. See note 10, above.

14. See J. D. Gates, S. Arabian, et al., note 1, above.

15. See note 14, above.

16. A. Gabbatt, D. Lovering, et al., "Two blasts at Boston Marathon kill three and injure more than 100," the *Guardian*, April 16, 2013, https://www.theguardian.com/world/2013/apr/15/boston-marathon-explosion-finish-line; see note 1, above; see Boston Marathon Terror Attack Fast Facts," note 9, above.

17. See note 5, above; see Boston Marathon Terror Attack Fast Facts," note 9, above; see A. Gabbatt, D. Lovering, et al., note 16, above.

18. See note 5, above.

19. See note 2, above; see note 5, above.

20. See note 9, above; see "Opening Statement by Mr. Weinreb," note 6, above .

21. See "Boston Marathon Terror Attack Fast Facts," note 9, above; see note 19, above.

22. See note 20, above.

23. See "Criminal Complaint," note 6, above; see note 10, above; see note 19, above.

24. See "Opening Statement by Mr. Weinreb," note 6, above; see note 19, above.

25. See note 24, above.

26. See note 23, above.

27. See note 23, above.

28. K. Cullen, "In Watertown, one brother's decision led to death of another," *Boston Globe*, March 16, 2015, https://www.bostonglobe.com/metro/2015/03/16/turn-makes-martyr/xWp8hj4Wx01mrKUglRF93J/story.html; see note 23, above.

29. See note 24, above.

30. See note 24, above.

31. See note 2, above; see note 10, above.

32. See "Boston Marathon Terror Attack Fast Facts," note 9, above; see note 23, above.

702

33. See note 32, above.

34. See note 2, above.

35. See note 10, above.

36. See note 2, above; see "Boston Marathon Terror Attack Fast Facts," note 9, above.

37. "Death Certificate—Tamerlan Tsarnaev," April 19, 2013, http://www.autopsyfiles.org/reports/deathcert/tsarnaev,%20tamerlan_dc.pdf; J. Bidgood, "Autopsy Says Boston Bombing Suspect Died of Gunshot Wounds and Blunt Trauma," the New York Times, May 4, 2013, https://www.nytimes.com/2013/05/05/us/autopsy-says-boston-bombing-suspect-died-of-gunshot-wounds-and-blunt-trauma.html.

38. See note 37, above.

39. See note 10, above; see K. Cullen, note 28, above.

40. See "Death Certificate—Tamerlan Tsarnaev," note 37, above.

41. Sontag, D. M. Herszenhorn, et al., "A Battered Dream, Then a Violent Path," the New York Times, April 27, 2013, https://www.nytimes.com/2013/04/28/us/shot-at-boxing-title-denied-tamerlan-tsarnaev-reeled.html; "Timeline: A look at Tamerlan Tsarnaev's past," CNN, April 22, 2013, https://www.cnn.com/2013/04/21/us/tamerlan-tsarnaev-timeline/index.html.

42. See note 41, above.

43. B. Chappell, "The Tsarnaev Brothers: What We Know About The Boston Bombing Suspects," National Public Radio, April 20, 2013, https://www.npr.org/sections/thetwo-way/2013/04/20/178112198/the-tsarnaev-brothers-what-we-know-about-the-boston-bombing-suspects; see note 5, above; see note 41, above.

44. See note 5, above; see D. Sontag, D. M. Herszenhorn, et al., note 41, above.

45. See D. Sontag, D. M. Herszenhorn, et al., note 41, above.

46. See note 45, above.

47. See note 45, above.

48. See B. Chappell, note 43, above; see note 45, above.

49. See note 48, above.

50. See note 45, above.

51. See note 6, above; see "Timeline: A look at Tamerlan Tsarnaev's past," note 41, above; see note 49, above.

52. H. Siddique, "Boston bombing suspect was put on terrorist database 18 months ago," the *Guardian*, April 25, 2013, https://www.theguardian.com/world/2013/apr/25/boston-bombing-suspect-terrorist-database; see "Timeline: A look at Tamerlan Tsarnaev's past," note 41, above; see note 49, above.

53. See note 52, above.

54. See "Timeline: A look at Tamerlan Tsarnaev's past," note 41, above; see note 44, above.

55. See note 54, above.

56. See note 41, above.

57. "Dzhokhar and Tamerlan: A profile of the Tsarnaev brothers," CBS News, April 23, 2013, https://www.cbsnews.com/news/dzhokhar-and-tamerlan-a-profile-of-the-tsarnaev-brothers/; "Dzhokhar Tsarnaev Biography," A&E Television Networks, original published date April 2, 2014, last updated July 31, 2020, https://www.biography.com/crime-figure/dzhokhar-tramaev.

58. See Dzhokhar and Tamerlan: A profile of the Tsarnaev brothers," note 57, above.

59. See B. Chappell, note 48, above.

60. See note 59, above.

61. See note 5, above; see note 58, above; see note 59, above.

62. See note 2, above; see note 58, above; see note 60, above.

63. See note 60, above.

64. See note 10, above; see note 58, above.

65. See note 60, above.

66. See "Dzhokhar Tsarnaev Biography," note 57, above.

67. M. Pearson, "Official: Suspect says Iraq, Afghanistan drove Boston bombings," CNN, April 24, 2013, https://www.cnn.com/2013/04/23/us/boston-attack; see "Opening Statement by Judy Clarke," note 6, above.

68. See note 10, above.

69. See note 10, above.

70. See note 10, above.

71. "Dzhokhar Tsarnaev Biography," A&E Television Networks, original published date April 2, 2014, last updated July 31, 2020, https://www.biography.com/crime-figure/dzhokhar-tramaev; see note 36, above.

72. "Judge Imposes Death Sentence for Boston Marathon Bomber," Department of Justice, June 26, 2015, https://www.justice.gov/opa/pr/judge-imposes-death-sentence-boston-marathon-bomber; see "Boston Marathon Terror Attack Fast Facts," note 9, above; see note 66, above.

73. "Boston bombing: Tsarnaev's death sentence could be reinstated," BBC, March 22, 2021, https://www.bbc.com/news/world-us-canada-56482800; A. Durkin Richer, "Court overturns Boston Marathon bomber's death sentence," Associated Press, July 31, 2020, https://apnews.com/article/sports-ri-state-wire-ma-state-wire-dzhokhar-tsarnaev-trials-af38a703ab88fe922629dcc254cb41df; "Boston Marathon bomber Dzhokhar Tsarnaev has death sentence overturned on appeal," ESPN, July 31, 2020, https://www.espn.com/olympics/trackandfield/story/_/id/29572538/boston-marathon-bomber-dzhokhar-tsarnaev-death-sentence-overturned-appeal; see "Boston Marathon Terror Attack Fast Facts," note 9, above.

74. See "Boston Marathon Terror Attack Fast Facts," note 9, above.

75. See A. Durkin Richer, and "Boston Marathon bomber Dzhokhar Tsarnaev has death sentence overturned on appeal," note 73, above.

76. See M. Pearson, note 67, above; see "Boston bombing: Tsarnaev's death sentence could be reinstated," note 73, above.

77. See note 45, above.

78. See note 60, above.

79. See M. Pearson, note 67, above.

80. See H. Siddique, note 52, above.

81. See "Timeline: A look at Tamerlan Tsarnaev's past," note 41, above; see note 60, above.

82. O. Dorell, "Mosque that Boston suspects attended has radical ties," *USA Today*, original published date April 23, 2013, last updated April

25, 2013, https://www.usatoday.com/story/news/nation/2013/04/23/boston-mosque-radicals/2101411/; L. Warren, "Bomber's ex-girlfriend revealed: High school sweetheart 'slapped' by Tamerlan calls him a 'bully' and a 'little tough guy,'" the *Daily Mail*, April 23, 2013, https://www.dailymail.co.uk/news/article-2313484/Boston-bombing-suspect-Tamerlan-Tsarnaevs-ex-girlfriend-Nadine-Ascencao-revealed.html; see "Opening Statement by Judy Clarke," note 6, above; see note 44, above; see "Dzhokhar and Tamerlan: A profile of the Tsarnaev brothers," note 54, above.

83. D. Kenner, "Who is Tamerlan Tsarnaev?" April 19, 2013, https://foreignpolicy.com/2013/04/19/who-is-tamerlan-tsarnaev/; see note 5, above; see note 81, above; see "Dzhokhar and Tamerlan: A profile of the Tsarnaev brothers," note 54, above; see L. Warren, note 82, above.

84. See note 54, above.

85. See "Opening Statement by Judy Clarke," note 6, above; see note 41, above.

86. See note 10, above.

87. See note 10, above.

88. See note 10, above.

89. See "Opening Statement by Judy Clarke," note 6, above.

90. See note 89, above.

91. See note 89, above.

92. See note 89, above.

93. "Boston bombing prosecutors rest case after gruesome autopsy testimony," CBS News, March 30, 2015, https://www.cbsnews.com/news/boston-marathon-bombing-prosecutors-rest-case-after-gruesome-autopsy-testimony/; see A. Durkin Richer, note 74, above; see note 79, above.

94. See note 89, above.

95. I. S. Sheehan, "Are Suicide Terrorists Suicidal? A Critical Assessment of the Evidence," *Innov Clin Neurosci* 11(9–10) (2014): 81–92, https://nasmhpd.org/sites/default/files/Suicide%20Terrorism%20

sheehan-are-suicide-terrorist-suicidal-a-critical-assessment-of-the-evidence.pdf.

96. G. Bruce, "Intrinsic and External Factors and Influences on the Motivation of Suicide Attackers," JMVH, 21(3), https://jmvh.org/article/motivation-of-suicide-attackers/; Y. Tanaka, "Japan's Kamikaze Pilots and Contemporary Suicide Bombers: War and Terror," *The Asia-Pacific Journal*, 3(7) (2005). https://apjjf.org/-Yuki-Tanaka/1606/article.html.

97. See Y. Tanaka, note 96, above.

98. "Suicide Bombers: Motivation, Recruitment, Indoctrination, and Effectiveness," Springer, https://link.springer.com/content/pdf/bfm%3A978-0-230-61650-9%2F5%2F1.pdf.

99. See note 98, above.

100. M. Bray, "Why young Muslims line up to die," CNN, August 18, 2003, https://www.cnn.com/2003/WORLD/asiapcf/southeast/08/17/martyr.culture/index.html; see G. Bruce, note 96, above; see note 98, above.

101. See note 98, above; see G. Bruce, note 96, above.

102. See note 98, above; see M. Bray, note 100, above.

103. V. Harmon, E. Mujkic, et al., "Causes & Explanations of Suicide Terrorism: A Systematic Review," *Homeland Security Affairs* 14, December 2018, https://www.hsaj.org/articles/14749; see note 10, above; see note 95, above; see note 101, above.

104. See note 10, above.

105. See note 95, above See G. Bruce, note 96, above; see M. Bray, note 100, above.

106. See M. Bray, note 100, above.

107. See note 10, above.

108. See note 10, above.

109. A. O'Neill, "U.S. ends Boston Marathon bomb case with grisly photos and testimony," CNN, March 31, 2015, https://www.cnn.com/2015/03/30/us/tsarnaev-boston-marathon-bombing-prosecution-ending/index.html; see K. Cullen, note 28, above; see note 89, above.

110. A. Jurberg, "Is 'Sex Sells' Still True?" Better Marketing, July 28, 2020, http://bettermarketing.pub/is-sex-sells-still-tru-35cd32dfc9db; "History of Advertising No. 87: The first ad with sex appeal," January 16, 2014, https://www.campaignlive.co.uk/article/history-advertising-no-87-first-ad-sex-appeal/1226933; see note 106, above.

111. A. Harel, "Profile of a Suicide bomber: Single Male, Average Age—21," Haaretz, August 24, 2001, https://www.haaretz.com/1.5405925; R. A. Hudson, "The Sociology and Psychology of Terrorism: Who Becomes a Terrorist and Why?" The Library of Congress, September 1999, https://fas.org/irp/threat/frd.html.

112. See A. Harel, note 111, above.

113. See G. Bruce, note 96, above.

114. See note 113, above.

32. *Tom Petty*

1. C. Payne, "Tom Petty's Final Concert: Watch Him Close With 'You Wreck Me' & 'American Girl,'" Billboard, October 3, 2017, https://www.billboard.com/articles/news/7982056/tom-petty-american-girl-last-concert-video-heartbreakers.

2. S. Whitten and L. Shaffer, "Tom Petty, iconic rock star, has died at age 66 after suffering cardiac arrest, manager says," CNBC, October 3, 2017, https://www.cnbc.com/2017/10/03/tom-petty-iconic-rock-star-has-died-at-age-66-after-suffering-cardiac-arrest-manager-says.html; see note 1, above.

3. "Watch Tom Petty's final live performance, recorded a week before his death," https://faroutmagazine.co.uk/tom-petty-final-performance-before-death-hollywood-bowl/; S. T. Levin, "Tom Petty family hope guitarist's death will raise awareness of opioid crisis," the *Guardian*, January 21, 2018, https://www.theguardian.com/music/2018/jan/20/tom-petty-died-from-of-accidental-drug-overdose-family-says.

4. See note 3, above.

5. See note 1, above.

6. See note 1, above.

708

7. "Tom Petty & the Heartbreakers' Final Concert," Best Classic Bands, https://bestclassicbands.com/tom-petty-final-concert-9-24-18/.

8. D. Kroll, "Hearbreaker: Tom Petty Died From An Accidental Overdose of Opioids And Benzodiazepines," *Forbes*, January 19, 2008, https://www.forbes.com/sites/davidkroll/2018/01/19/heartbreaker-tom-petty-died-from-an-accidental-overdose-of-medical-opioids/?sh=ec2920f71e44; "A Statement from the Petty Family," January 19, 2018, https://www.tompetty.com/news/statement-petty-family-1764366; A. Mandell, "Tom Petty Died of Accidental Drug Overdose, Coroner Says," *USA Today*, January 19, 2018, https://www.usatoday.com/story/life/people/2018/01/19/tom-petty-died-accidental-drug-overdose-coroner-says/1050228001/.

9. See "A Statement from the Petty Family," note 8, above.

10. See A. Mandell, note 8, above.

11. October 1, 2020, https://nightswithalicecooper.com/2020/10/02/three-years-later-tom-petty-remembered/.

12. K. Rife, "R.I.P. Tom Petty," https://www.avclub.com/r-i-p-tom-petty-1819079682; see note 11, above.

13. See note 10, above; see note 12, above.

14. See note 13, above.

15. See note 11, above.

16. See K. Rife, note 12, above.

17. See note 16, above.

18. See D. Kroll, note 8, above.

19. See note 18, above.

20. See note 9, above; see note 10, above; see note 18, above.

21. R. Ellis, "Tom Petty died of accidental drug overdose, medical examiner says," CNN, January 21, 2018, https://www.cnn.com/2018/01/19/health/tom-petty-cause-of-death/index.html; see note 10, above.

22. See note 18, above.

23. See note 18, above.

24. "Fentanyl," US National Institute on Drug Abuse, https://www.drugabuse.gov/drug-topics/fentanyl; M. Ghoshal and A. Haynes,

"Lethal High: Acetyl Fentanyl," *U.S. Pharmacist*, October 14, 2016, https://www.uspharmacist.com/article/lethal-high-acetyl-fentanyl; see note 9, above; see note 18, above; see R. Ellis, note 21, above.

25. See M. Ghoshal and A. Haynes, note 24, above.

26. R. Lewis, "Tom Petty's death is still a hard reminder for aging rockers about the downside of life on the road," *Los Angeles Times*, October 5, 2018, https://www.latimes.com/entertainment/music/la-et-ms-tom-petty-death-anniversary-20181006-story.html; see note 25, above.

27. See note 26, above.

28. H. A. Milman, "Prince," in *Forensics: The Science Behind the Deaths of Famous People*, (Bloomington, Indiana: Xlibris, 2020) 235–45; "Tom Petty Biography," A&E Television Networks, original published date April 1, 2014, last updated April 8, 2021, https://www.biography.com/musician/tom-petty; see R. Ellis, note 21, above; see note 25, above.

29. See H. A. Milman, note 28, above.

30. See note 28, above.

31. "Increases in fentanyl drug confiscations and fentanyl-related overdose fatalities," US Centers for Disease Control and Prevention Health Alert Network, October 26, 2015, http://emergency.cdc.gov/han/han00384.asp; see note 25, above.

32. See note 25, above.

33. See note 11, above; see note 18, above; see R. Ellis, note 21, above.

34. See note 11, above; see note 18, above.

35. See "Tom Petty Biography," note 28, above.

36. M. Sager, "Tom Petty: What I've Learned," *Esquire*, October 2, 2017, https://www.esquire.com/entertainment/music/a889/tom-petty-what-ive-learned-interview/.

37. See note 36, above.

38. "Tom Petty Knows 'How It Feels,'" National Public Radio, February 1, 2008, https://www.npr.org/2008/02/01/18580517/tom-petty-knows-how-it-feels.

39. B. Crandall, "10 Musicians who saw the Beatles standing there," CBS News, February 6, 2014, https://www.cbsnews.com/news/10-musicians-who-saw-the-beatles-standing-there/.

40. See note 39, above.

41. See note 35, above.

42. See note 16, above; see note 35, above.

43. See note 42, above.

44. See note 35, above.

45. See note 35, above.

46. See note 42, above.

47. D. Whitcomb, "Tom Petty died due to accidental drug overdose: coroner," Reuters, January 19, 2018, https://www.reuters.com/article/us-people-tompetty/tom-petty-died-due-to-accidental-drug-overdose-coroner-idUSKBN1F901T; see note 35, above.

48. See R. Lewis, note 26, above.

49. See note 9, above; see R. Ellis, note 21, above.

50. See note 48, above.

51. See note 48, above.

52. "Hip fracture," Mayo Clinic, https://www.mayoclinic.org/diseases-conditions/hip-fracture/symptoms-causes/syc-20373468.

53. See note 52, above.

54. See note 9, above.

55. "Fentanyl Patch," https://www.drugs.com/fentanyl.html.

56. See S. T. Levin, note 3, above; see note 11, above; see note 18, above; see R. Ellis, note 21, above.

57. See note 48, above.

58. S. Stedman, "Tom Petty's Family Says He Died of Accidental Overdose," *Variety*, January 19, 2018, https://variety.com/2018/music/news/tom-petty-accidental-overdose-autopsy-1202670558/; see D. Whitcomb, note 47, above; see note 18, above.

59. K. Grow, "Tom Petty's Cause of Death: Accidental Overdose," *Rolling Stone*, January 20, 2018, https://www.rollingstone.com/music/music-news/tom-pettys-cause-of-death-accidental-overdose-202789/.

60. See note 18, above.

61. See note 9, above; see S. T. Levin, note 3, above; see note 10, above; see R. Ellis, note 21, above.

62. H. A. Milman, "Elvis Presley," in *Forensics: The Science Behind the Deaths of Famous People* (Bloomington, Indiana: Xlibris, 2020) 61–72; H. A. Milman, "Anna Nicole Smith," in *Forensics: The Science Behind the Deaths of Famous People* (Bloomington, Indiana: Xlibris, 2020), 135–48; H. A. Milman, "Heath Ledger," in *Forensics: The Science Behind the Deaths of Famous People* (Bloomington, Indiana: Xlibris, 2020), 149–56; H. A. Milman, "Philip Seymour Hoffman," in *Forensics: The Science Behind the Deaths of Famous People* (Bloomington, Indiana: Xlibris, 2020) 203–10.

63. "Tom Petty Biography," https://www.imdb.com/name/nm0678816/bio.

64. See note 63, above.

65. See note 48, above.

33. Anthony Bourdain

1. "Anthony Bourdain's Fight with Addiction and Apparent Suicide," May 25, 2019, https://www.northpointrecovery.com/blog/anthony-bourdains-fight-with-addiction-and-apparent-suicide/.

2. J. Balsam, "What the last 12 months of Anthony Bourdain's life were like," Grunge, June 25, 2020, https://www.grunge.com/221167/what-the-last-12-months-of-anthony-bourdains-life-were-like/.

3. "Anthony Bourdain: Celebrity chef found dead at 61," BBC, https://bbc.com/news/world-us-canada-44414747; "Anthony Bourdain Biography," https://www.imdb.com/name/nm1113529/bio; see note 2, above.

4. See note 2, above.

5. D. Sharma, "How Did Anthony Bourdain Die? Heart-Breaking Details Reveal Cause of Death," *International Business Times*, June 10, 2018, https://www.ibtimes.co.in/

how-did-anthony-bourdain-die-heart-breaking-details-reveal-cause-death-771529; M. Margaritoff, "The Inside Story Of Anthony Bourdain's Death—And The Downward Spiral That Preceded It," July 8, 2021, https://allthatsinteresting.com/anthony-bourdain-death; E. Jensen and J. Deerwester, "Anthony Bourdain's Death: No narcotics in his system at time of death, official says," *USA Today*, June 22, 2018, https://www.usatoday.com/story/life/people/2018/06/22/anthony-bourdains-body-free-narcotics-time-death-report/725862002/; "Anthony Bourdain Biography," A&E Television Networks, original published date April 2, 2014, last updated September 1, 2020, https://www.biography.com/personality/anthony-bourdain; A. Adu, "'Gifted Storyteller' How did Anthony Bourdain die?" the *Sun*, https://www.the-sun.com/news/3052736/how-did-anthony-bourdain-die/; B. Stelter, "CNN's Anthony Bourdain dead at 61," CNN, June 8, 2018, https://www.cnn.com/2018/06/08/us/anthony-bourdain-obit/index.html; see note 2, above; see "Anthony Bourdain Biography," note 3, above.

6. See D. Sharma, M. Margaritoff, A. Adu, and B. Stelter, note 5, above.

7. See D. Sharma, note 5, above.

8. M. Ross, "Anthony Bourdain's 'addiction' to Asia Argento overtook last year of his life, new documentary says," the *Mercury News*, original published date July 14, 2021, last updated July 17, 2021, https://www.twincities.com/2021/07/14/anthony-bourdains-addiction-to-asia-argento-overtook-last-year-of-his-life-new-documentary-shows/.

9. See A. Adu, note 5, above; see note 7, above.

10. See note 9, above.

11. See note 1, above; see "Anthony Bourdain: Celebrity chef found dead at 61," note 3, above; see M. Margaritoff, note 5, above; see note 8, above; see note 9, above.

12. See M. Margaritoff, E. Jensen and J. Deerwester, and "Anthony Bourdain Biography," note 5, above.

13. See "Anthony Bourdain: Celebrity chef found dead at 61," note 3, above; see "Anthony Bourdain Biography," note 5, above.

14. See "Anthony Bourdain Biography," note 3, above.

15. J. McBride, "Anthony Bourdain Family: 5 Fast Facts You Need to Know," https://heavy.com/news/2018/06/anthony-bourdain-family-wife-parents-daughter/; "Anthony Bourdain Biography," https://thefamouspeople.com/profiles/anthony-michael-bourdain-740.php; see note 3, above; see E. Jensen and J. Deerwester, and "Anthony Bourdain Biography," note 5, above.

16. See J. McBride, note 15, above.

17. See note 16, above.

18. See note 16, above.

19. E. Chayes Wida, "Anthony Bourdain's brother opens up about the late chef's childhood and their family," June 21, 2019, https://www.today.com/food/anthony-bourdain-s-brother-talks-about-chef-s-greatest-accomplishment-t156651.

20. See E. Jensen and J. Deerwester, "Anthony Bourdain Biography," B. Stelter, and M. Margaritoff, note 5, above; see note 14, above; see "Anthony Bourain Biography," note 15, above.

21. See note 20, above.

22. See note 1, above; see note 2, above.

23. See note 1, above.

24. See note 1, above.

25. See note 2, above; see B. Stelter, note 5, above.

26. D. M. Bush and R. N. Lipari, "Substance Use and Substance Use Disorder by Industry," April 16, 2015, Substance Abuse and Mental Health Services Administration, https://www.samhsa.gov/data/sites/default/files/report_1959/ShortReport-1959.html; see note 1, above.

27. See note 1, above.

28. See note 1, above.

29. See "Anthony Bourdain Biography," and M. Margaritoff, note 5, above; see "Anthony Bourdain Biography," note 15, above; see note 25, above.

30. See note 1, above.

714

31. See note 1, above.

32. See note 1, above; see note 2, above.

33. See note 32, above.

34. See "Anthony Bourdain Biography," B. Stelter, and M. Margaritoff, note 5, above; see note 14, above; see "Anthony Bourdain Biography," note 15, above.

35. See B. Stelter, note 5, above.

36. See "Anthony Bourdain Biography," B. Stelter, and M. Margaritoff, note 5, above; see "Anthony Bourdain Biography," note 15, above.

37. See "Anthony Bourdain Biography," note 5, above; see "Anthony Bourdain Biography," note 15, above.

38. See "Anthony Bourdain Biography" and B. Stelter, note 5, above; see "Anthony Bourdain Biography," note 15, above.

39. See note 14, above.

40. See note 14, above.

41. See "Anthony Bourdain Biography," note 20, above.

42. See note 37, above.

43. See note 1, above; see "Anthony Bourdain: Celebrity chef found dead at 61," note 3, above; see note 41, above.

44. See B. Stelter, note 5, above.

45. See note 44, above.

46. See note 44, above.

47. See note 1, above.

48. See note 44, above.

49. See A. Adu, note 5, above.

50. J. Kegu, "Eric Ripert, who was with Anthony Bourdain in his final days, reflects on 20 years of friendship," CBS News, November 30, 2018, https://www.cbsnews.com/news/chef-eric-ripert-on-anthony-bourdain-death-friendship-and-le-bernardin/; see note 14, above; see note 43, above.

51. See note 50, above.

52. See note 14, above.

53. See note 1, above; see "Anthony Bourdain Biography" and M. Margaritoff, note 5, above; see note 44, above.

54. See M. Margaritoff, note 5, above; see note 44, above.

55. M. Wilstein, "The Dark Reality of Anthony Bourdain's Final Days," The Daily Beast, July 12, 2021, https://www.thedailybeast.com/anthony-bourdains-dark-final-days-revealed-in-new-documentary-roadrunner.

56. P. Sblendorio, "Anthony Bourdain discussed his mental health struggles during therapy session on 'Parts Unknown,'" *New York Daily News*, June 8, 2018, https://www.nydailynews.com/entertainment/tv/ny-ent-anthony-bourdain-parts-unknown-therapy-20180608-story.html; see note 1, above.

57. See M. Margaritoff, note 5, above; see note 56, above.

58. See "Anthony Bourdain: Celebrity chef found dead at 61," note 3, above.

59. See note 22, above.

60. See note 22, above; see P. Sblendorio, note 56, above.

61. See note 60, above.

62. "Suicide," US National Institute of Mental Health, https://www.nimh.nih.gov/health/statistics/suicide.

63. T. Dragisic, A. Dickov, et al., "Drug Addiction as Risk for Suicide Attempts," *Mater Sociomed.* 27(3) (2015): 188–91; see note 1, above.

64. "Does alcohol and other drug abuse increase the risk for suicide?" https://www.hhs.gov/answers/mental-health-and-substance-abuse/does-alcohol-increase-risk-of-suicide/index.html; see note 63, above.

65. "Thoughts of Suicide May Persist Among Nonmedical Prescription Opiate Users," US National Institute of Drug Abuse, March 4, 2013, https://archives.drugabuse.gov/news-events/nida-notes/2013/03/thoughts-suicide-may-persist-among-nonmedical-prescription-opiate-users; S. Janet Kuramoto, H. D. Chilcoat, et al., "Suicidal Ideation and Suicide Attempt Across Stages of Nonmedical Prescription Opioid Use and Presence of Prescription Opioid Disorders Among US Adults," *J Study Alcohol Drugs* 73(2) (2012): 178–84; see note 1, above.

66. "Suicide and Self-Harm Injury," US Centers for Disease Control and Prevention, https://www.cdc.gov/nchs/fastats/suicide.htm; see S. Janet Kuramoto, H. D. Chilcoat, et al., note 65, above.

67. See note 66, above.

68. M. Kumar, R. Mandhyan, et al., "Delayed Pulmonary Edema Following Attempted Suicidal Hanging—A Case Report," *Indian J Anaesthesia* 53(3) (2009): 355–57.

69. See note 68, above.

70. S. Reinberg, "Hanging Suicides Up in United States," https://www.medicinenet.com/script/main/art.asp?articlekey=165266; I. Gordon, H. A. Shapiro, et al., "Deaths usually initiated by hypoxic hypoxia or anoxic anoxia," *Forensic Medicine: A Guide to Principles*, 3rd edition (1988) 95–127.

71. M. Kumar, R. Mandhyan, et al., "Delayed Pulmonary Edema Following Attempted Suicidal Hanging—A Case Report," *Indian J Anaesthesia* 53(3): 355–57 (2009); C. E. Oswalt, G. A. Gates, et al., "Pulmonary edema as a complication of acute airway obstruction," *JAMA* 238(17) (1977): 1833–35; S. Mantha and S. M. Rao, "Noncardiogenic pulmonary edema after attempted suicide by hanging," *Anaesthesia* 45(11) (1990): 993–94; S. A. Lang, P. G. Dunca, et al., "Pulmonary edema associated with airway obstruction," *Can J Anaesth* 37(2) (1990): 210–18.

72. See "Anthony Bourdain: Celebrity chef found dead at 61," note 2, above; see M. Margaritoff, note 5, above.

73. See note 2, above; see note 8, above.

74. See note 2, above.

75. See note 2, above.

76. See P. Sblendorio, note 56, above.

77. See note 14, above.

78. See note 14, above.

34. *Aretha Franklin*

1. D. Boroff, "Singing his Praises: Who performed at Barack Obama's first and second inauguration?" the *U.S. Sun*, January 18, 2021, https://www.the-sun.com/news/2162883/barack-obama-inauguration-beyonce-aretha-franklin-jennifer-hudson/.

2. See note 1, above.

3. See note 1, above.

4. See note 1, above.

5. See note 1, above.

6. "One of Aretha Franklin's Iconic Performances: 'My Country, 'Tis of Thee' at 2009 Obama Inauguration," Inside Edition, August 16, 2018, https://www.insideedition.com/one-aretha-franklins-iconic-performances-my-country-tis-thee-2009-obama-inauguration-46000.

7. See note 6, above.

8. M. Fekadu and H. Italie, "'Queen of Soul' Aretha Franklin dies at 76," *Associated Press News*, August 16, 2018, https://apnews.com/article/aretha-franklin-music-north-america-ap-top-news-mi-state-wire-616951e51eaa4aa09f894b6ea9d9df44; J. Vejnoska, "Aretha Franklin sang for three presidents' inaugurations, including Jimmy Carter," August 16, 2018, https://www.ajc.com/news/aretha-franklin-sang-for-three-presidents-inaugurations/xSRcpNkJcRSdOj5IM3pXuL/; O. Blair, "Barack Obama Wants to Own Aretha Franklin's Inauguration Hat," *Elle*, August 22, 2019, https://www.elle.com/uk/life-and-culture/a28782930/barack-obama-aretha-franklin-inauguration-hat/; M. Kai, "Where's the Hat Headed? Obama Makes a Formal Request for Aretha Franklin's Inauguration Hat," the *Root*, August 23, 2019, https://www.theroot.com/where-s-the-hat-headed-obama-makes-a-formal-request-fo-1837496931; K. Coleman, "On this day in 2009: Aretha Franklin performs at Obama inauguration," January 20, 2021, https://michiganadvance.com/blog/on-this-day-in-2009-aretha-franklin-performs-at-obtama-inauguration/; M. Rothman, "Watch Aretha Franklin's iconic performance at President

Obama's 2009 inauguration," ABC News, August 16, 2018, https://abcnews.go.com/culture/story/watch-aretha-franklins-iconic-performance-president-obamas-2009-57219241; See ; see note 1, above; see note 6, above.

9. See O. Blair and M. Kai, note 8, above.

10. See M. Kai, note 8, above.

11. See note 10, above.

12. L. Respers France, D. Gilgoff, et al., "Aretha Franklin, the Queen of Soul, has died," CNN, August 16, 2018, https://www.cnn.com/2018/08/16/entertainment/aretha-franklin-dead/index.html; C. Morris, "Aretha Franklin, the Queen of Soul, Dies at 76," *Variety*, August 16, 2018, https://variety.com/2018/music/news/aretha-franklin-dead-dies-76-1202907265/; E. Chuck and A. Johnson, "Aretha Franklin, the 'Queen of Soul' whose reign spanned decades, dies at 76," NBC News, August 16, 2018, https://www.nbcnews.com/pop-culture/pop-culture-news/aretha-franklin-undisputed-queen-soul-dies-age-76-n822841.

13. See L. Respers France, D. Gilgoff et al., note 12, above.

14. G. Mitchell, "Aretha Franklin, Legendary 'Queen of Soul,' Dies at Age 76," Billboard, August 16, 2018, https://www.billboard.com/articles/news/obituary/7318784/aretha-franklin-dead; see M. Fekadu and H. Italie, J. Vejnoska, and K. Coleman, note 8, above; see E. Chuck and A. Johnson, note 12, above.

15. See M. Fekadu and H. Italie, note 8, above; see G. Mitchell, note 14, above.

16. See note 15, above.

17. See E. Chuck and A. Johnson, note 14, above.

18. See C. Morris, note 12, above; see note 13, above; see note 17, above.

19. L. Fisher and M. Rothman, "Aretha Franklin, 'Queen of Soul,' has died at 76," ABC News, August 16, 2018, https://abcnews.go.com/Entertainment/Culture/aretha-franklin-queen-soul-died-report/story?id=41677561; E. Gonzales, "Aretha Franklin Dies at 76 Years Old," *Harper's Bazaar*, August 16, 2018, https://www.harpersbazaar.

com/celebrity/latest/a22713438/aretha-franklin-death/; see note 18, above.

20. D. Clarendon, "Aretha Franklin Dead: Singer Dies at Age 76," *US Magazine*, August 16, 2018, https://www.usmagazine.com/celebrity-news/news/aretha-franklin-dead-queen-of-soul-dies-at-76/; see note 13, above.

21. T. Robbins, "Aretha Franklin, The 'Queen of Soul,' Dies At 76," National Public Radio, August 16, 2018, https://www.npr.org/2018/08/16/532687119/aretha-franklin-the-queen-of-soul-dead-at-76; see L. Fisher and M. Rothman, note 13, above; see G. Mitchell, note 14, above; see E. Gonzales, note 19, above.

22. D. Clarendon, "Aretha Franklin Dead: Singer Dies at Age 76," *US Magazine*, August 16, 2018, https://www.usmagazine.com/celebrity-news/news/aretha-franklin-dead-queen-of-soul-dies-at-76/; see M. Rothman, note 8, above; see note 13, above; see note 15, above; see C. Morris, note 18, above; see T. Robbins, note 21, above.

23. See note 13, above; see G. Mitchell, note 14, above.

24. Aretha Franklin Biography," A&E Television Networks, original published date April 2, 2014, last updated September 15, 2021, https://www.biography.com/musician/aretha-franklin; "Aretha Franklin Biography," https://www.thefamouspeople.com/profiles/aretha-louise-franklin-753.php; A. Codinha, "Aretha Franklin, America's Queen of Soul, Has Died," *Vogue*, August 16, 2018, https://www.vogue.com/article/aretha-franklin-obituary; see M. Fekadu and H. Italie, note 8, above; see note 17, above; see D. Clarendon, note 20, above; see note 21, above.

25. See M. Fekadu and H. Italie, note 8, above; see "Aretha Franklin Biography," and "Aretha Franklin Biography," note 24, above.

26. See "Aretha Franklin Biography," and "Aretha Franklin Biography," note 24, above.

27. See C. Morris, note 12, above; see note 25, above.

28. See note 13, above; see note 17, above; see L. Fisher and M. Rothman, note 19, above; see "Aretha Franklin Biography," and A. Codinha, note 24, above.

29. See T. Robbins, note 21, above.

30. See L. Fisher and M. Rothman, note 19, above; see "Aretha Franklin Biography," note 24, above.

31. See note 29, above.

32. See note 29, above.

33. See note 16, above; see note 17, above; see C. Morris, note 18, above; see E. Gonzales, note 19, above; see "Aretha Franklin Biography," note 24, above; see note 29, above.

34. See "Aretha Franklin Biography," note 24, above.

35. See M. Fekadu and H. Italie, note 8, above; see C. Morris, note 18, above; see note 34, above.

36. "Aretha Franklin Biography," https://www.imdb.com/name/nm0291349/bio; see note 12, above; see "Aretha Franklin Biography," note 24, above; see D. Clarendon, note 20, above; see note 29, above; see note 30, above.

37. See M. Fekadu and H. Italie, note 8, above.

38. See note 17, above; see A. Codinha, note 24, above; see note 26, above; see "Aretha Franklin Biography," note 36, above.

39. See note 37, above.

40. See note 37, above.

41. See note 13, above; see K. Coleman, note 14, above; see L. Fisher and M. Rothman, note 19, above; see "Aretha Franklin Biography" and A. Codinha, note 24, above; see note 37, above.

42. See note 34, above; see note 37, above.

43. See note 17, above; see A. Codinha, note 24, above.

44. See D. Clarendon, note 20, above; see note 25, above.

45. See G. Mitchell, note 14, above.

46. See note 13, above; see note 17, above; see L. Fisher and M. Rothman, note 19, above; see note 25, above; see note 31, above.

47. See C. Morris, note 12, above; see note 13, above; see L. Fisher and M. Rothman, note 19, above; see D. Clarendon, note 20, above; see note 37, above; see note 38, above.

48. See J. Vejnoska, note 8, above; see note 13, above; see K. Coleman, note 14, above; see "Aretha Franklin Biography," and A. Codinha, note 24, above; see note 37, above.

49. See J. Vejnoska, and M. Rothman, note 8, above; see C. Morris, note 12, above; see note 13, above; see note 17, above; see L. Fisher and M. Rothman, note 19, above; see A. Codinha, note 24, above; see note 25, above; see "Aretha Franklin Biography," note 36, above; see note 45, above.

50. See D. Clarendon, note 20, above; see "Aretha Franklin Biography," note 24, above.

51. See note 50, above.

52. See note 50, above.

53. See "Aretha Franklin Biography," note 24, above.

54. "Pancreatic Neuroendocrine Tumors (Islet Cell Tumors) Treatment—Patient Version," US National Cancer Institute, National Institutes of Health, https://www.cancer.gov/types/pancreatic/patient/pnet-treatment-pdq; "Pancreatic cancer," Mayo Clinic, https://www.mayoclinic.org/diseases-conditions/pancreatic-cancer/symptoms-causes/syc-20355421; "Pancreatic Neuroendocrine Tumor," Johns Hopkins Medicine, https://www.hopkinsmedicine.org/health/conditions-and-diseases/pancreatic-cancer/islet-cell-carcinoma.

55. "What Is a Pancreatic Neuroendocrine Tumor?" American Cancer Society, https://www.cancer.org/cancer/pancreatic-neuroendocrine-tumor/about/what-is-pnet.html; see note 54, above.

56. "Pancreatic cancer," Mayo Clinic, https://www.mayoclinic.org/diseases-conditions/pancreatic-cancer/symptoms-causes/syc-20355421.

57. See What Is a Pancreatic Neuroendocrine Tumor?" note 55, above; see "Pancreatic cancer," note 56, above.

58. "Neuroendocrine tumors," Mayo Clinic, https://www.mayoclinic.org/diseases-conditions/neuroendocrine-tumors/symptoms-causes/syc-20354132.

59. See note 58, above.

60. See note 57, above.

61. See note 1, above; see "Pancreatic Neuroendocrine Tumor," note 54, above; see note 57, above.

62. See "Pancreatic Neuroendocrine Tumor," note 54, above.

63. See note 1, above; see note 62, above.

64. C. Ro, W. Chai, et al., "Pancreatic neuroendocrine tumors: biology, diagnosis, and treatment," *Chin J Cancer* 32(6) (2013): 312–24.

65. See note 64, above.

66. See note 64, above.

67. "Survival Rates for Pancreatic Neuroendocrine Tumor," American Cancer Society, https://www.cancer.org/cancer/pancreatic-neuroendocrine-tumor/detection-diagnosis-staging/survival-rates.html.

68. H. Greenlee and E. Ernst, "What can we learn from Steve Jobs about complenetary and alternative therapies?" *Prev Med* 54(1) (2012): 3–4.

69. K. Harmon, "The Puzzle of Pancreatic Cancer: How Steve Jobs Did Not Beat the Odds—but Nobel Winner Ralph Steinman Did," *Scientific American*, October 7, 2011, https://www.scientificamerican.com/article/pancreatic-cancer-type-jobs/.

70. See note 68, above.

71. See note 68, above.

72. "Survival Rates for Pancreatic Cancer," American Cancer Society, https://www.cancer.org/cancer/pancreatic-cancer/detection-diagnosis-staging/survival-rates.html; see note 69, above.

73. "Celebrities with Pancreatic Cancer," https://www.webmd.com/cancer/ss/slideshow-celebrities-with-pancreatic-cancer.

74. See note 73, above.

75. G. Hauck, "Ginsburg v. cancer was a 'remarkable fight': RBG battled five bouts of cancer over two decades," *USA Today*, original published date September 19, 2020, last updated September 20, 2020, https://www.usatoday.com/story/news/health/2020/09/19/ruth-bader-ginsburg-pancreatic-cancer/5837919002/.

76. See note 75, above.

77. See note 75, above.

78. See note 75, above.

79. See L. Fisher and M. Rothman, note 19, above; see note 37, above.

80. See note 37, above.

81. See K. Coleman, note 14, above; see M. Rothman, note 22, above.

82. See note 37, above.

83. See note 81, above.

35   Jeffrey Epstein

1. G. Bruney, "Unpacking Donald Trump's Ties to Jeffrey Epstein, as Shown in Netflix's Filthy Rich," *Esquire*, June 5, 2020, https://www.esquire.com/entertainment/tv/a32784116/jeffrey-epstein-donald-trump-connection-friendship-explained/; C. Unger, "'He's a Lot of Fun to be With': Inside Jeffrey Epstein and Donald Trump's Epic Bromance," *Vanity Fair*, January 21, 2021, https://www.vanityfair.com/news/2021/01/jeffrey-epstein-and-donald-trump-epic-bromance; M. Gajanan, "Here's What to Know About the Sex Trafficking Case Against Jeffrey Epstein," *Time*, original published date July 8, 2019, last updated July 17, 2019, https://time.com/5621911/jeffrey-epstein-sex-trafficking-what-to-know/; C. Hallemann, "What We Do and Don't Know About Jeffrey Epstein," *Town & Country*, July 2, 2020, https://www.townandcountrymag.com/society/money-and-power/a28352055/jeffrey-epstein-criminal-case-facts/; G. Wallace, "Jeffrey Epstein's world of wealth and powerful friends," CNN, August 10, 2019, https://www.cnn.com/2019/07/08/politics/jeffrey-epstein-bio/index.html; E. Cranley and B. Goggin, "The life of Jeffrey Epstein, the convicted sex offender and well-connected financier who died in jail awaiting sex trafficking charges," Business Insider, August 10, 2019, https://www.businessinsider.com/jeffrey-epstein-life-biography-net-worth-2019-7.

2. See note 1, above.

3. See G. Bruney, C. Unger, M. Gajanan, C. Hallemann, and E. Cranley and B. Goggin, note 1, above.

4. See note 3, above.

5. J. K. Brown, "For years, Jeffrey Epstein abused teen girls, police say. A timeline of his case," *Miami Herald*, November 28, 2018, https://www.miamiherald.com/news/local/article221404845.html; "Jeffrey Epstein American Financier and Sentenced Child-Sex Offender," https://peoplepill.com/people/jeffrey-epstein; "Jeffrey Epstein Biography," A&E Television Networks, original published date December 5, 2019, last updated August 11, 2020, https://www.biography.com/crime-figure/jeffrey-epstein; see M. Gajanan, and E. Cranley and B. Goggin, note 1, above.

6. See M. Gajanan, note 1, above; see J. K. Brown, and "Jeffrey Epstein American Financier and Sentenced Child-Sex Offender," note 5, above.

7. See note 6, above.

8. See M. Gajanan, note 1, above; see J. K. Brown, note 5, above.

9. V. Bekiempis, "'His conduct left an impression that lingered': the life of Jeffrey Epstein," the *Guardian*, August 10, 2019, https://www.theguardian.com/us-news/2019/aug/10/jeffrey-epstein-life-profile; see G. Bruney, G. Wallace, C. Hallemann, and E. Cranley and B. Goggin, note 1, above; see "Jeffrey Epstein American Financier and Sentenced Child-Sex Offender," note 5, above.

10. A. Paybarah, "Epstein's Autopsy 'Points to Homicide,' Pathologist Hired by Brother Claims," the *New York Times*, original published date October 30, 2019, last updated October 31, 2019, https://www.nytimes.com/2019/10/30/nyregion/jeffrey-epstein-homicide-autopsy-michael-baden.html; J. Coaston, A. North, et al., "The life and death of sex offender Jeffrey Epstein, explained," January 16, 2020, https://www.vox.com/2018/12/3/18116351/jeffrey-epstein-case-indictment-arrested-trump-clinton; see G. Wallace, C. Hallemann, and E. Cranley and B. Goggin, note 1, above; see Jeffrey Epstein Biography," note 5, above; see note 6, above.

11. See G. Bruney, M. Gajanan, and G. Wallace, note 1, above; see "Jeffrey Epstein American Financier and Sentenced Child-Sex Offender," note 5, above.

12. "60 Minutes investigates the death of Jeffrey Epstein," CBS News, January 5, 2020, https://www.cbsnews.com/news/did-jeffrey-epstein-kill-himself-60-minutes-investigates-2020-01-05/; see G. Wallace, C. Hallemann, and E. Cranley and B. Goggin, note 1, above; see "Jeffrey Epstein American Financier and Sentenced Child-Sex Offender," and "Jeffrey Epstein Biography," note 5, above; see A. Paybarah, and J. Coaston, A. North, et al., note 10, above.

13. See V. Bekiempis, note 9, above.

14. See "Jeffrey Epstein American Financier and Sentenced Child-Sex Offender," M. Gajanan, C. Hallemann, G. Wallace, and E. Cranley and B. Goggin, note 1, above; see note 6, above; see "60 Minutes investigates the death of Jeffrey Epstein," note 12, above.

15. "Jeffrey Epstein Biography," https://history-biography.com/jeffrey-epstein/; K. Freifeld and S. N. Lynch, "Jeffrey Epstein autopsy report shows broken neck: sources," Reuters, August 15, 2019, https://www.reuters.com/article/us-epstein-autopsy/jeffrey-epstein-autopsy-report-shows-broken-neck-sources-idUSKCN1V50HW; see C. Hallemann, G. Wallace, and E. Cranley and B. Goggin, note 1, above; see "Jeffrey Epstein American Financier and Sentenced Child-Sex Offender," and "Jeffrey Epstein Biography," note 5, above; see J. Coaston, A. North, et al., note 10, above; see note 13, above.

16. E. Helmore, "Epstein case: judge agrees to keep documents on 2008 plea deal secret," the *Guardian*, July 27, 2019, https://www.theguardian.com/us-news/2019/jul/27/jeffrey-epstein-2008-documents-secret; see C. Hallemann, and E. Cranley and B. Goggin, note 1, above; see "Jeffrey Epstein American Financier and Sentenced Child-Sex Offender," note 5, above; see "Jeffrey Epstein Biography," note 10, above; see note 13, above.

17. J. Royston, "Inside Jeffrey Epstein's Prison Ordeal: Gangs, Suicide Watch and Extortion," *Newsweek*, https://www.newsweek.com/jeffrey-epstein-prison-gangs-suicide-extortion-feared-attack-mcc-spider-barry-levine-1540634.

18. See note 17, above.

19. D. Mangan, "'Missing' jail video from first Jeffrey Epstein suicide attempt has been found, prosecutors tell judge," CNBC, December 20, 2019, https://www.cnbc.com/2019/12/20/video-of-jeffrey-epstein-jail-suicide-attempt-is-found.html; see C. Hallemann, note 1, above; see "Jeffrey Epstein American Financier and Sentenced Child-Sex Offender," note 5, above; see "Jeffrey Epstein Biography," note 10, above; see "60 Minutes investigates the death of Jeffrey Epstein," note 12, above; see E. Helmore, note 16, above; see note 17, above.

20. See "Jeffrey Epstein American Financier and Sentenced Child-Sex Offender," note 5, above; see "Jeffrey Epstein Biography," note 10, above; see 60 Minutes investigates the death of Jeffrey Epstein," note 12, above; see K. Freifeld and S. N. Lynch, note 15, above; see E. Helmore, note 16, above.

21. D. Mangan, "'Missing' jail video from first Jeffrey Epstein suicide attempt has been found, prosecutors tell judge," CNBC, December 20, 2019, https://www.cnbc.com/2019/12/20/video-of-jeffrey-epstein-jail-suicide-attempt-is-found.html; J. K. Brown, "In latest Epstein deal, officers who slept while financier died plead guilty, avert trial," May 25, 2021, http://www.virginislandsdailynews.com/ap/in-latest-epstein-deal-officers-who-slept-while-financier-died-plead-guilty-avert-trial/article_1c05cc02-39c3-53c6-bcf9-e612cd02c255.html; see "Jeffrey Epstein American Financier and Sentenced Child-Sex Offender," note 5, above; see "60 Minutes investigates the death of Jeffrey Epstein," note 12, above.

22. M. R. Sisak, "Medical examiner dismisses doubts about Epstein autopsy," Public Broadcasting Service, October 30, 2019, https://www.pbs.org/newshour/nation/medical-examiner-dismisses-doubts-about-epstein-autopsy; see "Jeffrey Epstein American Financier and Sentenced Child-Sex Offender," note 5, above; see "Jeffrey Epstein Biography," note 10, above; see "60 Minutes investigates the death of Jeffrey Epstein," note 12, above; see K. Freifeld and S. N. Lynch, note 15, above; see J. K. Brown, note 21, above.

23. See C. Hallemann, G. Wallace, and E. Cranley and B. Goggin, note 1, above; see "Jeffrey Epstein American Financier and Sentenced Child-Sex Offender" and "Jeffrey Epstein Biography," note 5, above; see J. Coaston, A. North, et al., note 10, above; see "60 Minutes investigates the death of Jeffrey Epstein," note 12, above; see M. R. Sisak, note 22, above.

24. "Jeffrey Epstein: Blood Vessels in Eyes Popped During Hanging," August 15, 2019, https://www.tmz.com/2019/08/15/jeffrey-epstein-hanging-injuries-broken-neck-strangulation/; M. Hines, "What can a tiny bone tell us about Jeffrey Epstein's death?" *USA Today*, original published date August 15, 2019, last updated August 16, 2019, https://www.usatoday.com/story/news/health/2019/08/15/mystery-surrounds-hyoid-break-epstein-death-suicide-murder/2017579001/; see J. K. Brown, note 21, above.

25. See D. Mangan, note 19, above; see J. K. Brown, note 21, above.

26. See C. Hallemann, and G. Wallace, note 1, above; see "Jeffrey Epstein American Financier and Sentenced Child-Sex Offender," note 5, above.

27. See "Jeffrey Epstein American Financier and Sentenced Child-Sex Offender," note 5, above; see A. Paybarah, note 10, above.

28. B. McCandless Farmer, "Jeffrey Epstein's Autopsy: A Closer Look," CBS News, January 5, 2020, https://www.cbsnews.com/news/jeffrey-epstein-autopsy-a-closer-look-60-minutes-2020-01-05/; see "Jeffrey Epstein American Financier and Sentenced Child-Sex Offender," note 5, above.

29. See B. McCandless Farmer, note 28, above.

30. See note 29, above.

31. See note 29, above.

32. See note 29, above.

33. See "Jeffrey Epstein American Financier and Sentenced Child-Sex Offender," note 5, above; see K. Freifeld and S. N. Lynch, note 15, above; see note 29, above.

34. M. Hines, "What can a tiny bone tell us about Jeffrey Epstein's death?" *USA Today*, original published date August 15, 2019, last

updated August 16, 2019, https://www.usatoday.com/story/news/health/2019/08/15/mystery-surrounds-hyoid-break-epstein-death-suicide-murder/2017579001/; see M. R. Sisak, note 22, above.

35. M. R. Sisak, M. Balsamo, et al., "Medical examiner rules Epstein death a suicide by hanging," AP News, August 16, 2019, https://apnews.com/article/suicides-us-news-ap-top-news-bernard-madoff-new-york-city-a947e0d85d31496eb5bd9ff4994c9718; see note 27, above; see note 29, above.

36. See "Jeffrey Epstein American Financier and Sentenced Child-Sex Offender," note 5, above; see note 29, above.

37. See "Jeffrey Epstein Biography," note 5, above; see M. R. Sisak, note 22, above; see note 27, above.

38. See note 29, above.

39. A. A. Abouhashem, S. M. Bataw, et al., "Suicidal, homicidal and accidental hanging: Comparative cross sectional study in Aljabal Alkhdar Area, Libya," *Zagazig J. Forensic Med. & Toxicology* 19(1) (2020): 126–38.

40. M. A. Ali, T. N. Cheema, et al., "Hyoid Bone Fracture in Neck Strangulation: Five Years Meta-Analysis at Tertiary Care Hospital," Annals of Punjab Medical College 12(1) (2018): 4–7; see note 37, above.

41. See A. Paybarah, note 10, above; see M. R. Sisak, M. Balsamo, et al., note 22, above; see note 29, above.

42. See note 29, above.

43. H. K. Afridi, M. Yousaf, et al., "In Strangulation Deaths: Forensic Significance of Hyoid Bone Fracture," *Pakistan J Med Health Sci* 8(2) (2014): 376–78; H. Green, R. A. James, et al., "Fractures of the hyoid bone and laryngeal cartilages in suicidal hanging," *J Clin Forensic Med* 7(3) (2000): 123–26; see M. A. Ali, T. N. Cheema, et al., note 40, above.

44. See note 39, above.

45. See H. Green, R. A. James, et al., note 43, above.

46. See note 29, above.

47. See note 29, above.

48. K. Puschel, W. Holtz, et al., "Hanging: suicide or homicide?" *Arch Kriminol* 174(5–6) (1984): 141–53; see note 29, above.

49. See E. Cranley and B. Goggin, note 3, above; see "Jeffrey Epstein American Financier and Sentenced Child-Sex Offender," and "Jeffrey Epstein Biography," note 5, above.

50. "Jeffrey Epstein Biography," https://history-biography.com/jeffrey-epstein/; see "Jeffrey Epstein American Financier and Sentenced Child-Sex Offender," and "Jeffrey Epstein Biography," note 5, above; see note 13, above.

51. See "Jeffrey Epstein American Financier and Sentenced Child-Sex Offender," note 5, above; see "Jeffrey Epstein Biography," note 50, above.

52. See E. Cranley and B. Goggin, note 1, above; see note 50, above.

53. See M. Gajanan, and C. Hallemann, note 1, above; see note 13, above; see note 49, above.

54. See "Jeffrey Epstein Biography," note 5, above; see note 51, above.

55. See note 50, above.

56. See M. Gajanan, and C. Hallemann, note 1, above; see note 52, above.

57. See "Jeffrey Epstein American Financier and Sentenced Child-Sex Offender," note 5, above.

58. See M. Gajanan, and C. Hallemann, note 1, above; see note 50, above.

59. See note 57, above.

60. See note 54, above.

61. See note 54, above.

62. See "Jeffrey Epstein Biography," note 5, above; see note 57, above.

63. See note 62, above.

64. See note 54, above.

65. See note 54, above.

66. See note 51, above.

67. See M. Gajanan, note 1, above; see note 62, above.

68. See note 62, above.

69. See note 57, above.

70. See note 57, above.

71. L. Voytko, "Excerpt: 'The Spider' Spotlights How Trump's Presidency Helped Expose Jeffrey Epstein," *Forbes*, October 18, 2020, https://www.forbes.com/sites/lisettevoytko/2020/10/18/spider-book-excerpt-how-trumps-presidency-helped-expose-jeffrey-epstein/?sh=321164fb408f; see note 62, above.

72. See C. Unger, note 2, above.

73. See note 39, above.

74. See note 39, above.

75. See note 39, above.

76. C. Méheut, "Ex-Modeling Agent and Epstein Associate Found Dead in a Paris Jail," *The New York Times*, February 19, 2022, https://www.nytimes.com/2022/02/19/world/europe/brunel-epstein-prince-andrew-giuffre.html.

36.   Naya Rivera

1. "Lake Piru," https://explorelakepiru.com/.

2. M. Watts, "Harrison Ford Is Under FAA Investigation for Plane Operation Blunder — Yes, Again," *Newsweek*, April 29, 2020, https://www.newsweek.com/harrison-ford-under-faa-investigation-plane-operation-blunder-yes-again-1501008; see "Lake Piru," note 1, above.

3. See note 1, above.

4. "Complaint—Josey Hollis Dorsey v. County of Ventura et al.," Superior Court of the State of California for the County of Ventura, November 17, 2020, https://www.courthousenews.com/wp-content/uploads/2020/11/DorseyVenturaCty-COMPLAINT.pdf.

5. "Ventura Sheriff Press Conference Transcript on Death of 'Glee' Actress Naya Rivera," https://www.rev.com/blog/transcripts/ventura-sheriff-press-conference-transcript-on-death-of-glee-actress-naya-rivera; "Naya Rivera," https://thefamouspeople.com/profiles/naya-rivera-15666.php; see note 4, above.

6. See note 4, above.

7. See note 4, above. See "Ventura Sheriff Press Conference Transcript on Death of 'Glee' Actress Naya Rivera," note 5, above.

8. "Naya Rivera's Full Autopsy Report Reveals Devastating Details About the Day She Died," September 11, 2020, https://www.justjared.com/2020/09/11/naya-riveras-full-autopsy-report-reveals-devastating-details-about-the-day-she-died; see note 4, above.

9. See note 4, above.

10. See note 7, above.

11. See note 7, above.

12. See note 7, above.

13. See "Ventura Sheriff Press Conference Transcript on Death of 'Glee' Actress Naya Rivera," note 5, above.

14. See note 7, above.

15. See note 13, above.

16. See note 13, above.

17. "Autopsy confirms Naya Rivera's death by accidental drowning," CBC, July 15, 2020, https://www.cbc.ca/news/entertainment/naya-rivera-autopsy-1.5650155.

18. "Naya Rivera's Full Autopsy and Toxicology Report Uncovers New Details," September 11, 2020, https://www.accessonline.com/articles/naya-riveras-full-autopsy-and-toxicology-report-uncovers-new-details; see note 17, above.

19. See note 13, above.

20. "Naya Rivera Biography," https://www.imdb.com/name/nm0729369/bio; see "Naya Rivera's Full Autopsy and Toxicology Report Uncovers New Details," note 18, above.

21. See note 18, above.

22. C. Harvery-Jenner, "Naya Rivera's autopsy confirms her cause of death as drowning," *Cosmopolitan*, July 15, 2020, https://www.cosmopolitan.com/uk/reports/a33319799/naya-rivera-cause-death/.

23. A. Dalton, "Autopsy report: Naya Rivera called for help as she drowned," Associated Press, September 11, 2020, https://apnews.com/article/naya-rivera-accidents-california-archive-lakes-c26cab1

196aa1245ab8b19d08d972943; see "Naya Rivera's Full Autopsy and Toxicology Report Uncovers New Details," note 18, above.

24. See "Naya Rivera's Full Autopsy and Toxicology Report Uncovers New Details," note 18, above.

25. See note 24, above.

26. See note 24, above.

27. "Naya Rivera," https://ethnicelebs.com/naya-rivera; S. Prideaux, "'Glee' actress Naya Rivera's rise to fame: from child star to symbol of hope," July 14, 2020, https://www.thenationalnews.com/arts-culture/television/glee-actress-naya-rivera-s-rise-to-fame-from-child-star-to-symbol-of-hope-1.1049099; see "Naya Rivera Biography," note 20, above.

28. "City of Santa Clarita," https://www.santa-clarita.com/home/showdocument?id=2132.

29. See "Naya Rivera," note 5, above; H. Yasharoff and C. Henderson, "'Heaven gained our sassy and angel': Naya Rivera's family speaks out after 'Glee' actress' drowning," *USA Today*, original published date July 13, 2020, last updated July 15, 2020, https://www.usatoday.com/story/entertainment/celebrities/2020/07/13/naya-rivera-search-lake-piru-glee-actress/5426865002/; see "Naya Rivera Biography," note 20, above; see S. Prideaux, note 27, above.

30. See "Naya Rivera," note 5, above; H. Yasharoff and C. Henderson, "'Heaven gained our sassy angel': Naya Rivera's family speaks out after 'Glee' actress' drowning," *USA Today*, original published date July 13, 2020, last updated July 15, 2020, https://www.usatoday.com/story/entertainment/celebrities/2020/07/13/naya-rivera-search-lake-piru-glee-actress/5426865002/; see S. Prideaux, note 27, above.

31. A. Rosenbloom and A. Morin, "Why Naya Rivera Says Working on Step Up: High Water Reminds Her of Glee," March 20, 2019, https://www.eonline.com/news/1025075/why-naya-rivera-says-working-on-step-up-high-water-reminds-her-of-glee.

32. See note 31, above.

33. See note 31, above.

34. L. Parker, "11 Famous Singers Rejected by 'American Idol'," *Rolling Stone*, February 23, 2015, https://www.rollingstone.com/music/music-news/11-famous-singers-rejected-by-american-idol-108997/; see "Naya Rivera," note 5, above; see "Naya Rivera Biography," note 20, above.

35. G Edwards, "Naya Rivera: 'Glee' Bad Girl Aims for the Pop Charts," *Rolling Stone*, November 7, 2013, https://www.rollingstone.com/movies/movie-news/naya-rivera-glee-bad-girl-aims-for-the-pop-charts-247985/; see "Naya Rivera," note 5, above.

36. J. Steinberg, "Naya Rivera Filled with Glee," https://web.archive.org/web/20090908162752/http://starrymag.com/content.asp?ID=4317&CATEGORY=INTERVIEWS.

37. See note 36, above.

38. See "Naya Rivera Biography," note 20, above.

39. See note 38, above.

40. See note 38, above.

41. See note 38, above.

42. See note 38, above.

43. See note 38, above.

44. See "Naya Rivera," note 5, above.

45. See note 44, above.

46. O. Singh, "Authorities are 'confident' that the body found at Lake Piru is 'Glee' star Naya Rivera," *Insider*, July 13, 2020, https://www.insider.com/naya-rivera-dead-2020-7; see note 44, above.

47. See H. Yasharoff and C. Henderson, note 29, above; see O. Singh, note 46, above.

48. B. Haring, "Naya Rivera Autopsy Report Released, Says 'Glee' Actress Called Out For Help," Deadline, September 11, 2020, https://deadline.com/2020/09/naya-rivera-autopsy-report-claims-glee-actress-shouted-for-help-1234575761/; see note 4, above; see note 23, above.

49. O. Niland, "Naya Rivera's Official Cause of Death Was An Accidental Drowning," BuzzFeed, July 14, 2020, https://www.buzzfeednews.com/article/olivianiland/naya-rivera-cause-of-

death-was-accidental-drowning; see note 13, above; see note 22, above; see H. Yasharoff and C. Henderson, note 29, above.

50. See S. Prideaux, note 27, above.

51. See O. Singh, note 46, above; see note 50, above.

52. H. A. Milman, "Natalie Wood," in *Forensics: The Science Behind the Deaths of Famous People* (Bloomington, Indiana: Xlibris, 2020), 73–84.

53. H. A. Milman, "Whitney Houston," in *Forensics: The Science Behind the Deaths of Famous People* (Bloomington, Indiana: Xlibris, 2020), 187–202.

54. See note 44, above.

55. See note 44, above.

56. See note 38, above.

57. See note 38, above.

58. See note 17, above.

59. See note 17, above.

60. See O. Niland, note 49, above.

61. See note 22, above.

62. See B. Haring, note 48, above; see note 50, above.

63. "Autopsy report—Cory Monteith," https://www2.gov.bc.ca/assets/gov/birth-adoption-death-marriage-and-divorce/deaths/coroners-service/reports/investigative/monteith-cory-allan-michael.pdf; see A. Dalton, note 23, above; see note 50, above.

64. See "Autopsy report—Cory Monteith," note 63, above.

65. See A. Dalton, note 23, above; see note 50, above.

66. "Music Legends Who Lived Fast and Died at 27," History, original published date September 13, 2018, last updated April 2, 2019, https://www.history.com/news/music-legends-who-lived-fast-and-died-at-27-slideshow.

37. Conclusions

1. "15th Report on Carcinogens," US National Toxicology Program, Department of Health and Human Services, December 21, 2021.

2.   See note 1, above.

3.   "Environmental Carcinogens and Cancer Risk," US National Cancer Institute, US National Institutes of Health, https://www.cancer.gov/about-cancer/causes-prevention/risk/substances/carcinogens.

4.   L. Surugue, "Cult leaders: What makes people like David Koresh so successful at getting people to follow them?" International Business Times, January 23, 2017, https://www.ibtimes.co.uk/cult-leaders-what-makes-people-like-david-koresh-so-successful-getting-people-follow-them-1555073.

5.   See note 6, above.

6.   See note 6, above.

7.   See note 6, above.

8.   See note 6, above.

9.   W. Jacobs, "Fatal amphetamine-associated cardiotoxicity and its medicolegal implications," Am J Forensic Med Pathol 27(2):156-60, (2006).

10.   H. A. Milman, "Sam Kinison," (*Forensics: The Science Behind the Deaths of Famous People*, pp 103-112, Xlibris, 2020).

11.   A. Vigderman, "A Timeline of School Shootings Since Columbine," August 9, 2021, https://www.security.org/blog/a-timeline-of-school-shootings-since-columbine/.

12.   E. Chuck, A. Johnson, et al., "17 killed in mass shooting at high school in Parkland, Florida," NBC News, original published date Feb. 14, 2018, last updated Feb. 15, 2018, https://www.nbcnews.com/news/us-news/police-respond-shooting-parkland-florida-high-school-n848101; J. Hanna, D. Andone, et al., "Alleged shooter at Texas high school spared people he liked, court document says," CNN, May 19, 2018, https://www.cnn.com/2018/05/18/us/texas-school-shooting/index.html; N. Chavez, E. Grinberg, et al., "Pittsburgh synagogue gunman said he wanted all Jews to die, criminal complaint says," CNN, October 31, 2018, https://www.cnn.com/2018/10/28/us/pittsburgh-synagogue-shooting/index.html.

13. M. Martin and E. Bowman, "Why Nearly All Mass Shooters Are Men," National Public Radio, March 27, 2021, https://www.npr.org/2021/03/27/981803154/why-nearly-all-mass-shooters-are-men.

14. See note 13, above.

15. See note 13, above.

16. J. Peterson and J. Densley, "Op-Ed: We have studied every mass shooting since 1966. Here's what we've learned about the shooters," Los Angeles Times, August 4, 2019, https://www.latimes.com/opinion/story/2019-08-04/el-paso-dayton-gilroy-mass-shooters-data.

17. See note 16, above.

18. See note 16, above.

19. See note 16, above.

20. See note 16, above.

21. S. Chokshi, "Why Spree Killers Kill Themselves," Wired, December 18, 2012, https://www.wired.com/2012/12/why-spree-killers-kill-themselves/.

22. S. Ferro, "How Often Do Mass Shooters Die In Their Attacks?" September 17, 2013, https://www.popsci.com/science/article/2013-09/how-often-do-mass-shooters-die-their-attacks/.

23. See note 22, above.

24. S. Chokshi, "Why Spree Killers Kill Themselves," Wired, December 18, 2012, https://www.wired.com/2012/12/why-spree-killers-kill-themselves/; see note 22, above.

25. See S. Chokshi, note 24, above.

26. See note 25, above.

27. A. Preti, "School Shooting as a Culturally Enforced Way of Expressing Suicidal Hostile Intentions," J Am Acad Psychiatry Law 36:544-550 (2008).

28. See note 27, above.

29. See note 27, above.

30. See note 27, above.

INDEX

A

Abou-Foul, Ahmad K, 14
abrasion, 229, 231, 269, 315, 363, 370, 426, 475, 505
acetaminophen, 46, 207, 455, 457–58, 473
acetyl fentanyl, 397–98, 401, 455
acid, aminobutyric, 456
Acosta, Alexander, 424
acute epiglottitis, 9
acute myocardial infarction, 165, 288, 475–76, 496
acute respiratory failure, 15, 476
adenosine triphosphate (ATP), 46, 476
adrenaline, 300
Akin, Lane, 139
alcohol, 30, 39, 41–42, 47, 78–79, 82–84, 90, 122, 129, 133, 143–45, 157, 164, 174, 182, 193–95, 199–201, 207–8, 217–20, 233–34, 265, 271, 281, 283, 311, 327, 332, 372–73, 401, 406–7, 410, 442, 444, 449–50, 456–57, 462, 480–81, 486, 493, 496, 498, 504, 506
alcoholism, 195, 199–201, 281, 410, 444, 450
Alex (Johnny Carson's wife), 306
Alexander, John, 209
Alexandra (tsarina), 34, 45
Alexei (Tsarina Alexandra's son), 34, 45
Alexis, Constantine, 51
Allen, Steve, 304
alopecia, 331
alpha-1-antitrypsin deficiency, 312, 477
alpha particles, 333, 338–39, 477
alprazolam, 397–98, 401, 456
alveoli, 88, 155, 311–12, 354, 476, 478, 490, 497, 509

American Association of Neurological Surgeons, 53
American Revolution, 12, 386
Ames, Ed, 310
amphetamine, 73, 79, 83–84, 221,
437, 449, 456
Amrozi, 392
amygdala, 67, 478
anaerobic respiration, 46, 478
Anastasia, Umberto, 49–50, 52,
447
Anastasia Crime Family, 49–50
Anderson, Brian, 237, 239
Anderson, Michael E., 322
Anderson, Robyn, 236
Andy (Gibb, M.'s younger brother), 283
aneurysms, 291, 300
angina, 89, 317, 473, 478
angiogram, 288
anhidrosis, 105, 453, 479
antecubital fossa, 269, 479
anticoagulants, 288
antimony, 4, 141, 463, 472
Anti-Terrorism Department. *See*
Federal Counterintel-
lignece Service (FSK), 335
Antommarchi, Francesco, 19–24
aorta, 64, 77–78, 84, 118, 142,
155, 229, 232, 269, 280,
291, 316, 362, 479
aortic dissection, 288–89, 291–92,
445–46, 479
Applewhite, Marshall, 203–4,
206, 208–15, 447
Argento, Asia, 411
Armstrong, A. James, 125
Arnott, Archibald, 20
arrhythmia, 77–79, 84, 183, 219,
296, 300–301, 318–19,
331, 371, 373, 447, 449,
460–61, 479, 523, 525, 527

arsenic, 27–32, 329, 444, 457,
480
arteriosclerosis, 183, 206, 209,
480
arthritis, 348, 353
Ascencao, Nadine, 388
aspirin, 99, 102–3, 453, 455, 457,
463, 493, 521
asthma, 77–79, 82–83, 184, 463,
501, 519
asthmatic attack, 77–78, 83
astrocytoma, 64, 66, 480
atherosclerosis, 53, 168, 189–90,
219, 229, 269, 300, 362,
371, 373, 397, 399,
445–46, 481
constrictive coronary, 206,
209
Attew, Dean, 326
Augustine (G. Washington's
father), 10
Austin State Hospital, 63
autopsy, x–xii, 6, 21–24, 31, 39,
41, 43, 52–53, 62–66, 68,
76–79, 82–84, 88–89, 94,
99–104, 106, 117, 120,
122, 140, 143–44, 155–57,
164, 172–75, 183–84,
196, 206, 208, 213, 219,
221, 228, 234, 245–46,
255, 260, 268, 270, 278,
280–81, 289, 295–96, 307,
314, 316, 318, 331, 334,
348, 361, 363, 370–71,
373, 383, 397, 399, 404–5,
415, 426–29, 437–38,
449, 453, 522, 703, 706,
725–28, 732–35
Auyb, Bill, 436
avulsion, 362, 481

B

Baden, Michael, 427
Bailey, David, 173
Baird, Zoë, 154, 160
Baker, Cliff, 162
Baker, Susan, 411
Baldwin, Marceline, 123
Barbara (Ramone's wife), 268
barbiturates, 83, 120, 207, 215,
    457–58, 470, 518
Bargneti, Elsa, 55
barium, 141
Barker, Creighton, 9
Barker, Stuart, 353
Baselt, Randall C., 173
Baskin, Helen, 90
Baxter, John Clifford, 321
Baxter Springs Whiz Kids, 197
The Beatles, 257, 261–64, 399,
    711
Bee Gees, 277, 279, 282–83, 286
Belushi, John, 168, 220
Benadryl. *See* diphenhydramine,
    463
benign reactive lymphoid hyper-
    plasia, 229, 481
benzodiazepine, 171, 221, 254,
    397, 399, 447, 456–58,
    462, 464, 467–68, 472–73,
    709
benzoylecgonine, 183, 296, 458
Berezovsky, Boris, 336–37
Berman, Alan L., 161
Berman, Richard, 425
Bernstein, Leonard, 306
Berra, Yogi, 193
Berry, Chuck, 185
Betty Ford Center, 182, 194
Beyer, James C., 155
Biden, Joe, 252
Billy (Mantle's son), 199

bionic man. *See* Knievel, Evel
Bissel, Pelham St. George, III, 58
Black, Albert, Jr., 131
Blackbourne, Brian D., 161, 206
black box warning, 233
Blakely, Philip, 113
bleeding, 4, 6, 8, 23–24, 45, 315,
    481, 506
blood, x, 4, 6–7, 13–14, 35,
    38–39, 46, 64–65, 78–79,
    88–89, 93, 100, 120,
    143–44, 157, 174, 183,
    188, 207, 221, 230, 233,
    291, 296, 301, 311, 330,
    332, 346, 363, 382, 419,
    429, 465–66, 476, 478,
    480, 482–83, 486, 488–90,
    494–98, 501–2, 504,
    511–12, 515–16, 518–19,
    527–28
blood alcohol concentration
    (BAC), 78, 438, 456, 481
blood-brain barrier, 100, 482
blood clots, 100, 144, 168, 286,
    300, 372, 524
bloodletting, 2–6, 13, 15, 482
blood loss, 6–7, 291, 498
blood replacement, 14
Bobbitt, Lorena, 71
Bocchino, Joseph, 50
Bonanno, Joe, 56
Bonaparte, Napoleon, 17–32, 444,
    450
Boston Marathon, 379, 381–82,
    385–89, 392, 448, 705, 707
    bombers. *See* Tsarnaev,
        Tamerlan; Tsarnaev,
        Dzhokhar
    bombing, 379, 381–82,
        385–89, 392, 448, 705,
        707
Boswell, Charles, 125

Boteler, Blake, 134
Bourdain, Anthony, 403–9, 411–12, 447, 712–17
Braddock, Edward, 11
Braden, Elizabeth "Lisa," 158
brain, xi, 6, 40, 43, 52–53, 63–67, 71, 77, 89, 98, 100–101, 118–20, 142, 156–57, 178, 188, 220, 230–33, 259, 270, 315–16, 332, 354, 362, 373, 410, 456, 459, 461–62, 464–73, 478, 480, 482, 484–85, 487–88, 492, 495, 500–501, 507, 514, 516, 518, 521–24, 528
    frontal region of, 233, 523
    temporal region of, 523
brain injury, traumatic, 100
brain tumors, 67–68, 72–73, 100, 495
Branch Davidians, 133–40, 142, 144–51, 249, 448
Brancheau, Dawn, 357–62, 364–65, 367–68, 449
Breitbart, Andrew, 369–78, 446
    Righteous Indignation: Excuse Me While I Save the World, 376
Brennan, Ian, 441
Brickell, James, 6
Bricklayers Arms, 81
Brocklehurst, R. J., 47
bronchitis, 354, 485, 519
Bronfman, Edgar, 431
Brothers, Joyce, 305
Brown, Brooks, 235–36
Brown, Gustave Richard, 4, 13
Brown, Stuart L., 67
Bruce, Gregor, 393
Bruce Lee: A Life (Polly), 104
Brunel, Jean-Luc, 433
Buford, Bill, 149

Bunds, David, 146
Bureau of Alcohol, Tobacco, and Firearms (ATF), 133
Burrows, Nick, 224
Burton, Bill, 323
Burton, Richard, 262
Bush, George, 414
Bush, George H. W., 310
butalbital, 207–8, 458

C

caffeine, 296, 437, 458–59, 480
calomel, 4, 21, 30, 459
Campbell, David, 270
Campbell, Linda, 63
cancer, 21, 23, 30, 199–200, 206, 210, 213, 258–59, 264–65, 279, 362, 420–21, 441, 444, 449, 480, 486, 495–96, 498–99, 506, 510, 512, 527, 723
    colorectal, 286, 486
    gastric, 24, 26, 28, 30–32, 444, 493
    head and neck, 496
    liver, 195–96, 201, 213, 444, 506, 526
    lung, 258, 261, 265, 444, 509
    oropharyngeal, 257, 264–65, 510
    pancreatic, 414, 419–21, 444, 504, 511–12, 722–23
Candy, John, 163–69, 445–46
cannabis, 98, 100–103, 409, 453, 459, 465–66
cantharides, blisters of, 3–4, 7, 15, 458
capillaries, 427, 482, 487, 498, 515
Caputo, Dennis, 88
carbon dioxide, 42, 89, 216, 311, 478, 483, 487, 511, 518–19

Carbon Monoxide, 143
carcinoma
    undifferentiated hepatocellu-
        lar, 195–96, 200, 526
    verrucous, 279, 513, 527
cardiac arrest, 277, 280, 330, 396,
    426, 483, 708
cardiomegaly, 188, 373, 483
cardiomyopathy, 446, 483
cardiopulmonary resuscitation
    (CPR), 315, 396, 483, 527
cardiotoxicity, 221, 247, 447, 736
carfentanil, 343, 459
Carlson, Dylan, 174
Carlson, Matt, 273
Carlson, Susan, 247
Carlson, Tucker, 377
Carr, David, 375
Carrillo, Juan M., 370
Carson, Johnny, 303–12, 352, 444
Carter, Jimmy, 418
Carter, Tim, 115–16
Cartmell, Mike, 128
Cary, Jacob, 238
Cary, Nathaniel, 331
Case, Ross E., 124
catecholamine, 300
Cause of Death, xi, 10, 22, 24,
    28, 43, 52–53, 68, 79, 90,
    100–103, 106, 144, 158,
    165, 175, 184, 196, 208,
    221, 230, 234, 247, 261,
    270, 281, 289, 296, 308,
    319, 333–34, 348, 364,
    373, 383, 399, 405, 415,
    420, 427, 430, 438, 447,
    450, 453, 484, 496, 504,
    517, 522, 711–12, 732, 734
Cavalli, Franco, 259
Cavanaugh, Linda, 247
CBS, 92, 309
cecum, 280, 484, 502

Celexa. *See* citalopram
cellular respiration, 27
Centers for Disease Control and
    Prevention (CDC), 104,
    167, 398, 710, 717
central nervous system, 65, 84,
    208, 442, 447, 456–57,
    461, 466, 468–70, 482,
    484, 492, 516
cerebral edema, 98, 100–106,
    280, 450, 453, 484
cerebral hemisphere, 156, 232–33,
    485, 495
cerebral ischemia, 410, 485, 504
Cheatham, Michael L., 15
Chenar, Coleman de, 63
Cherry Garcia, 191
chloral hydrate, xi, 114, 460
Chloroquine, 119, 460
cholesterol, 188–89, 470, 480–81,
    496, 515
Chow, Raymond, 98–99, 104,
    108–9
Chris (Candy's son), 163, 166,
    405
Christopher, Sybil, 262
chronic obstructive pulmonary
    disease (COPD), 307, 354,
    444, 476, 485, 490
Ciesynski, Mike, 174
cigarette smoke, 190, 449
Cipro. *See* ciprofloxacin
ciprofloxacin, 328, 460–61
cirrhosis, 53, 196, 200–201, 269,
    281, 372, 450, 485–86, 506
cisatracurium, 254, 461
citalopram, 397, 461
Clark, Flaherty, 366
Clarke, Judy, 386, 704, 706
Clay, Cassius. *See* Muhammad Ali
clinicians, goal of, 285
Clinton, Bill, 153, 158–59, 418,

421

Clinton, Hillary, 421

Close, Del, 223

Cobain, Kurt, 85, 171–79, 442, 447

cocaine, 84, 95, 165, 168, 174, 182–83, 186–87, 189–91, 219–21, 291, 295–96, 299–301, 401, 406–7, 409, 446–47, 458, 461–62, 468, 472, 480

codeine, 89, 462

cognitive enhancers, 178

cognitive impairment, 178

Cohen, John, 241

Colfer, Chris, 442

Colloff, Pamella, 148

Columbine High School, 225, 233, 235–37, 240–41, 447–48

massacre at, 227, 241, 447

Columbine shooters, 241

Commission (crime syndicate), 55

commune, 112–14

confirmatory tests, x, 486

congestive heart failure, 93, 167, 371–72, 486, 496

Connolly, John, 66

Constitutional Convention, 12

contusion, 231, 363, 370, 373, 426, 487

Cooke, Nick, 213, 215–16

Coppola, Anthony, 50

Corbett, Valerie, 80

Cordell, Eugene, 124

Costas, Bob, 199

Costello, Frank, 56

Craik, James, 2–5, 7–8, 13–16

cranium, 140, 230, 487

Creer, Dean, 328

Crete, 122

Crookes, William, 524

Crotchford Farm, 75

Cullen, Dave, 239

Cullen, William, 8

cult, 125, 128, 146, 151, 211–13
        leader, 447–48, 736

Cummings, John, 272–74

Curie, Marie, 338

Curran, John, 387

Curtis, Martha Dandridge, 2, 12

cyanide, 37, 41, 45, 47, 117, 120–21, 487

cyanide intoxication, 119, 132

cyanide poisoning, 42, 46–48, 115

Cyanocarbonate, 42, 487

cynanche trachealis, 8, 488

cytochrome c oxidase, 46, 488

D

Daddy Grace (founder of United House of Prayer for All People), 124

Daly, John, 346

Damamme, Jean-Claude, 28

Dana (Petty's wife), 396

Danforth Report, 150

D'Angelo, Rio, 203

Davis, Clive, 421

Davis, Don, 215

Deadheads, 182

death, x–xii, 6–7, 9–10, 12, 15, 20, 24, 27–30, 32, 39, 41, 43, 46, 48, 52–53, 56, 60–62, 65, 68, 77–79, 83–85, 89–90, 94, 98, 101–6, 109, 114–15, 119–22, 131, 139, 142–46, 155–58, 161, 164–65, 173–75, 179–80, 183–84, 196, 202, 205, 207–9, 219–21, 233–34, 245–47, 250–51, 260–61, 266, 270, 279, 281, 284, 289–92, 295–96, 301,

307–8, 312, 315–19,
332–34, 348, 354, 362–64,
373, 383, 387, 389–90,
397–99, 401–2, 404–5,
408, 410–11, 415, 420,
427–30, 437–38, 442–50,
452–54, 456, 458, 460,
462, 464, 466, 468–70,
472–73, 475, 483–85, 495–
96, 503–4, 506–7, 516–17,
520, 522–23, 527–28, 702,
708, 711–13, 717, 725–28,
731–32, 734
  by drowning, 84, 184, 363,
    366, 436, 440–41, 449,
    732
  firearm, 174
  from heart-related events,
    445–46
  manner of, xi, 506
  sudden, 522
death penalty, 252–53
death tape, 116
death touch, 109
delta-9-tetrahydrocannabinol
  (THC), 459, 467
Densley, James, 451
depression, xi, 65, 89, 153,
    157, 160, 208, 221, 247,
    269–70, 397–99, 401,
    409–10, 442, 447, 456,
    458, 460–62, 464–66,
    468–69, 472–73, 479, 488,
    516, 518
de Rocquigny du Fayel, Christian,
    404
Dershowitz (former professor at
    Harvard Law School), 432
DesLauriers, Richard, 381
despropionyl fentanyl, 397–98,
    462
DeWit, Susanne, 359

diabetes, 94, 157, 187–88, 348,
    353, 457, 465, 470, 488,
    492, 504, 510, 514, 526
diabetic coma, 186
diabetic ketoacidosis, 157,
    488–89
diazepam, 115, 173, 254, 437, 462
Dick (Carson's younger brother),
    307
Dick, Elisha Cullen, 4, 8, 13–16,
    307
Dilantin. See phenytoin
Dillon, Frederick, 46
diphenhydramine, 120–21, 221,
    463
diphtheria, 9
Diverticulosis, 372, 489
Divine, M. J., 124–25
Donahue, Timothy, 421
Dorsey, Ryan, 439
Doyle, Clive, 135, 137–38, 151
Dozier, William, 108
drowning, 39, 43, 77–79, 83–84,
    104, 255, 269, 358, 363–
    64, 436–38, 449, 732–33
Drudge, Matt, 375
drug intoxication, 101–2, 208
drug paraphernalia, 88, 268, 295
drugs, ix–xi, 65, 79, 84, 94, 96,
    98, 102, 104, 119–20, 129,
    157, 164, 168, 171, 174,
    177–78, 182–84, 186,
    207–8, 218–19, 233–34,
    246, 253–55, 296, 300–
    301, 316–17, 363, 397–98,
    406, 437, 442, 446, 450,
    455–58, 460–64, 467–73,
    486, 494–95, 502, 512,
    516, 521, 524
  half-life of, 495
  illicit, 78, 84, 190, 219, 446,
    449

Dulany, Benjamin Tasker, 2
Duma, 34–35
duodenum, 23, 489, 493, 504, 517
Dylan, Bob, 263, 400
dysentery, 11, 489, 512
dysphagia, 7, 490

E

edema, 101, 219, 490
Edenberg, Howard J., 201
Eighth Amendment, 253, 256
Elba, 26, 28
elements, four basic, 482
Elias, Brian, 397
Elliot, Cass, 167
embalmed, 65, 117, 278
embalming, 23, 122, 490
embalming process, 118–19, 490
Embery, Joan, 305
emetic tartar, 20, 463, 472. *See also* tartar emetic
Emmy, 290, 309
emphysema, 88–89, 280–81, 307–8, 311–12, 354, 397, 444, 477, 485, 490, 519
endocarditis, 491
endocrine, 143, 155, 269, 281, 362, 372, 419–20, 491, 507, 512
endocrine system, 155, 269, 281, 362, 372, 491
endothelin-1, 189
Enron Corporation, 313, 320–24
enteropathy, intestinal ischemic, 503
Ephron, Nora, 304
epiglottitis, 10, 16, 444, 491
epinephrine, 300, 370, 463
Epstein, Jeffrey, 423–33, 447, 724–28
Epstein-Barr virus, 200
Equagesic, 99, 101–4, 453, 463

Erdelyi, Thomas, 272
Erickson, Gary, 183
Evel Knievel's Motorcycle Dare-devils, 350
Evel Knievel Syndrome, 355
Evolutionary Level Above Human, 214
executions, botched, 254–55
Exodus Recovery Center, 172
extremist groups, 251, 385, 388, 390

F

faith healings, 124, 129
Falchuk, Brad, 441
familial pulmonary fibrosis, 354, 492
Farahany, Nita A., 72
Farley, Charles, 221
Farley, Chris, 217–20, 222–23, 447
fatty liver, 219, 450, 492, 506
Federal Counterintelligence Service (FSK), 335
Federal Security Service (FSB), 325, 336–37, 385, 388
Feldman, J., 370
fentanyl, 254, 398, 401, 447, 455–56, 460, 462, 464, 709
fentanyl transdermal patches, 397, 400–401
fibrosis, 155, 229, 232, 492
Fienberg, David, 403
Filkins, James, 104, 453
Fisher, Carrie, 221
Fiske, Robert B., Jr., 154, 161
Flavor Aid, 112, 115
Fleming, Alexander, 16, 469
Floyd, Richard, 355
flunitrazepam, 171, 464
fluoxetine, 219, 221, 464
fluvoxamine, 233–34, 238,

464–65
foramen magnum, 156, 492
Ford, Paul Leicester, 6
Ford, Whitey, 193
forensic analysis, xii, 118, 453
forensics, ii, ix, xi–xii, 427, 710,
712, 735–36
forensic toxicologists, ix–x, 173
forensic toxicology, ix
formaldehyde, 65, 119, 490, 493
Foroud, Tatiana, 201
Forshufvud, Sten, 26
Foster, Vince, 153, 160
Foster, Vincent W., Jr., 153–55,
158–61, 447
Franklin, Aretha, 413–21, 444,
718–20
Freeh, Louis J., 154
French, Elizabeth, 2
Fricke, David, 275
fruit punch, poisoned, 112,
120–21, 132
fundus, 280, 493
Funston, Lindi, 307
Fuselier, Dwayne, 240

G

Gail (Maeder's daughter), 212
Galea, Sandro, 174
Galloway, Ben, 228
Gambino, Carlo, 57
gamma aminobutyric acid, 456,
462, 468
gamma rays, 333
Garafolo, Mary, 145
Garcia, Jerry, 181–84, 186–88,
191, 445
gastritis, 42, 493–94
gastroenteritis, 328, 494
gastroesophageal reflux disease
(GERD), 317, 494
gastrostomy, 494

gastrostomy site, 280
Gates, Bill, 282
Gekko, Gordon, 323
Genovese, Vito, 56–57
Genta, Robert, 23
George (Lois's son), 146
Geraldine (Liston's wife), 87
Gibb, Barry, 282, 285–86
Gibb, Maurice, 277–86, 444
Gibb, Robin, 278, 281, 285–86
Gillespie, Paula, 360
Gingrich, Newt, 377
Ginsburg, Ruth Bader, 154, 420
glabella, 141, 494
glairy mucus, 77
glioblastoma multiforme, 66, 495
Glioma, 64, 73, 495
glottis, 8, 495
glucose, 188, 372, 465
Golden Harvest, 97–98, 108
Goldsberry, Don, 365
Golovlev, Vladimir, 342
Good, Victor, 237
Grasso, Arthur, 50
Grateful Dead, 182, 185, 187, 190
gray matter, 178
Great War, 33
Green, Michael, 95
Greenberg, Alan, 430
Greenwade, Tom, 197
Greer, Jim, 275
Griffin, Ted, 365
Grisman, David, 186
Gross, Diane, 368
Guinier, Lanie, 160
Guinn, Jeff, 120
gunpowder residue, 40, 118, 122,
143
gunshot wounds, 40, 43, 50,
52–53, 63–64, 68, 119,
121–22, 132, 139–41,
143–44, 156, 158, 173,

175, 228, 230, 232, 234,
322, 382–83, 447, 450,
452, 703
Gutfeld, Greg, 377
Guyana, 46, 112–13, 116–17,
126–27, 448

H

Hackett, Buddy, 57
Haddock, Mary, 76
hair, 27–29, 32, 39, 44, 50, 57–58,
81, 108, 111, 181, 211,
218, 228, 231, 262, 315,
328, 331–33, 339, 359,
361, 481
Hale-Bopp comet, 204
half-life, 338, 495, 515
Halpern, Charna, 220, 222–23
Hamas, 390
Hanger, Charles, 244
hanging
accidental, 428, 433, 475
homicidal, 428, 499
judicial, 410, 433, 504
suicidal, 427–28, 433, 447,
523
Hanna, Jack, 368
Hansen, Eric, 314
Hanvey, Dusty, 294
Hare, Robert, 240
Without Conscience, 240
Harel, Amos, 392
Harkin, Nicole, 189, 299
Harris, 226–28, 231, 233–40,
447–48
Harris, Eric, 225–28, 231,
233–40, 447–48
Harrison, Brian, 109
Harrison, George, 257–58,
260–63, 265, 400, 444
Harrison, John, 333
Harry, Deborah, 274

Hart, Mickey, 186–87, 190
Hartrell, Dick, 80
Hartshorne, Nikolas, 172
Hartzler, Joseph, 249
Harvey, Craig, 268
hashish, 98, 465
Hatfield, Bobby, 293–99, 301,
445–46, 449
heart, 22, 34, 37, 53, 63–64, 68,
77–79, 84, 93, 100–101,
118, 142, 155, 168, 183,
187, 189–90, 229, 281,
288, 295–96, 299–301,
307, 314, 316–18, 332,
371–72, 446, 449, 463,
471, 473, 476, 479–80,
483, 491, 496, 500–501,
507–8, 513–16, 522–23,
526–27
heart attack (*see also* myocardial
infarction), 57, 79, 84, 142,
155, 165–68, 184, 189,
219, 280–81, 288, 296,
299, 301, 312, 316–17,
319, 372, 416, 444–47,
461, 475, 481, 496, 502,
508, 515, 524
heartburn, 317
heart disease, 53, 89, 166–68,
187, 189–90, 281, 290,
312, 317, 378, 444–46,
478, 496, 501, 507, 510
ischemic, 301
heart failure, 90, 93–94, 167,
183, 188–89, 334, 371–73,
445–46, 483, 486, 496–97,
507, 523
heart failure cells, 372, 497
heart ventricles, 479, 497
Heatly, Maurice Dean, 70
heatstroke, 105, 479, 497
Heaven's Gate, 203–7, 211–16,

447

Heavyweight Boxing Champion of the World, 87

Hébert, Curtis L., Jr., 323

Helicobacter pylori, 31

Helpern, Milton, 52

hemophilia, 34, 45, 497

Hemorrhagic shock, 15, 497

hemosiderin laden macrophages, 372, 498

Henneberry, David, 382

hepatitis, 195–96, 200–201, 347, 444, 471, 498, 506
  chronic, 19, 22, 24, 450

hepatocellular carcinoma. *See* cancer, liver

Herman, Mark, 89

Hermogenes (bishop of Saratov), 44–45

heroin, 88–89, 95, 175–78, 182–83, 187, 189, 191, 220–21, 270–71, 274, 401, 406–7, 409, 442, 447, 455–56, 466, 472

Hinckley, John W., Jr., 71

hip fracture, 396, 400, 711

histamine, 463, 471

Hodgkin's lymphoma, 199–200, 498–99

Hoffenberg, Steven, 431

Hoffman, Philip Seymour, 221, 402, 712

Holiday Inn Express, 215

Holland, Sonny, 349

homicidal strangulation, 427

homicide, xi, 43, 53–54, 89, 121–22, 144, 156, 173, 329, 334, 383, 410, 427–28, 433, 443, 447, 499, 506, 730

Hooker, Chris, 238

Hope, Bob, 306

Hospice care, 260, 415, 499

Hospira, Inc., 253

House of David, 147

Houston, Whitney, 84, 440, 735

Houteff, Victor, 146

Huffington, Arianna, 375

human papillomavirus (HPV), 264, 499

humerus, 362, 500

humors, four basic, 482

Humphrey, Charles, 215

Hunter, Michael, 167

Hustmyre, Chuck, 134

hydrocodone, 207–8, 466, 473

hydrogen cyanide, 45, 338, 500, 516

Hyma, Bruce A., 278

Hyman, Jeffrey, 272

hyoid bone, fractures in, 428–29, 500, 729

hypertension, 188

hyperthermia, 105, 500

hypertrophy, 300–301, 371, 501

hypotension, xi, 6, 501

hypovolemic shock, 498

hypoxia, 46, 410, 501

I

Ibn al-Khattab (Islamist leader), 342

idiopathic pulmonary fibrosis (IPF), 347–48, 353–54, 444, 492, 501–2

ileum, 280, 502

immunoassays, x

immunologic toxicology screen, 502

improvised explosive device (IED), 380, 389

ImprovOlympic, 220–22

infarct, 481, 502

innominate bone, 142, 502

insanity defense, 71, 503
insulin, 188, 419, 465, 488, 526
Intercontinental Assets Group
    Inc., 431
International Agency for Research
    on Cancer (IARC), 31, 445
International Association of Ma-
    chinists, 59
International Longshoremen's
    Association, 54
intestinal ischemic enteropathy,
    503
intestinal malrotation, 503
Investigation and Prevention of
    Organized Crime, 336
"Invictus," 245
ionizing radiation, 333
Irina (princess, Nicholas II's only
    niece), 36
ischemic enteropathy, 279, 281,
    503

J

Jackson, James, 9
Jagger, Mick, 81–82
jaundice, 18, 471, 504
Jeffrey, Keith, 41
jejunum, 280, 489, 502, 504
Jen (Candy's daughter), 166, 169
J. Epstein & Company, 431
Jett, John, 367
JFK, 166
Jim Jr. (Jones, J.'s son), 116
Jobs, Steve, 420, 723
Joel, Billy, 293
John (Farley's brother), 218
Johnson, Lyndon Baines, 59
Johnson, Micah, 72
Johnson-Dare, Jill, 314
Jones, Brian, 75–85, 111–30, 132,
    180, 449–50
Jones, David, 134

Jones, D. R., 117
Jones, Jim, 111–25, 127–31, 141,
    447–48, 450
Jones, Peter, 311
Jones, Rachel, 147
Jones, Scott, 83
Jonestown massacre, 111, 114–16,
    127, 131
Josey (Rivera and Dorsey's son),
    436, 440
Joslyn, Dick, 212
Judgment Day, 239–40
judicial execution, 247
justifiable homicide, 68, 383, 443

K

Kastle, Tim, 238
Kathy (Whitman's wife), 60
Keele, N. Bradley, 67
Kennedy, John F., 95
Kennedy, William, 154
Kerensky, Alexander, 34
ketones, 157, 504
Keys, T. E., 9
Khashoggi, Adam, 431
King, Carol, 414
King, Larry, 414
King, Martin Luther, Jr., 126, 417
Klebold, 226–29, 234–41, 447–48
Klebold, Dylan, 225–29, 231–32,
    234–41, 447–48
Klintmalm, Goran, 195
Knievel, Evel, 345–56, 444, 450
Knotts, Don, 292
known human carcinogen, 31,
    445, 480
Koenigs, Michael, 67
Kohl, Laura Johnston, 112
Kondaurov, Alexei, 341
Koran, 390
Koresh, David, 133–50, 249, 448,
    450, 736

Kosorotov, Dmitrii, 39
Kovtun, Dmitry, 326–27, 339–42
Krischer, Barry, 424
Kulbacki, Rob, 228
kung fu, 107
Kurfirst, Gary, 267
Kurtzman, Robert A., 314, 317

L

Labash, Matt, 376
lacerations, 229–30, 363, 505
Lacinak, Thad, 366
Lake, Simeon T., III, 324
Lalich, Janja, 212–13
Lanegan, Mark, 172
Langer, Jacob C., 285
Langford, Don, 97, 102, 453
Lankford, Adam, 451
Lansky, Meyer, 57
Lanza, Adam, 241
laparotomy, 280, 285, 505
Lapp, Joshua, 228
Lappin, Warden Harley, 245
laryngeal diphtheria, 8, 505
laryngitis, 9, 505, 519
larynx, 5, 8–9, 118, 155, 281,
    495–96, 500, 505, 508,
    521, 524
Lasaga, Jose I., 130
latency period, 32, 506
Lawrence (Washington's
    half-brother), 10
Lawson, Janet, 75
Lay, Ken, 313–14, 316–20, 323,
    445
Lazenby, George, 98
Lazovert, Stanislaus de, 36–37,
    41–42
lead, 19, 26, 130, 139, 141, 149,
    157, 171, 183, 188, 190,
    196, 205, 210, 239, 261,
    272, 282, 297–98, 329,
    400, 448, 483, 485, 488,
    494, 497–98, 503, 507,
    519, 527–28
Lear, Tobias, 2
Lederman, Gil, 259–60
Ledger, Heath, 402
Lee, Bruce, 97–99, 101–7, 109,
    450, 453
Lee, Henry C., 161
Lee, Joseph, 288
Lee, Tom, 384
Lennon, John, 261
Leno, Jay, 312
Leon, Lisa, 105
Letterman, David, 305–6
leukemia, 329, 506
Leung, Lam King, 101
Lewis, Fielding O., 9
Lewis, Jerry, 304
Lewis, Richard, 163
Lewy body dementia, 65
Limarev, Yevgeny, 326
Lincoln, Abraham, 243
Linda (Lay's wife), 247, 313, 322
Lindsay, John, 310
Lipscomb, Jerry, 207
Liston, Sonny, 87–96, 444, 446
Liston, Tobe, 90
Listyev, Vlad, 336
Litvinenko, Alexander, 325–42,
    447
liver cirrhosis, 195, 485
liver metastasis, 420
Lobotomy: Surviving the Ra-
    mones (Ramone, D.), 273,
    275
Lockett, Clayton D., 254
Lofgren, Nils, 400
Logue, Jennifer, 189
Lois (Roden's wife), 146
Longwood, 18
Lopez, Santana. *See* Rivera,

Naya, 439, 441
Lopez, Santana (character of
    Naya River in *Glee*), 439
Lotysch, Matthew, 290
Love, Courtney, 171, 177
Lowe, Hudson, 23
loyalty tests, 112, 114
Luciano, Charles "Lucky," 54
Luciano Crime Family, 56
Lugovoy, Andrei, 326–27, 339–42
Lulu (Gibb's first wife), 283
Lurie, John, 409
Lycette, R. R., 99–102
Lyle, David, 356
Lynch, Larry, 135
Lynne, Jeff, 263, 400
Lynott, Phil, 274

M

Madhusoodanan, Subramoniam,
    68
Maeder, Alice, 212
Magruder, Kathleen, 323
malaria, 15, 119, 460, 471, 519
Malaya Nevka River, 38
Manes, Mark, 236
Mangano, Philip, 56
Mangano, Vincent, 55
Mangano Crime Family, 55–56
Mann, Barry, 298
Mannheim, Lou, 323
mannitol, 98, 466
Mantle, Mickey, "Time in a Bot-
    tle," 194, 201
Maranzano, Salvatore, 54–55
Marchand, Louis-Joseph, 23
Mari, Francesco, 30
Maria (Rasputin's daughter), 42
marijuana, 81, 88, 102–3, 174,
    185, 401, 459, 465–67. *See
    also* cannabis; hashish
Maris, Roger, 193

Markel, Howard, 9, 13
Markov, Georgi, 343
Marshall, Marty, 91
martial artist, 97
Martin, Leotis, 93
Martin, Sheila, 147
Martin, Steve, 169
Martin, Thomas E., 126
Martin, Wayne, 135
martyrs, 391–93
Maslin, Janet, 166
Mason, Jackie, 304
massacre, 73, 111, 115, 127,
    130–31, 225, 234, 237–41,
    447–48, 450
Masseria, Joe "the Boss," 54
mass shooting, 241, 451, 736–37
Matsch, Richard, 245–46
Matteson, Catherine, 135
Mayo Clinic, 29, 258, 317, 711,
    722
McCartney, Paul, 261
McGee, James, 136
McMahon, Ed, 303
McNeil, Legs, 271, 275
McVeigh, Timothy, 234, 243–50,
    448
Medley, Bill, 293–94, 297–98
medulla oblongata, 231, 507
Meng, Dun, 381
mental disorder, 410
meprobamate, 99, 102–3, 463,
    467
Merchant, Larry, 95
mercury, 15, 329, 467, 501, 713
Mertz, Michael, 255
mesentery, 332, 507
metabolic acidosis, 46, 507
MI6, 40–41, 337
Michaels, Lorne, 222
midazolam, 2, 254–56, 467
Midler, Bette, 304

Millennium Hotel, 326–27, 339
Milne, A. A., 75
Mobley, Fannie, 129
Moika Palace, 36, 38, 47
Moldeo, Don, 159
Moliére (poet), 13
mononucleosis, infectious, 200
Monroe, Marilyn, xi
Monteith, Cory, 442
Moore, Annie, 121
Moore, Carey Dean, 254
Morens, David M., 9, 14
Morgan, Fran, 60
Morgan, John, 60
morphine, 89, 173, 175, 183,
        219–20, 270–71, 343, 398,
        455, 459, 462, 464, 466,
        468, 473
Morse, Stephen, 72
Moscone, George, 127
Muhammad Ali, 92–93, 95, 729
Muhammad Ali. *See* Clay, Cas-
        sius, 92–93, 95, 729
Mulcahy, Mary, 421
multifocal myocardial fibrosis,
        183, 507
multiple endocrine neoplasia type
        1 syndrome, 419, 507
murderers, mass, 132, 447–48,
        450–52
Murder Inc., 55–56
Murphy, Ryan, 441
Murrow, Edward R., 306
muscles, breathing, 519
muzzle imprint, 118, 122
myocardial infarction, 508
myocardium, 77, 508
Mystic, Russian, 33

N

Naipaul, Shiva, 113
Nalchik, 335–36

naloxone, 270, 466, 468–69, 473
nannygate, 154
Napoleonic Code, 25
narcan. *See* naloxone
nasal pharynx, 230, 508
Nasser, Tom, 295
Nathwani, Amit, 330
National Crime Syndicate, 55
National Institute on Drug Abuse
        (NIDA), 177, 709
National Public Radio (NPR),
        255, 407, 451, 703, 710,
        720, 737
National Toxicology Program
        (NTP), 31, 445
Navalny, Alexei, 343
Ndumele, Chiadi, 189
Nebraska, 254, 304, 308, 320
Nembutal. *See* pentobarbital
Nettles, Bonnie, 210–11
neuroendocrine cancers, 419
neurofibromatosis type 1, 420,
        508
neuroscience, 71–72
neutrons, 338, 477, 509
nevus, 229, 509
Newton, Wayne, 310
Next Level Above Human, 211
Nicholas II (tsar), 34, 36
Nichols, Stacy, 359
Nichols, Terry, 249
Nielson, Patricia, 237
Nirvana, 171, 176–77
nitric oxide, 189, 509
Nixon, Richard, 310
nodule, penile verrucous, 513
Noesner, Gary, 135, 139
norcocaine, 296, 468
Novichok nerve gas, 343, 510

O

Obama, Barack, 381, 413, 415,

418, 421–22, 718
Obama, Michelle, 421
obese, 164, 166–67, 189, 219–20, 254, 370, 510
obesity, 30, 77, 94, 167–68, 188–89, 446, 470, 483, 492, 506, 510
Obregón, Ana, 431
occipital bone, 141, 156, 510
Ochberg, Frank, 240
O'Dwyer, William, 55
Oglesbee, Terra, 239
Ohio, 253, 294, 317, 347, 368
Oklahoma, 253
Oklahoma City Bombing, 234, 244, 251, 448
Olivia (Harrison's wife), 258, 260
Olson, John, 323
O'Meara, Barry, 18
Operation Trojan Horse, 134
opioid, 89, 207, 219–21, 254, 269–70, 301, 317, 343, 397–99, 401, 404, 410, 447, 455–56, 458–59, 462, 464, 466, 468, 472–73, 518, 708–9, 716
Orbison, Roy, 263, 400
oropharynx, 257, 510–11
O'Shea, Teri Buford, 126, 130
osteomyelitis, 197, 511
O'Toole, George, 387
oxycodone, 397–98, 401, 456, 468
oxygen, 6, 14, 16, 46, 63–64, 77, 89, 93, 100–101, 114, 168, 190, 288, 299, 301, 311, 316, 348, 354, 410, 464, 466, 472, 476, 478–79, 481–83, 485, 490, 496–98, 500–501, 503, 508, 511, 515–16, 518–19, 522, 525

P

Paar, Jack, 304
pancreas, 64, 118, 143, 155, 188, 230, 232, 269, 315, 372, 419–20, 465, 491, 507, 511–12, 526, 528
exocrine cells, 419
islet cells, 419, 507
pancreatic ductal adenocarcinoma, 419–20, 512
Pancreatic neuroendocrine cancer, 419–20, 512
pancuronium, 469. *See also* pancuronium bromide
pancuronium bromide, 246
Pancytopenia, 330, 512
Panto, Peter, 55
Papas, Alex, 214
Parks, Rosa, 417
Park Sheraton Hotel, 49–50, 57–58
pathogen, 2, 512
Patrushev, Nikolai, 336
Patterson, Floyd, 91–92
Pavarotti, Luciano, 420
Pavlovich (lieutenant, first cousin of Tsar Nicholas II), 36
Pearson, Muriel, 148
pectus excavatum, 229, 513
Peerwani, Nizam, 140, 150
penicillin, 15, 197, 279, 469
pentobarbital, xi, 119–20, 253–54, 256, 469–70
Peoples Temple, 111–13, 125–31, 448
members of, 116
peptic ulcer, 232, 513
pericardium, 22, 513
peripheral neuropathy, 330, 514
peritoneum, 332, 507, 514
peritonitis, 371, 514, 528

Petechiae, 514
petechial hemorrhages, 427–28
Peter (Harrison's brother), 261
Peter (Lee's older brother), 99
Peters, Kenneth, 366
Peterson, Jillian, 451
phagocytic cells, 498
phantom punch, 93
pharmaceuticals, benzodiazepine
    class of, 456, 462, 464,
    467, 472
pharynx, 230, 505, 508
Phenergan. *See* promethazine
phenobarbital, 207, 470
phentermine, 437, 470
phenytoin, 98, 470
Phoenix, River, 220
Pick-Jones, Antoinette, 130
Pitts, Byron, 247
Piva, Larissa, 128
plaque, 53, 77, 118, 142, 155,
    190, 206, 232, 269, 280,
    316, 361, 480–81, 496, 515
plasma, 14, 466, 515
pleural adhesions, 22, 515
Poehler, Amy, 223
Poh-hwye, Eugene Chu, 99
poison, ix–x, 36–37, 39, 41–42,
    46–47, 101, 114, 340, 342,
    457, 480
poisoning, 27, 29, 326, 342–43,
    410, 517
    arsenic, 26–28, 30, 480
Politkovskaya, Anna, 338
Pollak, Joel B., 374, 377
Pollock, Mindy, 227
Polly, Matthew, 104, 453
    Bruce Lee: A Life, 104
polonium, 330, 332–34, 338–40,
    515
polypharmacy, 208, 399, 402,
    447, 449, 516

Populus, Gustave, 164
postmortem fermentation, 144
postmortem redistribution, x,
    174–75, 516
potassium chloride, 246, 254, 471
potassium cyanide, 35, 37, 40–43,
    46–47, 114, 471, 487, 516
poultice, 473–74
Praskovya (Rasputin's wife), 44
Presley, Elvis, 318, 399, 402
Preti, Antonio, 452
Prikazchikov, Yuri, 327
Profaci, Joe, 56
promethazine, 114, 471
prophylaxis, 119
Prozac. *See* fluoxetine, 464
Prussian blue, 329–30, 516
pseudotubercles, 22, 517
psychiatrists, 65–67, 73, 239,
    449–50, 452
psychological autopsy, 429, 517
psychological operation, 137
psychopaths, 240
pulmonary edema, 255
punctate hemorrhages, 77
Purishkevich, Vladimir, 35–36, 40
Putin, Vladimir, 334, 336, 338,
    340, 342
putrefaction, 117, 144
pylorus, 23, 493, 517

Q

Queen of Soul, 413, 417, 421,
    718–20
quinine, 15, 471
quinsy, 7–9, 517–18

R

radioactivity, 329, 331–32, 338,
    340–41
radioisotope, 331, 338–39, 341,

495

radiosurgery, stereostatic, 259, 265

radiotherapy, cobalt, 259, 265

Ramone, Dee Dee, 267–69, 271–72, 274–75, 447, 450

Lobotomy: Surviving the Ramones, 273, 275

Ramones, 267–75, 447, 449–50

Ramsay, Gordon, 408

Raskin, Jeffrey, 285

Rasputin, Grigori, 33–40, 42–48, 447

Rattlesnakes, 282

Rawlins, George, 2

Rayner, Oswald, 40

Reagan, Ronald, 71, 310

Rector, Russ, 368

regulation D, 518

Reisbord, David, 103

Reiterman, Tim, 112

Reles, Abe, 55

Reno, Janet, 137

respiratory arrest, xi, 208, 470

respiratory depression, 89, 221, 247, 270, 398–99, 442, 447, 456, 458, 462, 464, 466, 468–69, 472–73, 516, 518

respiratory failure, 354, 518

Restoril. *See* temazepam

Richards, Keith, 81–82

Richardson, James T., 128

Ride, Sally, 420

Righteous Brothers, 293–95, 297–99

Righteous Indignation: Excuse Me While I Save the World (Breitbart), 376

Ripert, Eric, 404

Risenhoover, John, 134

Ritter, John, 287–90, 292, 446–47

Rivera, Naya, 435–41, 449, 731–34

Sorry Not Sorry: Dreams, Mistakes, and Growing Up, 439

Rivers, Joan, 305

Road to Jonestown: Jim Jones and the Peoples Temple, the (Guinn), 120

Rock, Chris, 222

Rock and Roll Hall of Fame, 264, 267, 293, 299, 400, 418

Roden, Ben, 146

Rodzianko, Michael, 34

Rogin, Gilbert, 91

Rohypnol. *See* flunitrazepam, 464

Rolling Stones, 75, 81–82, 172, 176, 275, 711, 734

Romanov, Dmitri Pavlovich, 35

Rose, Naomi, 367

Rose Law Firm, 154, 159

Ross, Kyle, 237

Royal London Hospital, 331, 347

Russell, Katherine, 385

Ryan, Leo, 113

S

Sachs, Albert, 76

Sadat (president), 310

Sage, Byron, 134, 138, 149

Sailing, Mark, 442

Saint-Denis, Louis-Étienne, 20

Sainz, Mario, 373

Saltz, Leonard, 420

Sampson, Barbara, 427

Sanborn, Jill, 252

Sanders, William "Dave," 227

Sando, Arthur, 369, 378

Scaramella, Mario, 326

Schaber, Lynne, 359

Scheele, Carl Wilhelm, 45

schistosomiasis, 22, 519

756

Schneider, Steve, 144
School, Dalton, 430
Schwartz, Sierra, 386
Schwarzenegger, Arnold, 305
Scully, Rick, 205
Scurvy, 18, 519
SeaWorld Orlando, 357–59,
    364–67, 449
SeaWorld trainers, 358, 360
Sebring, Jay, 108
Second City, 163, 165, 168, 218,
    221, 223
Securities and Exchange Commis-
    sion, 321
sepsis, 331, 520
septic shock, 15, 520
septum, 371
Serenity Knolls Treatment Center,
    182, 187
Service, Robert, 342
Shamu (female orca), 364–65
Sheila (Foster's sister), 153
siderophages, 497
Simmons, Mark, 366
Simon, Neil, 292
Simon, Ron, 306
Sinatra, Frank, 402
Skilling, Jeffrey, 320
Skripal, Sergei, 343
sleep apnea, 354, 520
Smith, Anna Nicole, 402, 712
Smith, Don, 91
Smith, Douglas, 42
Smithsonian Institution, 355, 408
smoking, 30, 167–68, 187, 265,
    300, 304–5, 312, 443,
    509–10
socialism, 113, 116, 123–24
sodium thiopental, 246, 253, 255,
    472
Sommerville, Angus, 79
Song, Luke, 414

soot, 142
Sorry Not Sorry: Dreams, Mis-
    takes, and Growing Up
    (Rivera), 439
Spade, David, 222
Spanish fly beetle, 3
Spector, Phil, 298
speedball, 220–21, 447, 472
sphenoid sinuses, 363, 521
Spielberg, Steven, 166
squamous cells, 264, 521
Starr, Kenneth W., 161
Staten Island University Hospital,
    259–60
Steen, Rob, 94–95
Stein, Alexandra, 448
Stengel, Casey, 193
Stephan (Jones, J.'s biologi-
    cal son), 116, 120, 124,
    128–29, 132
Stephany, Joshua D., 361
stereotactic radiosurgery, 521
Stevens, Alois, 90
St. Helena, 17–18, 27–29, 32
Stoen, Tim, 126–27
Stokoe, John, 19
stomach ulcer, 20, 521
Stone, Oliver, 166
stridular suffocates, 8, 521
stroke, 100, 300, 348, 354, 461,
    476, 485, 495, 500, 522,
    524
Strummer, Joe, 272
Substance Abuse and Mental
    Health Services Adminis-
    tration, 406
sudden unexplained death in
    epilepsy (SUDEP), 104,
    453, 522
suicide, xi, 45–46, 122, 131, 157–
    58, 161–62, 171–73, 175,
    177, 209, 213–16, 228,

234, 322, 329, 334, 404–5,
      409–11, 425, 427–28,
      430, 433, 437, 443, 447,
      451–52, 488, 506, 517,
      523, 707, 716, 729–30
  altruistic, 131, 477
  death from, 447
  fatalistic, 131, 492
  mass, 46, 112, 131, 203, 206,
      212, 215, 448
  revolutionary, 114–16
suicide bombers, 390–92, 707
Sukhotin, Sergei Mikhailovich, 36
Summerall, Pat, 194
Sun, Lowell, 388
suppuration, 8, 523
Susann, Jacqueline, 310
Swayze, Patrick, 222, 420
sweating, 105
Swift, Benjamin, 331
system, respiratory, 519

T

tachycardia, 30, 460, 523, 527
Tamerlan, Tsarnaev, 381–83
Tanaka, Yuki, 390
tartar emetic, 4, 30, 463, 472. *See
      also* emetic tartar
Teare, Donald, 102–3, 453
temazepam, 397–98, 401, 472
terrorism, 250–52, 335, 388,
      706–8
  domestic, 250–52
  ethnonationalist, 250
  far-right extremist, 250–51
  religious, 250
Terrorist Identities Datamart En-
      vironment (TIDE), 388
terrorists, 343, 388, 390–92, 452,
      706
tests, confirmatory toxicology,
      486

Texas, 23, 60, 66, 133–34, 145,
      195, 209, 241, 249, 252,
      313, 448, 736
thallium, 326, 329–30, 516–17,
      524
thallium (Crookes), 329–30, 524
thallium poisoning, 329–30, 516
the tower, 61–62, 70–71, 73, 450
Thibodeau, David, 138, 147, 150
Thompson, Ojetta Rogeriee, 387
Thornton, William, 5
Thorogood, Frank, 75–76, 83
thromboembolism, 372, 524
thrombosis, 300, 524
thyroid cartilage, fractures of,
      428–29, 500, 524
Tilikum, 358–61, 365–68
Tilikum (male orca), 358–61,
      365–68
"Time in a Bottle" (Mantle), 194,
      201
Ting-Pei, Betty, 98, 101, 103
tolerance, 120, 128, 456, 464, 524
Tom Petty and the Heartbreakers,
      395, 399
Tompkins, Cuck, 358, 367
Topoleski, Jan, 358
Torres, Harrys, 195
torsades de pointes, 30, 525
total blood volume, 6–7
toxicology testing, xii, 6, 43, 65,
      68, 79, 89, 103, 119, 122,
      144, 157, 164, 175, 184,
      196, 207–8, 219, 221, 234,
      260, 270, 295–96, 307,
      318, 334, 348, 373, 399,
      405, 415, 429, 438
trace evidence, ix
tracheobronchial tree, 64, 143,
      525
tracheotomy, 5, 14–15, 525
tranquilizer, 99, 114, 120, 171,

173, 221, 397, 447, 463, 467
Travelgate, 154, 160
trazodone, 154, 157, 473
Trebek, Alex, 420
trichloroethanol, 460
triglyceride, 188–89
trismus, 7, 526
Tristan, Charles, 28
Trixie (Garcia's daughter), 187
troponin, 189
Trump, Donald, 251
Trynka, Paul, 83
Tsarnaev, Dzhokhar, 380, 382–83, 386–87, 389–93, 704–6
Tsarnaev, Tamerlan, 379–93, 448, 703–6
Tsarnaev brothers, 381
Tsepo, Roman, 343
tuberculosis, 10, 22, 517
tumor, 66–68, 72, 232, 420, 507–8, 521, 523, 528
tumors, pancreatic neuroendocrine, 512, 723
Twenty-Seven Club, 85, 180, 442
Tylenol. *See* acetaminophen

U

unidentified flying object (UFOs), 203, 211, 214
University of Texas, 60–63, 69–70
University of Texas Southwestern Medical Center, 23, 31
Upshaw, Gene, 420
urine, x, 65, 79, 119, 143, 157, 183, 221, 233–34, 330, 372, 458, 486, 502, 519

V

Valium. *See* diazepam

vasoconstriction, 299–300
vasovagal shock, 410
Vaughan, Wendy, 324
Ventre, Jeffrey, 367
ventricles, 479, 497, 522, 525–27
ventricular fibrillation, 77, 460, 479, 526–27
ventricular tachycardia, 30, 460, 527
verapamil, 296, 473
verrucous, 279, 513, 527
    carcinoma, 279, 513, 527
    nodule, 279, 513
Versed. *See* midazolam
vertigo, 437, 527
Vicious, Sid, 274
Vicodin, 207, 398, 473
Vine, Calvin, 205–6
violence, 72, 249, 404, 448, 451
violent extremists, domestic, 250–52
Virchis, Andres, 328–29, 338
Virginia, 1, 3, 8, 10–12, 16, 154, 251–52, 271
vitreous humor, 157, 528
volvulus, 279, 444, 528
von Hippel Lindau syndrome, 419, 528

W

Waco siege, 133, 139
Wagner, Robert, 440
Walken, Christopher, 440
Walker, Jimmy, 298
Walker, Pinkney, 320
Wall, Marina, 325, 341
Wallace, Mike, 306
Wallenborn, White McKenzie, 8–9
Wall of Sound, 298
Walters, Eric, 365
Warren, Edith, 209

Washington, George, 1–2, 4–7, 9–10, 12–13, 15, 444
waterboarding, 255
Watkins, Sherron, 321
Watts, Charlie, 81–82
Weaver, Randy, 249
Weil, Cynthia, 298
Weiner, Anthony, 376
Weinreb, William, 383, 386, 389, 392, 702
Weinstein, Harvey, 411
Wells, Walter A., 9
Wembley Stadium, 345, 352
Wende, Stephen, 314
Wepner, Chuck, 93
West, Louis Jolyon, 213
Weston, Dan, 295
Wexler, Jerry, 414, 417
Wexner, Leslie, 431
wheat-bran poultices, 5, 473
white matter, 77
White Nights, 112
Whitman, Charles J., 59–70, 73, 118, 142, 155, 229, 248, 280, 315, 332, 361, 448–50
Whitmer, Gretchen, 251
Wide World of Sports, 346, 351–52, 355
Wilder, Jessica, 360
wildnil. *See* carfentanil
Wilkes, G. A., 47
Williams, Pat, 353
Williams, Robin, 65
Willius, F. A., 9
Wilmore, Chuck, 123
Wilmore, Phyllis, 111
Wilson, Leslie, 113, 116

Winant, Louise, 209
Wineberger, Jean, 49
Wing Chun, 107
Winslow, Robert, 126
Without Conscience (Hare), 240
Wohlin, Anna, 75–76
Wolpin, Brian, 421
Wood, Kimba, 160
Wood, Natalie, 440
World Health Organization (WHO), 31, 445
World War I, 33
wound
    entrance, 40, 118, 122, 141, 143–44, 156, 230, 232
    exit, 118, 141, 143–44, 156, 230, 232
Wray, Christopher, 252
Wu, Peter, 98, 102, 453
Wyman, Bill, 81

X

Xanax. *See* alprazolam

Y

Yandarbiev, Zelinkhan, 342
Yip Man, 107
Young, Jeffrey, 387
Yulia (Skripal's daughter), 343
Yussupov, Felix, 35–38, 41–43
Yvonne (Gibb, Maurice's second wife), 284

Z

Zivot, Joel, 255